Social and Behavioral Aspects of PHARMACEUTICAL CARE

Edited by

Nathaniel M. Rickles, PharmD, PhD, BCPP
Assistant Professor of Pharmacy Practice and Administration
School of Pharmacy
Northeastern University
Boston, MA

Albert I. Wertheimer, PhD, MBA
Director, Center for Pharmaceutical Health Services Research
School of Pharmacy
Temple University
Philadelphia, PA

Mickey C. Smith, PhD
Emeritus Professor
School of Pharmacy
University of Mississippi
Oxford, MS

JONES AND BARTLETT PUBLISHERS
Sudbury, Massachusetts
BOSTON   TORONTO   LONDON   SINGAPORE

World Headquarters

Jones and Bartlett Publishers
40 Tall Pine Drive
Sudbury, MA 01776
978-443-5000
info@jbpub.com
www.jbpub.com

Jones and Bartlett Publishers
Canada
6339 Ormindale Way
Mississauga, Ontario L5V 1J2
Canada

Jones and Bartlett Publishers
International
Barb House, Barb Mews
London W6 7PA
United Kingdom

Jones and Bartlett's books and products are available through most bookstores and online booksellers. To contact Jones and Bartlett Publishers directly, call 800-832-0034, fax 978-443-8000, or visit our website www.jbpub.com.

Substantial discounts on bulk quantities of Jones and Bartlett's publications are available to corporations, professional associations, and other qualified organizations. For details and specific discount information, contact the special sales department at Jones and Bartlett via the above contact information or send an email to specialsales@jbpub.com.

The authors, editor, and publisher have made every effort to provide accurate information. However, they are not responsible for errors, omissions, or for any outcomes related to the use of the contents of this book and take no responsibility for the use of the products and procedures described. Treatments and side effects described in this book may not be applicable to all people; likewise, some people may require a dose or experience a side effect that is not described herein. Drugs and medical devices are discussed that may have limited availability controlled by the Food and Drug Administration (FDA) for use only in a research study or clinical trial. Research, clinical practice, and government regulations often change the accepted standard in this field. When consideration is being given to use of any drug in the clinical setting, the healthcare provider or reader is responsible for determining FDA status of the drug, reading the package insert, and reviewing prescribing information for the most up-to-date recommendations on dose, precautions, and contraindications, and determining the appropriate usage for the product. This is especially important in the case of drugs that are new or seldom used.

Production Credits

Publisher: David Cella
Associate Editor: Maro Asadoorian
Senior Production Editor: Renée Sekerak
Production Assistant: Jill Morton
Senior Marketing Manager: Barb Bartoszek
Associate Marketing Manager: Lisa Gordon
Manufacturing and Inventory Control
    Supervisor: Amy Bacus

Composition: Arlene Apone
Cover Design: Kristin E. Parker
Cover Image: © Tito Wong/ShutterStock, Inc.
Printing and Binding: Malloy, Incorporated
Cover Printing: Malloy, Incorporated

Library of Congress Cataloging-in-Publication Data
Social and behavioral aspects of pharmaceutical care / [edited] by Nathaniel M. Rickles, Albert I. Wertheimer, and Mickey C. Smith. -- 2nd ed.
    p. ; cm.
 Includes bibliographical references and index.
 ISBN-13: 978-0-7637-6408-1
 ISBN-10: 0-7637-6408-6
 1. Pharmacy--Social aspects. 2. Pharmacy management. 3. Pharmacist and patient. I. Rickles, Nathaniel M. II. Wertheimer, Albert I. III. Smith, Mickey C.
 [DNLM: 1. Pharmaceutical Services. 2. Drug Therapy--psychology. 3. Health Behavior. 4. Pharmacists--psychology. 5. Professional-Patient Relations. 6. Social Medicine. QV 737 S6775 2010]
 RS92.S638 2010
 615.5'8--dc22
                                        2008047471
6048

Printed in the United States of America
13 12 11 10 09   10 9 8 7 6 5 4 3 2 1

Dedication

I would like to dedicate this book to my wife and soul mate, Jenny Rickles, for her persistence, enthusiasm, and unconditional support for all that I strive to do. I also owe much to my parents, Susan and Haskell Rickles, for giving me the guidance and nurturance to pursue my dreams.

NATHANIEL RICKLES

To Joaquima and Lia.

ALBERT WERTHEIMER

Contents

Foreword

When Medicare was introduced in 1965, drug coverage was not seen as essential, and it was not until the Medicare Prescription Drug Improvement and Modernization Act of 2003 that pharmaceuticals gained coverage. In 1965, prescription drugs, other than the antimicrobials, were not as important as they are today, and drugs cost considerably less. It would be unthinkable today to develop a new healthcare program that did not include prescription drugs as an indispensable component. As pharmaceuticals have become increasingly important, expenditures have risen, from $53 billion in 1993 to more than $200 billion in 2005. Government actuaries estimate that expenditures for prescription drugs will be almost half a trillion dollars by 2016, constituting more than one eighth of total health expenditures.

In a similar vein, the social and behavioral aspects of pharmaceutical practice were not seen as particularly important in the early 1960s, although there were some visionary leaders at schools of pharmacy such as at Wisconsin and Ohio State University who foresaw the future and began developing programs that incorporated growing social and behavioral knowledge into pharmacy education. The *First Edition* of this book was the initial comprehensive effort to introduce young pharmacists to the wide range of issues that had an impact on the quality of health care and that would have growing relevance as pharmaceutical practice assumed a more central role in modern health care. Each subsequent edition has sought to deepen the discussion, building on the latest research findings, so that newly educated pharmacists are prepared thoughtfully to adopt expanded roles in our changing healthcare system.

There have been important emerging developments in almost all aspects of pharmaceutical practice, from drug development, testing, approval, and marketing to the role of pharmacists in hospitals and communities. Pharmacists are now less likely to be small entrepreneurs in mom-and-pop pharmacies and more likely to have significant roles in dispensing, monitoring, and advising as an indispensable part of the healthcare team. Pharmacy practice roles continue to evolve, with many more drugs, complex drug regimens, and drug interactions with adverse effects, as well as difficulties retaining patients on even simple drug regimens. In many areas of care, motivating patients to adhere to needed medication regimens, to use their drugs properly, and to avoid harmful combinations of substances constitutes a major aspect affecting quality of care and good outcomes. The social psychology of medication use makes clear that solving such problems requires an understanding of the illness and treatment models that drive patient behavior and that may contradict biomedical models.

The growing pervasiveness and importance of pharmaceuticals is accompanied by much public misinformation, confusion, and patient experimentation based on naive theories of how their bodies respond to medications. Social and behavioral aspects of pharmacy have growing relevance in dealing with these problems, which contribute to many injuries and deaths. Understanding the larger healthcare system and its dynamics also contributes to preventing system errors, particularly those dealing with the administration of pharmaceuticals in hospitals, nursing homes, and other medical facilities.

In recent years pharmacists have taken increasing responsibility in almost every aspect of health care, with the aggregation of patients in large health plans, health maintenance organizations, and medical groups. As attention is directed to improved management of chronic disease and maintaining health through preventive action, pharmacists contribute to monitoring, advising, and assisting patients to keep them properly informed and motivated and to help them arrange their regimens in ways that minimally interfere with their everyday valued activities. In these organizational settings, pharmacists also assist in evaluating and administering drugs, setting pharmaceutical policies, and helping shape drug formularies. Given the hurried pace of medical practice and primary care in the community, patients often look to their neighborhood pharmacist to help them understand and cope with a drug regimen their doctors failed to explain. As retail medicine grows, further new opportunities for pharmaceutical practice will become apparent.

Almost everyone agrees that there are serious problems with our healthcare system and that major changes are needed. Many see a major challenge in improved chronic disease management, new ways of delivering primary care services, and the development of more effective teamwork at all levels of care. Broadly educated pharmacists bring strong assets to such teamwork, making it more possible to provide care that is patient oriented, evidence based, technically outstanding, and consistent with high aspirations and public expectations.

The editors and authors of this book present an important and far-reaching set of social and behavioral perspectives that can help shape many aspects of evolving patient care and pharmacy practice. Such understanding, it is hoped, will contribute to an improved system of practice and care that is adaptive to the healthcare needs of the public and the dynamic nature of medical knowledge and technology.

DAVID MECHANIC
Director, Institute for Health,
Health Care Policy and Aging Research
Rutgers University

Preface

Although this is the *Second Edition* of this book, it is actually the *Fifth Edition* of a book that changed titles with the last edition. In 1974 the *First Edition* of *Pharmacy Practice: Social and Behavioral Aspects* was published by the University Park Press, which was subsequently purchased and merged into a larger publishing firm. The *Second Edition* was published by Williams and Wilkins, and the *Third Edition* by the Haworth Press. What would have been the *Fourth Edition* had a slight name change at the request of the publisher, and it became *Social and Behavioral Aspects of Pharmaceutical Care* in 1996. Now, 13 years later, the present textbook is the *Second Edition* under this same title and is being published by Jones and Bartlett Publishers.

This newly revised and updated edition brings to the contemporary pharmacy practitioner or student a combination of some well-established principles from the social and behavioral sciences along with newer findings and examples of cases and reports of applications of these principles in practice. Ever since the earliest mention of social pharmacy in the late 1960s, there has been a growing body of literature within pharmacy and in the other health sciences helping the pharmacy community reach a deeper understanding of patient behavior and its relationship to treatment outcomes.

What are some important changes since the last edition? First, the present edition is somewhat slimmer than the *First Edition* of this title. This is in part a response to students' desire for fewer pages, more focused discussions on the psychosocial aspects of medication use, and less overlap between chapters. As a result, we removed several chapters in the prior edition that focused on specific pharmacy sites, clinical issues, and clinical populations. We hope these changes will make the book easier to read and broader in scope for those interested in general pharmacy practice issues but less focused on specific clinical applications.

Second, this edition contains a significant focus on public health concepts. The decision to incorporate a greater emphasis on public health is a reaction to a growing focus in pharmacy practice on community-based health education and prevention. One can see this change in focus by the addition of the following six chapters: Chapter 2 on social epidemiology, Chapter 4 on international perspectives on health disparities, Chapter 5 on health promotion and evaluation, Chapter 8 on organizational change, Chapter 21 on psychosocial aspects of medication errors, and Chapter 22 on ethical issues influencing public policy initiatives.

Third, we have also added two chapters that focus on the involvement of caregivers and facilitating behavioral change. Both chapters provide additional perspectives on the medication-use process that had not been included in prior editions.

Several chapters are similar to the 1996 edition because they represent core applications of social and psychological theory to pharmacy practice. Long ago, it was established that patients are people, not objects, and that their opinions, biases, cultures, and trust influence their collaborations with pharmacists and other healthcare professionals. By understanding how these attitudes toward healthcare professionals, medicines, illness, stigma, and privacy influence patient behaviors, we are in a better position to influence beneficial behaviors toward treatment success. This edition will help the reader think of ways in which all patients and their environments present unique challenges regarding medication use, and how organizations and social systems affect patient experiences with medications.

The textbook is organized into four main parts. The first part includes five chapters that focus on describing how health and illness behaviors intersect across individual and societal perspectives given the known empirical and theoretical literature on health behavior and behavioral change. The second and largest part in the book explores more specifically the different alternatives and experiences that individuals and social systems use when engaging in treatment options. This part of the book takes the reader through patient access to a variety of healthcare services that can complement medication use. Chapters in this part consider how pharmacy practice has evolved and factors affecting the provision of various pharmacy services. Across these chapters, there is significant consideration of both individual, interpersonal, and systemic factors that contribute to the structure, function, and evaluation of the medication-use process.

The third part builds on the prior parts' foundations on general considerations affecting pharmaceutical care and explores the challenges of providing care to specific patient populations. The last and smallest part in the textbook examines specific psychosocial dimensions of macro-level problems facing pharmacy practice as we move deeper into the 21st century. In future editions, we suspect we will need to devote a proportionately greater number of pages to this part as our society gains experience tackling the psychosocial complexities concerning such issues as the growing use of health technologies and pharmacogenomics.

A great deal of material is presented in the following pages, and it is probably not realistic to expect any reader of this material to be able to master and apply everything presented. The editors hope that some of the concepts and techniques presented here will assist readers in their journey toward reaching a stronger understanding of the complex and dynamic interactions between patients, their medications, their behaviors, and the healthcare environment. We hope these chapters will challenge readers to continually ask questions, to find answers, and to explore ways to change the pharmacy profession so it can best optimize the provision of pharmaceutical care and meet the drug therapy needs of all patients throughout the world.

We welcome feedback regarding the book and how it has changed approaches to pharmacy practice. We hope the journey through these chapters is enjoyable and thought provoking.

NATHANIEL M. RICKLES
ALBERT I. WERTHEIMER
MICKEY C. SMITH

Acknowledgments

The completion of this textbook would not have been possible without the dedication and hard work of several individuals. The editors would like to thank Dave Cella, the publisher at Jones and Bartlett, for his support throughout the process of bringing the textbook to completion. The editors would also like to thank both Maro Asadoorian, associate editor, and Jill Morton, production assistant, for their tireless efforts to help move the book through its various phases from receipt of chapters to verification of copyright, copyediting, and achieving final copy. Their positive encouragement, diligence to detail, and persistence helped simplify the editing process considerably and keep us all on track. We are all indebted to Jenny Rickles, who helped in several stages of editing and preparing the chapters for completion. Her excellent organizational skills and dedication were critical to the completion of this book. Dr. Rickles thanks Jeffrey Olshan for his editorial assistance on several chapters. Dr. Rickles would also like to give special thanks to Dean John R. Reynolds of the Northeastern University School of Pharmacy for supporting Dr. Rickles' time and effort on the book.

NATHANIEL M. RICKLES
ALBERT I. WERTHEIMER
MICKEY C. SMITH

About the Editors

Nathaniel ("Nate") M. Rickles, PharmD, PhD, BCPP, is an assistant professor of pharmacy practice and administration in the Department of Pharmacy Practice at the School of Pharmacy at Northeastern University. Nate received his BS in psychology and chemistry from Dickinson College, his PharmD from the University of the Sciences in Philadelphia, and his MS and PhD in the social and administrative sciences from the School of Pharmacy at the University of Wisconsin–Madison. Nate also completed a psychiatric pharmacy practice residency at the University of Texas and is board certified in psychiatric pharmacy practice. His primary research interests are to develop, implement, and evaluate intervention programs that improve pharmacist collaboration with patients and other professionals, patient medication adherence, and patient safety. Dr. Rickles also explores educational methods to improve the teaching of communication skills and issues of patient safety. He has published in several peer-reviewed publications and presented at multiple local, national, and international meetings. In addition, Dr. Rickles has received grants from corporations, the federal government, and a national foundation.

Albert I. Wertheimer, PhD, MBA, is the director of the Center for Pharmaceutical Health Services Research at the School of Pharmacy at Temple University. He is the former director of outcomes research and management at Merck & Company, Inc., in West Point, Pennsylvania, and the former vice president of First Health Services (PBM) in Richmond, Virginia. Dr. Wertheimer has held academic appointments as dean of the Philadelphia College of Pharmacy and graduate studies director at the University of Minnesota. He has served as a consultant to governmental and international agencies, such as the World Health Organization, the U.S. Congress, and the

World Bank, as well as to pharmaceutical manufacturers, managed care organizations, and professional societies. Dr. Wertheimer is the author or coauthor of more than 300 journal articles and the author or editor of 27 chapters and 25 books. Dr. Wertheimer has lectured and consulted in more than 55 countries. His current research interests are outcomes research, pharmacoeconomics, quality of life evaluation inquiries, and international drug use.

Mickey C. Smith, PhD, is professor emeritus in the School of Pharmacy at the University of Mississippi. He is a highly acclaimed researcher/writer with an international reputation in the field of pharmaceutical marketing. He has published over 400 articles in over 100 different research and professional journals. Other various awards include the Research Achievement Award from the Academy of Pharmaceutical Sciences, the Rho Chi national lecture award, the first-ever Lyman Award, and the first-ever Distinguished Educator Award from the American Association of Colleges of Pharmacy. His research interests range from health planning and health economics to the sociological aspects of pharmacy.

Contributing Authors

Ilene Abramson, PhD
Adjunct Professor
Lawrence Technological University
College of Arts and Sciences
Southfield, Michigan

H. John Baldwin, PhD
Associate Dean
Nova Southeastern University
College of Pharmacy, Health
    Professions Division
Fort Lauderdale, Florida

Ashley J. Beard, PhD, MPH
Pharmaceutical Policy Research Fellow
Harvard Medical School
Department of Ambulatory Care
    and Prevention
Boston, Massachusetts

Jennifer Beard, PhD, MPH
Assistant Professor
Boston University
School of Public Health, Center for
    International Health
Boston, Massachusetts

Paul Bissell, PhD
Deputy Director of Section, Senior
    Lecturer (Non-Clinical)
University of Sheffield
Section of Public Health
Sheffield, United Kingdom

Susan J. Blalock, PhD, MPH
Associate Professor
University of North Carolina
School of Pharmacy, Division of
    Pharmaceutical Outcomes and Policy
Chapel Hill, North Carolina

**Nicole J. Brandt, PharmD, CGP,
    BCPP, FASCP**
Associate Professor
University of Maryland
School of Pharmacy, Peter Lamy Center
Baltimore, Maryland

Nicky Britten, PhD
Professor
Universities of Exeter and Plymouth
Peninsula Medical School
Exeter, Devon, England

Patricia J. Bush, PhD
Professor Emeritus
Georgetown University
School of Medicine
Washington, DC

Stephen Joel Coons, PhD
Professor
University of Arizona
College of Pharmacy
Tucson, Arizona

Marcus Droege, PhD
Assistant Professor
Nova Southeastern University
College of Pharmacy, Health
      Professions Division
Fort Lauderdale, Florida

Stacie B. Dusetzina, BA
Graduate Teaching Assistant
University of North Carolina
School of Pharmacy, Division of
      Pharmaceutical Outcomes and Policy
Chapel Hill, North Carolina

Kevin C. Farmer, PhD
Associate Professor
University of Oklahoma
College of Pharmacy, Clinical and
      Administrative Sciences Department
Oklahoma City, Oklahoma

Elizabeth Flynn, PhD
Associate Research Professor
Auburn University
School of Pharmacy, Center for Pharmacy
      Operations and Designs
Auburn, Alabama

Sally-Anne Francis, PhD
Honorary Senior Lecturer
University of London
School of Pharmacy, Department of
      Practice and Policy
London, England

Robert I. Garis, PhD, MBA
Associate Professor
Creighton University
School of Pharmacy and
      Health Professions
Omaha, Nebraska

Kent E. M. Groves, PhD, CChem
Adjunct Professor
Dalhousie University
College of Pharmacy
Halifax, Nova Scotia, Canada

Katri Hämeen-Anttila, PhD
Postdoctoral Researcher
University of Kuopio
Department of Social Pharmacy
Kuopio, Finland

Gregory J. Higby, PhD
Executive Director
University of Wisconsin–Madison
School of Pharmacy, American Institute of
      the History of Pharmacy
Madison, Wisconsin

Karen S. Hudmon, DrPH
Associate Professor
Purdue University
School of Pharmacy and
      Pharmaceutical Sciences,
      Department of Pharmacy Practice
West Lafayette, Indiana

Jeffrey A. Johnson, PhD
Professor
University of Alberta
School of Public Health
Edmonton, Alberta, Canada

Jan Kavookjian, PhD, MBA
Assistant Professor
Auburn University
Harrison School of Pharmacy,
      Pharmacy Care Systems
Auburn, Alabama

Anna Knapp, MPH
Program Manager
Boston University
School of Public Health, Center
    for International Health
    and Development
Boston, Massachusetts

Sean T. Leonard, PhD
Assistant Professor/Psychometrician
Nova Southeastern University
College of Pharmacy, Health
    Professions Division
Fort Lauderdale, Florida

John M. Lonie, EdD
Associate Professor
Long Island University
Arnold and Marie Schwartz College of
    Pharmacy and Health Sciences
Division of Social and
    Administrative Sciences
Brooklyn, New York

Neil J. MacKinnon, PhD, FCSHP
Associate Director for Research
    and Associate Professor
    College of Pharmacy
Associate Professor
Dalhousie University
School of Health Services Administration,
    Department of Community Health
    and Epidemiology
Halifax, Nova Scotia, Canada

**Linda Gore Martin, PharmD,
    MBA, BCPS**
Associate Professor
University of Wyoming
School of Pharmacy, Department of
    Social and Administrative Pharmacy
Laramie, Wyoming

Candace Miller, ScD, MHS
Assistant Professor
Boston University
School of Public Health, Center for
    International Health and
    Development, Department of
    International Health
Boston, Massachusetts

Richard L. O'Brien, MD, FACP
Professor
Creighton University Medical Center
Center for Health Policy and Ethics
Omaha, Nebraska

Denise L. Orwig, PhD
Assistant Professor
University of Maryland
School of Medicine, Department of
    Epidemiology and Preventive
    Medicine, Division of Gerontology
Baltimore, Maryland

John Pappan, MA, MS
Research and Teaching Assistant
Long Island University
Arnold and Marie Schwartz College of
    Pharmacy and Health Sciences
Brooklyn, New York

Lourdes G. Planas, PhD
Assistant Professor
University of Oklahoma
College of Pharmacy, Department of
    Clinical and Administrative Sciences
Oklahoma City, Oklahoma

Jeremy Popek, PharmD
Staff Pharmacist
Walgreens
Springfield, Missouri

Paul L. Ranelli, PhD
Professor
University of Minnesota
College of Pharmacy, Department
    of Pharmacy Practice and
    Pharmaceutical Sciences
Duluth, Minnesota

Jenny O. Rickles, MPH, CPHQ
Quality Improvement Analyst
Dana-Farber Cancer Institute
Boston, Massachusetts

Nathaniel M. Rickles, PharmD,
    PhD, BCPP
Assistant Professor
Northeastern University
School of Pharmacy, Department
    of Pharmacy Practice
    and Administration
Boston, Massachusetts

Kraig L. Schell, PhD
Associate Professor
Angelo State University
Department of Psychology, Social
    Sociology, and Social Work
San Angelo, Texas

Ingrid Sketris, PharmD, MPA (HSA)
Professor
Dalhousie University
College of Pharmacy
Halifax, Nova Scotia, Canada

Felicity Smith, PhD
Professor
University of London
School of Pharmacy, Department of
    Practice and Policy
London, England

Janine Morgall Traulsen, PhD
Associate Professor
University of Copenhagen
Section of Social Pharmacy, Department of
    Pharmacology and Pharmacotherapy
Copenhagen, Denmark

Brenda Waning, MPH
Assistant Professor
Boston University
School of Public Health, Center for
    International Health
Boston, Massachusetts

Albert I. Wertheimer, PhD, MBA
Director
Temple University
School of Pharmacy, Center
    for Pharmaceutical Health
    Services Research
Philadelphia, Pennsylvania

Salisa Westrick, PhD
Assistant Professor
Auburn University
Harrison School of Pharmacy, Department
    of Pharmacy Care Systems
Auburn, Alabama

PART I

Interpretation of the Health Problem and Need for Treatment

The first five chapters of *Social and Behavioral Aspects of Pharmaceutical Care* focus on individuals' interpretations of their health problems and their need for treatment. These five chapters focus on describing health and illness behaviors from both individual and societal perspectives and within the context of both the empirical and theoretical literature on health behavior and behavioral change. Chapter 1 defines health and illness behavior. To obtain a more global perspective on health and illness behavior, Chapter 2 explores the nature and frequencies of illnesses throughout the world. Chapter 3 builds on the first chapter by bringing together multiple theoretical concepts of how individual health and illness behaviors operate within the context of an individual's interaction with the social systems around him or her. Chapter 4 examines how individuals are affected by health and social systems that do not adequately meet their health needs. Chapter 5 investigates models of how individuals and communities can improve health behaviors that ultimately help meet the health needs identified in Chapter 4. These chapters connect with each other as building blocks for thinking about how individuals and social systems react and interact with one another in response to illness. Such multilevel foundations of health and illness behaviors are important for the pharmacy professional as a way to better understand the factors that affect the general experiences and opportunities of patients throughout the world.

SECTION A

Concepts of Health and Illness

CHAPTER 1

Definitions and Meaning of Health and Illness

Marcus Droege, PhD, Sean T. Leonard, PhD, and H. John Baldwin, PhD

THE GENESIS OF SOCIAL PHARMACY

Arguably, no other health profession has been challenged with changes as profound and momentous as the profession of pharmacy in recent history. A significant transformation involving a professional shift in focus from the product to the patient has occurred, pharmacists have assumed new roles as patient care providers, and pharmacy education has faced formidable challenges subsequent to this evolution, particularly the transition to the doctor of pharmacy as the first professional degree.

A basic understanding of historical events that have shaped contemporary pharmacy education reveals edifying insights into the pharmacist's role in society today. Pharmacy educators formed the Millis Study Commission in 1975 in an attempt to align (or realign) pharmacy education with the contemporary drug-related needs of patients.[1] The commission set out to revise pharmacy curricula that were historically oriented to basic sciences and devise a road map to the profession's future. The Millis Commission, convened by the American Association of Colleges of Pharmacy (AACP), had a significant impact on contemporary pharmacy education, and many believe that pharmacy education today has been shaped by the numerous recommendations of the commission. The commission was charged with addressing the perceived lack of "insight and foresight" in pharmacy education pertaining to the role of the pharmacist as an integral member of the healthcare team. In addition to the many recommendations related to the need for an outcomes-based pharmacy curriculum, student recruitment, and a six-year doctor of pharmacy degree as a first professional degree, the commission's recommendations were for "curricula with less knowledge of science and more knowledge of patients and well people."[1] De-emphasizing the basic science focus of pharmacy curricula while focusing more on knowledge about how people make decisions about their health was deemed to be an important early step toward the differentiation of pharmacists while they are still students. Pharmacy education at the time was perceived to be all about drugs and not about people, an emphasis in stark contrast with the need for a qualified practitioner possessing the skills and knowledge necessary to identify, resolve, and prevent patients' drug therapy problems.

The patient-oriented view required pharmacy curricula to include topics such as the social and behavioral aspects of healthcare delivery and communication skills. Discussion about curricular change and the Millis Commission report coincided with the creation of graduate programs and a disciplinary focus area in the social and administrative sciences as they pertain to pharmacy. These social pharmacy programs deal with the full scope of problems of pharmacy and medicines in society.

DEFINITIONS OF HEALTH AND ILLNESS

Health and illness are central themes of human existence, with various definitions and interpretations spanning all cultures. Addressing concerns arising from ill health receives much attention in virtually every society around the world, and substantive resources are devoted to the education of health professionals. The raison d'être for any healthcare professional to practice in his or her respective field can be found in the very existence of health and illness along a continuum of definitions. In fact, the conceptualization of health and illness delineates the wide-ranging spectrum of practitioner activities across disciplines. Decisions about someone's healthcare needs, irrespective of who makes this determination, drive interventions. In the case of pharmacy, practitioner responsibilities can be found in the identification, resolution, and prevention of drug therapy problems, which should logically coincide with the focus of pharmacy education.

Given the universality, prevalence, and frequency of illness and disease for both individuals and society, it perhaps seems strange that they are considered to be abnormal conditions. One could argue, as René Dubos has, that disease and sickness are normal, whereas health is the abnormal condition.[2] However, it is socially necessary for each individual within a society to contribute to that society for the society to flourish. Thus, each person has one or more roles that define who that person is, what he or she does, and what is expected of him or her—for example, student, spouse, wage earner, parent. These roles have two characteristics of relevance to this discussion, namely, the societal expectations of an individual occupying a particular role and the reciprocal nature of any role.

A review of the literature reveals that definitions of health and illness vary largely on the basis of cultural background. *Disease* is a medical term, meaning there is a pathologic change in the structure or function of the body or mind. The World Health Organization's 1947 definition of health, "a state of complete physical, mental, and social well being, not merely the absence of disease or infirmity," reflects this mechanistic view of the body in which ill health is treated as the mechanical failure of some part of one or more systems of the body and the medical task is to repair the damage.[3] At the same time, however, the definition expands the role of healthcare providers beyond the traditional role of treating disease.

Illness is the response of the person to a disease; it is an abnormal process in which the person's level of functioning is changed. Talcott Parsons's 1972 definition of *health*, "the state of optimum capacity of an individual for the effective performance of the roles and tasks for which he has been socialized," expands earlier definitions to address the social needs of individuals—that is, normal role functioning.[4] This shift from an individualistic toward a more collectivistic view of the effects of health and illness had far-reaching consequences for healthcare practitioners because they were no longer limited to treating disease but could engage in preventive measures.

THE SOCIAL DIMENSION OF PHARMACY

Just as individual actions collectively form and affect the society in which individuals live, so too society affects the actions of individuals. Sociology is the social science that examines the organization and mores of a society, and sociologists study a variety of issues with which pharmacy is concerned , such as professions and role theory.

Sociology is a social science focused on theory, whereas pharmacy can be viewed as a field of application, taking concepts and facts from other fields and applying them to practice. As stated earlier, pharmacy education has tended to focus on chemical and biological sciences, with little input from the social sciences. It was not until the mid-1960s that the seminal papers on social pharmacy topics were published in the pharmacy literature. Harding and Taylor discussed the social dimensions of pharmacy and pointed out that our actions as healthcare professionals are embedded in a social context. Societal change and increased risk averseness have prompted providers of health care to rethink their professional roles and define their activities as an "exemplar of social action."[5]

A major theme in sociology has been the process of becoming a patient. It has been suggested that the sick role be the focus of medical sociology. Certainly the patient may be considered as a central concept in any discussion of health care, the role of pharmacists, or medication use. Perhaps the best known and most cited characterization of the concept of "patient" is that of Talcott Parsons, a sociologist interested in social systems and the development of societies.[6] To oversimplify, all societies consist of "actors" with multiple roles, each with a complementary role, adhering to a common or normative set of characteristics, and having reciprocal expectations. Each role has associated rights and obligations. The rights of a particular role are the responsibilities of its complementary role. There is some degree of tolerance for deviance from the norm. However, every society must have some means for enforcement of what Parsons calls the "societal normative order." As stated earlier, it is socially necessary that each individual within a society contribute to that society for the society to flourish, and illness or sickness is a deviation from what is considered normal. Consequently, the sick role is a method of social control over illness as a deviant behavior. There are two rights inherent in the sick role: the right to not be responsible or blamed for the condition and the right to be excused from normal role responsibilities; the two obligations or responsibilities are to seek competent help and to "want to get well."

Another sociologist, Edward A. Suchman, formulated illness behavior as consisting of five stages: symptom experience, assumption of the sick role, medical care contact, dependent patient, and recovery or rehabilitation (Table 1-1).[7] Each stage necessitates a decision by the "could-be patient" and illustrates the importance of the "lay referral" system, made up of family and friends, which constitutes the complementary role to the sick role.

At the symptom experience stage, the initial stage of illness behavior, the decision is made that something is wrong, or not normal. There are three aspects to this stage: physical experience, cognitive aspects, and emotional response. The most common physical experience indicating that something is wrong is pain. Cognitively, the experience is interpreted based on what the physical manifestations are, their severity, and the course they take, as well as previous personal experience or knowledge about the

TABLE 1-1 Suchman's Model of the Stages of Illness Experience
1. Symptom experience
2. Assumption of the sick role
3. Medical care contact
4. Dependent patient
5. Recovery or rehabilitation
Adapted from Suchman EA. Stages of illness and medical care. J Health Hum Behav 1965;6:114-28.

signs. Symptoms are recognized and defined in terms of their interference with normal role functioning. The emotional response includes fear, concern, or anxiety. When symptoms are extremely severe, felt to be serious, and perceived to interfere with other role responsibilities, the most common first inclination is to seek medical care, with a smaller number considering self-medication. However, even then there is a tendency to delay seeking treatment and engage in self-denial, at least until one has discussed the symptoms with a layperson, typically a relative and most frequently a spouse.

Healthcare practitioners distinguish between signs and symptoms of disease. *Signs* are measurable changes of physiologic functioning and are detectable using diagnostic procedures, often involving medical instruments and diagnostic methods (e.g., stethoscope, glucometer). Many times, signs have little to no meaning to patients and may not even be noticed by them. *Symptoms*, however, are inherently subjective and not easily quantifiable. In most cases, patients will notice symptoms (e.g., pain, fatigue, nausea) as an expression of ill health, and a practitioner will seek to get a sense of the nature of the symptoms by asking the patient to, for example, rate pain during an examination. Healthcare professionals rely on patients reporting symptoms during an examination because they will use both signs and symptoms in formulating a hypothesis of a likely diagnosis.

An acute illness has a rapid onset of symptoms and lasts only a relatively short time, whereas characteristics of chronic disease often include permanent change to the body's functioning. Chronic disease causes, or is caused by, irreversible alterations in normal anatomy and physiology. Although a cure is possible in most cases of acute illness, chronic diseases tend to require special patient education for rehabilitation as well as long periods of care or support.

Symptom experience varies widely from individual to individual, as does the description of symptoms along the continuum of acute versus chronic conditions. A key determining factor is the "return to normal" and the ability to assume normal role functioning without permanent change. In most cases, chronic symptoms result in sustained changes in a person's life. In addition, patients will likely be able to communicate the underlying cause (disease) of which the symptoms are a consequence. This is in contrast to an acute illness, where patients are often unaware of the underlying cause of their symptoms and will in most cases rely on expert practitioners to combine signs and symptoms as evidence for disease.

The assumption of the sick role stage is when the individual makes the decision that he or she is sick. As the individual seeks information and advice and relief of symptoms, the individual's lay referral system is paramount because few individuals are sufficiently confident to decide on their own that they are sick. Also, consistent with Parsons's formulation, sickness excuses them from their normal role obligations and imposes concurrent obligations on these significant others. Thus, the sick individual seeks permission (technically, "provisional validation" or "provisional legitimization") from these individuals to be sick and excused from his or her normal responsibilities. In almost all cases, the sick individual follows the advice given by his or her discussant.

At the medical care contact stage, the sick individual contacts a professional within the healthcare system, seeking advice and permission to be sick from a "scientific" rather than a lay source, that is, an authoritative definition or diagnosis of his or her condition, a proposed treatment, and official sanctioning or "legitimization" to be sick. If legitimization is denied, the individual is expected to return to his or her normal role activities. This stage may continue if the sick individual is not satisfied with the initial physician's diagnosis or recommended treatment; for example, the individual may begin to "doctor shop." Interestingly, a significant minority of treated individuals indicate that they never received a diagnosis or prognosis from the physician. The most common treatment is medication, with the physician writing one or more prescriptions for the diseased or ill person.

At the dependent patient stage, a decision is made to transfer control to the physician and accept and follow the prescribed treatment. The most important aspects of this stage are that (1) only at this stage does the sick individual become a patient, (2) most patients believe, or claim, that they adhere to the physician's treatment, and (3) the family and "lay referral system" continue to play an important role. Most patients do not accept the patient role easily because they are reluctant to give up their normal roles, but they may see that the only way to health and a return to these roles is to surrender their autonomy to the professional and lay caregivers. Also significant are the variety of barriers—social, administrative, logistical, psychological—that may easily affect the treatment process.

Of course, it is not always desirable to be assigned to the role of patient, or one who suffers from an illness. For example, until relatively recently homosexual individuals in the United States could be diagnosed with a mental illness. It was not until 1973 that the American Psychiatric Association voted to change the diagnostic system to allow homosexuality to be considered normal.[8] Before that time a diagnosed homosexual could be assigned to the sick role and consequently lose social rights and privileges. He or she could be committed to psychiatric institutions, arrested and detained as a "sexual deviant" for engaging in homosexual behavior, and so on.[9]

It is important for the student of pharmacy to recognize that the nature of sexuality did not somehow change in the early 1970s—rather, the social context and values surrounding sexual orientation changed. Homosexual orientation had been medicalized as an illness by Western clinicians for nearly a century, and some historians have argued that this reflects a pervasive bias within Western medicine against nonconventional sexual expression.[10] This bias may have its origins in moral or religious values about what is "right" and proper, yet the values are expressed in the form of a clinical diagnosis. In this way, diagnoses can be used as a social tool to regulate behavior. The personal values of the clinician may intersect or even conflict with standards of clinical practice, as may be observed in the assertion by some pharmacists that their moral or religious values prohibit them from dispensing certain kinds of contraceptive medications.

The final stage of illness, recovery or rehabilitation, requires a decision to relinquish the patient role. Because of the patient's desire (and responsibility) to return to health, this decision is generally easy in comparison to the necessary decisions at other stages. Also at this point, either or both the healthcare professional and the lay caregivers withdraw their legitimization of the patient's right to be excused from normal role responsibilities, and the patient is expected to resume his or her old roles or, in chronic conditions or disability, accept a long period of convalescence or rehabilitation or a new role as an invalid.

Both Suchman's and Parsons's formulations have withstood the test of time during the last four to five decades. It must be noted, however, that Suchman validated his formulation based on a well-defined sample of people who had experienced a specific episode of illness and passed through all five stages. There is no requirement that all five stages be involved, nor are specific time frames associated with each phase, which may be brief or lengthy. Suchman pointed out that for the ill person, social concerns seem to predominate over medical or health concerns and that responses to minor illness would seem to be even more likely to be governed by social rather than medical concerns. Additionally, Suchman dealt with people with acute conditions or an acute episode of a chronic condition. However, Suchman also points out that individuals have a natural tendency to underestimate (dismiss, ignore, disregard, or deny) symptoms that are neither severe nor incapacitating. Because many chronic diseases are characterized by a lack of symptoms, or seemingly minor, virtually unrecognizable symptoms, they are more easily denied and people are therefore unlikely to seek early medical care.

Indeed, this same characteristic would appear to be an explanation for some types of nonadherence, together with the natural responsibility to want to return to a healthy status and normal role functioning. The classic example is high blood pressure and patient nonadherence to blood pressure medications that serve as a constant reminder that one is sick, despite the lack of overt symptoms.

The recovery and rehabilitation stage also holds special significance for those with chronic conditions. Because the ill person is expected to do everything possible to return to health, yet chronic conditions by definition mean that there is no cure, special strain is put upon both the ill person and the lay caregiver. Frequently this seems to be resolved by a redefinition of what is "normal" for the afflicted individual. The classic example is patients with diabetes, who most frequently are able to control the disease with medication and, despite the continued reminders (regular medication, blood glucose readings) and relatively minor lifestyle changes (diet, exercise), generally are able to resume their previous social roles with only minor, if any, restrictions.

The sick role, as formulated by Parsons, carries within it an inherent potential conflict. The ill person has the right to be excused from normal role responsibilities while at the same time has the responsibility to seek competent help and do everything possible to return to health and resume normal role responsibilities. For some people, the care and attention they receive when sick, coupled with being excused from doing things they would normally be expected to do (e.g., in the case of children, going to school when they are unprepared for an upcoming test or have not done the expected homework), is an attractive proposition. These people accept the rights of illness but seek to avoid the responsibility. Thus, these people adopt the "negative sick role."

Relinquishing the sick role appears to cause most people less difficulty than assuming it.[11] Convalescence, although not enjoyable, proceeds smoothly in most cases and ends with the patient's return to his or her former well status. Although there may be some concern about picking up where one had left off, this is not a problem for most people.

Succinctly stated, health and illness exist along a continuum, are inherently constrained by interference with social action, and are much less objective than most people recognize.

CULTURAL AND CONTEXTUAL FACTORS IN HEALTH AND ILLNESS

There is much to be learned about health and illness in the process of becoming a healthcare professional. Even in training programs that last for years, there may be relatively little time devoted to recognizing that definitions of health and illness are subjective in many ways. It may be tempting for students to assume that the diagnoses they learn in training are objective, free from bias, and durable over time. The most common philosophical approach to these issues reflected in medical schools and textbooks has been described as naïve normalism, in which illness connotes abnormal functioning and health is suggestive of "normal" functioning.[12] However, the actual definition of "normal" is hardly clear, and in fact may be largely subjective and influenced by prevailing cultural factors.

For example, what constitutes a disease or illness in one culture may be considered normal and healthy in another. In Germany, low blood pressure is often interpreted as an illness, whereas in the United States it typically is not. An individual in Germany with this condition may be permitted to assume the sick role: he or she may be excused from some social responsibilities and receive treatment from healthcare professionals. Yet if the same individual were part of a different culture, he or she might not be afforded the sick role. Similarly, interpretations of a disease state may vary as well. Students may be surprised to learn that a fairly large proportion of adults (as many as 40%) are colonized by *Helicobacter pylori*, yet relatively few of these individuals develop duodenal and peptic ulceration.[13] Therefore the mere presence of *H. pylori* in a patient does not necessarily mean that he or she is "sick."

Clinicians are afforded social status and power by virtue of their training and expertise, which means that their personal values are often given great weight—even when those values and opinions are not informed by their professional training or scientific findings. We can expect that when there are significant, widespread changes in social values within a culture, then definitions and standards for health and illness will also be in some way affected.

This may be a humbling point for healthcare professionals to accept: the nature of our role and work is not strictly objective, and our current understandings of health and illness will likely change over time. It is sound advice to new students that one ought to avoid the temptation of being overly confident in one's knowledge and work. A tragic example from history is the fact that the genocide perpetrated by the Nazis during World War II was to some extent facilitated by healthcare professionals.[14] Physicians and other healthcare professionals were recruited by the Nazi party to medicalize the process of killing socially undesirable people: the sick and feeble were "euthanized" in hospitals, sterilization was forced upon certain social and cultural groups, and physicians routinely evaluated new arrivals to concentration camps to determine their fitness for work (where the alternative to work was execution). By giving the process of genocide a medical façade, the Nazi social and political agendas were more easily disguised and adopted on a large scale. Of course, this was only possible because some healthcare professionals adopted the Nazi value system (and extreme biases) as their own. History warns healthcare professionals that we are not immune to having our expert knowledge swayed and distorted by larger social forces.

This lesson may be especially relevant to today's pharmacists. There is considerable controversy surrounding the marketing of medications to laypersons, and how advertisements about medications contribute to the social context in which pharmacists practice. Large pharmaceutical companies have been accused by some of either creating or exaggerating the prevalence of diseases and symptoms to persuade people that they may "need" medication treatment. The controversy has largely focused on psychiatric conditions, such as attention deficit disorder, but also has extended to diagnoses such as restless leg syndrome, irritable bowel syndrome, and the medical treatment of menopause. The argument is that marketing efforts by pharmaceutical companies have perpetuated the widespread belief that "there is a pill for everything" and therefore there has been a proliferation of new disease states and symptoms that merit medication treatment.

It can be observed that there are some common conditions that do not have medication treatments available (e.g., celiac disease), yet these are not as well known within the lay public as diagnoses that carry with them known medication treatments. Also, it is not unusual to group nonmedication treatments collectively as "alternative therapies" even when those treatments (such as psychotherapy, occupational therapy, behavioral modification, etc.) demonstrate equal or better responses. It is also interesting to note that symptoms of an illness (such as "fatigue") are portrayed in many advertisements as being as "serious" as the illness itself and that associations between symptoms and diseases are overstated—for example, implying that a vaccine for the human papilloma virus is essentially a vaccine for cervical cancer or asserting that depression is a medical condition. Although the diagnosis of major depressive disorder has been substantiated as a disease, the lay use of the term *depression* tends to be situational and usually refers to less severe emotional experiences (e.g., hearing distressing news) that generally do not satisfy the diagnostic criteria.

The controversy about pharmaceutical marketing is ongoing, and we certainly cannot offer the reader any firm conclusions about it, yet we can point out that the existence of this controversy demonstrates that definitions of health and illness do not exist in a vacuum. Even business and economic forces influence our interpretations of what is healthy and what is pathologic.

It is interesting that people may define health and illness in ways that are different from clinicians. For example, it has been found that older adults who have multiple health problems may still describe themselves as "healthy." On the other hand, some people define themselves as suffering from a medical condition in which the nature of the "illness" is poorly defined or subjectively understood. This is best observed in the ubiquity of the word *addiction* in Western society, where addiction implies a biological or medical condition or both. When one is "addicted" to something, he or she may be afforded the sick role and thereby be partially or fully excused from responsibility for his or her actions because of uncontrollable biological forces. Addiction has been applied to alcohol and other substances, but more recently has also been used to explain behaviors that do not involve a known substance, such as addictions to shopping, television, the Internet, sexual behaviors and pornography, gambling, and so on. Such definitions of addictions are controversial among clinicians and researchers, yet it is not at all unusual to encounter laypersons who use these terms to explain their own or someone else's behavior.

Body image is another area in which the medicalization of common problems and concerns may be observed. Standards of beauty change over time; several centuries ago, women with large ("Rubenesque") physiques were considered more attractive than slender women. In modern Western civilization that standard for beauty has essentially reversed, and perhaps it is no coincidence that drugs and medical procedures that alter physical appearance have become increasingly popular. Elective surgery (such as liposuction) and other cosmetic procedures are rendered largely within a medical context: procedures are performed by professional clinicians, and recipients of elective cosmetic procedures may undergo surgery, receive prescription medications, and even be identified by clinicians as "patients"—yet they typically are not defined as "ill," "sick," or being "in need of treatment." There is literature suggesting that most people are in some way disappointed with their physical appearance (it is normal to be dissatisfied with some feature of one's own appearance), but whether or not this constitutes a medical problem has yet to be substantiated.

Nonetheless, modern pharmacists will recognize that concerns about body image pervade Western culture, and that increasingly people are turning to either medical or pseudomedical solutions. A new term in the pharmacy lexicon is *lifestyle drugs*, which are not always medically necessary yet may be prescribed for other (e.g., cosmetic) reasons. Lifestyle drugs may include those that decrease wrinkles in skin, promote hair growth, and so forth. Examples of pseudomedical solutions include advertisements for "nutritional supplements" that look surprisingly like advertisements for prescription medications and offer guarantees of weight loss and increased sexual performance.

Thus, it can be seen that individuals interact with healthcare professionals for diverse reasons, and the nature of those interactions is shaped by numerous external forces, such as culture, society, morality, and economics. Further, definitions of health and illness are not limited to clinical interactions: an individual can define himself or herself as "sick" without any formal clinical diagnosis or can define himself or herself as "healthy" even in the presence of a formal diagnosis. Suffice it to say that objectively understanding health and illness is remarkably complicated, even though clinicians routinely interact with patients as though there were little or no subjectivity involved in the process.

We have been building up to a point that by now should make intuitive sense: as a pharmacist, it is both prudent and necessary to consider clinical interactions of all kinds as a type of social experience. Social experiences are not strictly objective, and consequently even the most skilled and competent pharmacist is susceptible to making errors during clinical interactions. Being mindful of the social context in the practice of pharmacy can help one reduce the risk of errors and thereby enhance the quality of treatment.

In this sense of the word, *errors* are not limited to medical errors. Rather, the concept refers to the universal problem that human perception is not reliably objective: nobody is perfect. Sociologists, social psychologists, and other social scientists can tell us much about the ways in which we are prone to perceiving social experiences inaccurately. Although the list of perceptual errors and distortions that all of us are susceptible to is quite long, we can benefit from focusing upon a few.

The fundamental attribution error (FAE) is also known as either personality over-attribution or correspondence bias.[15,16] It has been defined in different ways, but essentially the FAE is the tendency to overlook situational factors in favor of more durable personality traits when explaining human behaviors. In short, the FAE is the tendency to believe that someone's observed behavior is entirely representative or descriptive of who they are as a whole person. The problem with such sweeping conclusions is that behavior changes significantly according to its context, and in reality, most people are very complex and their behaviors are determined by multiple factors.

For example, imagine that you are working in a community pharmacy and are confronted with a frustrated patient. The patient complains about the costs of his pain medications and about having to wait for the prescription to be filled. The FAE may lead you to conclude, "This is the kind of person who complains about everything—he's just an irritable person and nothing will satisfy him." These are attributions about the patient's personality, which is durable and unlikely to change. The reality may be that this patient is actually very reasonable and likeable in most other contexts—it's just that right now, he is in pain and distress. These are situational factors. You might not fully appreciate the FAE until a time when you are in pain and distress while waiting for treatment, at which point you become frustrated and demanding toward your caregivers. The FAE might lead you to believe that you are normally a patient, calm individual, except that now you are in a frustrating situation.

Practically everyone is susceptible to the FAE, and it has a clear implication for clinicians. As a pharmacist, you will be interacting with patients when they are sick, and being sick commonly induces distress. That is, being sick is a situational factor that may influence behavior, yet the behavior you observe among your patients may not be at all descriptive of their entire personalities. The individual who presents to you as irritable and demanding at the pharmacy counter may, under most other contexts, be quite calm and patient.

Similar to the FAE is confirmatory bias, in which one's attention is focused upon supporting initial impressions about someone else—even to the exclusion of disconfirming evidence. There was a case in which a patient attempted to fill a prescription that the pharmacy did not have on hand; when informed of the problem, the patient complained and demanded to speak to the pharmacy manager. The pharmacy manager first met with her staff, who advised her that "this patient is slurring his words and is probably drunk." Upon meeting with the disgruntled patient, the pharmacy manager fell victim to the confirmatory bias: she operated from the first impression that this patient was intoxicated, and disregarded the patient's assertions to the contrary. It turned out that the patient was dysarthric due to a cerebral vascular accident and was not intoxicated at all. This part of the patient's medical history might have been revealed had the pharmacy manager assessed him more objectively. Another way of expressing the thinking behind the confirmatory bias is "Don't confuse me with the facts—my mind is made up." The lesson here is to be wary of operating too strongly from first impressions.

Other sources of bias frequently come into play as clinicians interact with patients, and so it is not surprising to learn that clinicians are often more confident in their assessments of patients than they are accurate in those assessments.

SUMMARY

Both Parsons's concept of the sick role and Suchman's theory of illness behavior have stood the test of time. But times have changed, and patient–pharmacist interactions are increasingly influenced by social forces. Because future roles are expected to expand and direct patient care is predicted to increase, an understanding of the patient as well as of social and behavioral aspects of pharmaceutical care is highly pertinent to today's practicing pharmacist. It is important to acknowledge the inherently subjective nature of health care and healthcare delivery despite the presumed objectivity that is implied in today's science-driven approach. As pharmacists provide direct patient care, there is a responsibility of the profession to recognize the dynamic social context of healthcare practices.

Culture and norms have changed and become more complex over time. Major changes include the following: the recognition of the patient's right to make decisions about his or her treatment; an emphasis on preventive medicine and wellness; recognition of nonadherence; acknowledgment that traditional Western medicine is only one choice for the ill person, and that people tend to use both conventional medicine and alternative therapies concurrently or in a complementary fashion; an increase in the use of health insurance, including federal and state programs; the emphasis on cost containment by third parties, including health maintenance organizations and managed care; the change from a preponderance of acute conditions to chronic conditions; emphasis on self care; direct-to-consumer advertising; lifestyle drugs; the proliferation of allied health professionals and paraprofessionals; and demographic changes, including the aging of America. Each of these changes is associated with a social dimension relative to pharmacy practice and will be addressed in subsequent chapters of this text.

REFERENCES

1. Worthen DB, ed. The Millis Study Commission on Pharmacy: a road map to a profession's future. Binghamton, NY: Pharmaceutical Products Press, 2006.
2. Dubos R. Mirage of health: utopias, progress and biological change. London: Allen and Unwin, 1960.
3. Doyal L. What makes women sick: gender and the political economy of health. New Brunswick, NJ: Rutgers University Press, 1995.
4. Parsons T. Definitions of health and illness in the light of American values and social structures. In: Jaco E, ed. Patients, physicians, and illness. 2nd ed. New York: Free Press, 1972.
5. Harding G, Taylor K. Social dimensions of pharmacy: (1) the social context of pharmacy. Pharm J 2002;269:395-7.
6. Parsons T. The social system. London: Routledge & Kagan Paul, 1951.
7. Suchman EA. Stages of illness and medical care. J Health Hum Behav 1965;6:114-28.
8. American Psychiatric Association. Position statement on homosexuality and civil rights. Am J Psychiatry 1973;131:497.
9. Pratt J. The rise and fall of homophobia and sexual psychopath legislation in postwar society. Psychol Public Policy Law 1998;4:25-49.
10. Bullough VL. Science in the bedroom: a history of sex research. New York: Harper Collins, 1994.
11. Baldwin HJ, Cosler LE, Schulz RM. Opinion leadership in medication information. Communication Q 1987;35:84-102.
12. Sadegh-Zadeh K. Fuzzy health, illness, and disease. J Med Philos 2000;25:605-38.
13. Cherry MJ. Polymorphic medical ontologies: fashioning concepts of disease. J Med Philos 2000;25:519-38.
14. Lifton RJ. The Nazi doctors: medical killing and the psychology of genocide. New York: Harper Collins, 1986.
15. Jones EE, Harris VA. The attribution of attitudes. J Exp Social Psychol 1967;3:1-24.
16. Ross L. The intuitive psychologist and his shortcomings: distortions in the attribution process. In: Berkowitz L, ed. Advances in experimental social psychology. Vol. 10. New York: Academic Press, 1977.

CHAPTER 2

Social Epidemiology

Candace Miller, ScD, MHS, Brenda Waning, MPH, Jennifer Beard, PhD, MPH, and Anna Knapp, MPH

Society enters the body in many ways. From the dawn of civilization, throughout history and time and across geography and place, the society within which we live has influenced health and illness. Whereas *epidemiology* is the discipline that studies the distribution and causes of disease, *social epidemiology* is the discipline focused on the societal factors that determine the patterning of disease within and across populations. Social epidemiologists seek to explain how society "gets into the body" and to identify complex patterns of morbidity and mortality that vary based on societal structure, cultural norms, and socioeconomic position (Table 2-1). For example, why are some groups more likely to suffer from cardiovascular disease, human immuno-deficiency virus (HIV) infection, or cancer? Why are some patients more or less likely to adhere to various treatment regimens? What factors buffer some groups from harm or increase access to and effectiveness of pharmacologic interventions?

Social epidemiologists argue that we are not all created equal. On the contrary, economic, political, social, and other processes and structures determine the different and unequal distribution of resources and services that promote health, buffer against illness, and cure disease. Throughout the world, the highest socioeconomic classes have the highest-quality shelter, health care, and schools, whereas the lowest classes often struggle with reduced access to affordable food, adequate housing, health care, and protection from environmental hazards. Modern social epidemiologists argue that throughout history, social elites have inequitably organized societies through laws, policies, and cultural norms in order to protect or benefit their position. As a result, persisting inequalities based on gender, class, age, sexual orientation, race and ethnicity, and other characteristics are the rule, rather than the exception.

TABLE 2-1   Various Factors at Different Levels That Interact to Influence Health Status

Structural	Social	Individual
Legal Structures	**Social Capital**	**Individual Characteristics**
Laws	Trust	Sex
Law enforcement	Norms	Age
		Race/ethnicity
Policy Environment	**Community**	Disability
Economic policy	Access to health care	Psychosocial
Health and education policy	Community groups	Biology
Social policy	Schools and workplaces	Heredity
Agricultural, transportation,	Institutions	
trade, etc., policies	Risks and protections	**Behaviors**
		Hygiene
Demographic Change	**Cultural Context**	Sexual activity
Urbanization	Beliefs, patterns of behavior	Diet and exercise
Migration	Traditions	Care practices
Aging of population	Gender roles	
		Socioeconomic Position
Institutions	**Social Networks**	Income
Government	Social influence	Education
Legislative system	Engagement	Occupation
Judicial system	Access to resources	
Regional and international	Support	
bodies and laws		
	Physical Environment	
	Weather	
	Natural resources	
	Hazards	

Our bodies are directly and indirectly influenced by where we live, our parents' (and their parents') economic status, our mothers' prenatal care, our education, the stressors we face, the resources we can access, and the support we enjoy or lack within our communities. In addition, government policies and laws that regulate taxes, pollution, trade, drug prices, welfare support, food supplies, the economy, employment, access to and quality of health insurance, and other important factors also affect health and disease. Morbidity and mortality are not random, but geographically and socially patterned to render some people winners and others losers.

Social epidemiology can be conceptualized along a scale of biological organization, in which molecular biology focuses on the level of molecular particles; cell biology concentrates on the cellular level; physiology focuses on the organ level; clinical research occurs at the individual level; and finally, epidemiology occurs at the level of the individual, family, community, and society.[1] Social epidemiologic inquiry occurs at the levels of the individual and the society simultaneously, without overlooking genetics and biomedical causation.[2]

HISTORY

For centuries, physicians, scientists, activists, philosophers, and laypeople have sought to understand the causes of disease in populations. This has always been a political process, largely led by elite social classes and dominant global powers. Thus, including social causes of disease in the public discourse has been a difficult, arduous journey transcending centuries and continents.

In the 17th century, efforts to understand and predict disease motivated the documentation of disease symptoms, outbreak patterns, and patient outcomes. For example, in the 1600s, the first Bills of Mortality were compiled, creating what is now a modern-day death registry, listing characteristics of individuals and providing details on who died of what. In London, John Graunt (1620–1674), an early statistician, set out to understand who was dying during outbreaks of the bubonic plague in order to set up an early warning system and prevent death. He noted differences in death rates based on sex and residency and completed a seminal work in vital statistics called the *Natural and Political Observations Upon the Bills of Mortality*.

By the 1700s, there was a greater understanding of the specific causes of disease. A French physician, Louis René Villerme (1782–1863), recognized elevated levels of illness that appeared work related, thus identifying social class and work conditions as crucial determinants of health or disease. Villerme found that wealth was inversely associated with risk of mortality, short stature, illness, and deformities, leading him to argue that longevity is not fixed, but based on economic conditions that can be influenced by government policy. Villerme's findings were not well received, however, because he called for regulation within the workplace and protection for the poor—perhaps at the expense of businesses.

By the mid-1800s, physicians and others argued that miasma, or bad air and emanations from decaying matter, caused outbreaks of cholera. Observing that deaths were commonly clustered among the poor, proponents of the theory of miasma argued that the lower classes had terrible hygiene, which poisoned the air. Reducing death required people to be less filthy. This theory contrasted with the work of John

Snow (1813–1858), who methodically covered the streets of London collecting statistics documenting the location of outbreaks. Snow identified contaminated water from communal pumps as the source of cholera. Contaminated water was more common in poorer neighborhoods, where infrastructure was of lower quality.

In 1844, Friedrich Engels (1820–1895), a German social scientist, further described the working conditions of factory workers in England. Through direct observation, Engels witnessed horrible working conditions and identified the relationship between these conditions and disease, motivating him to write *The Condition of the Working Class in England in 1844*. Engels described long hours without breaks, dingy facilities, repetitive duties, and environmental hazards, writing:

> All of these adverse factors combine to undermine the health of the workers. Very few strong, well-built, healthy people are to be found among them. . . . They are for the most part, weak, thin and pale. . . . Their weakened bodies are in no condition to withstand illness and whenever infection is abroad they fall victims to it. Consequently they age prematurely and die young. This is proved by the available statistics of death rates.[3]

The documentation of and attention to the impact of society on the body lost traction as the concept of *germ theory* became popular in the 1860s. Germ theory identifies single causal agents, such as *Salmonella typhi*, as the cause of disease—in this case, typhoid fever. Whereas many scientists, physicians, and funding agents rallied around germ theory, early social epidemiologists argued that lifestyle, behaviors, hygiene, and socioeconomic status, which affect nutrition and shelter, were more important than exposure to germs. They noted that once exposed, susceptibility to disease and mortality from the specific virus was dependent on social status, noting that the poor were less able to fight off even minor infections.

The causal model connecting the combined influence of host, environment, and agent emerged in the 1920s to 1930s. This model asserts that the human host is constantly besieged by viral, bacterial, or other disease-causing agents that are repelled by an uncompromised immune system. Therefore, unhealthy environmental characteristics can compromise this natural protection and allow the entry of the agent into the host. This theory gave rise to the disciplines of genetics and cellular biology. Although the causal model furthered our understanding of the influence of environmental agents on the body, the lines of scientific inquiry it prompted ignored the role of social environment on disease.

In the early 1940s, Salvador Allende, who would later go on to become the president of Chile, wrote *The Structure of National Health*, linking illness and socioeconomic status. Allende argued that social change and efforts toward creating a more egalitarian society are the only effective approach to solving health problems. "It is impossible," he wrote, "to give health and knowledge to a people who are malnourished, who wear rags, and who work at a level of unmerciful exploitation."[4] Allende urged wage and land reform, rent control, reorganization within the Chilean Ministry of Health, and control of pharmaceutical production to allow generic drugs. Allende was one of the first socialist presidents in Latin America and was at odds with the capitalist societies of the West. He identified national development as a critical determinant of health, a theory that laid the early groundwork for the creation of the Human Development Index in 1990 by Amartya Sen and Mahbub ul Haq (Fig. 2-1).[5]

By the 1950s and 1960s, chronic diseases such as cancer and heart disease were becoming more frequent, particularly in more developed countries where infectious diseases were better controlled. Over the last 60 years, clinicians and epidemiologists treating and monitoring these conditions gradually came to understand that chronic diseases are caused by a combination of biological, social, and behavioral exposures leading to the creation of differential risk patterns for various populations.

This new branch of epidemiology, focused on the health impact of social conditions and social status as key determinants of morbidity and mortality, emerged in the 1960s and 1970s using statistics and classic epidemiology to investigate the relationship between social structure and disease vulnerability. By the end of the 20th century, the concept of social causation of disease gained traction, leading to increased funding for research and new journals such as *Social Science and Medicine*. Today, social epidemiology integrates concepts and methods from anthropology, biology, biostatistics, medicine, political science, public health, psychology, sociology, and other disciplines.

KEY CONCEPTS IN SOCIAL EPIDEMIOLOGY

The World Health Organization published the projected number of deaths from various causes for 2030 (Fig. 2-2). According to these projections, nearly 11 million people will die of cancer per year globally, more than 9 million from heart disease, and about 6 million per year from HIV/AIDS. To reduce disease-specific mortality, complementary strategies for prevention, management, and treatment of diseases linked to the geographic distribution of disease, risk levels of diverse populations, and the proximal, distal, and fundamental causes of disease are needed.

If we envision disease as a river, proximal causes are downstream, or the end results, of the more upstream, distal, or fundamental causes. We know that, for example, the proximal or immediate causes of heart disease include elevated blood

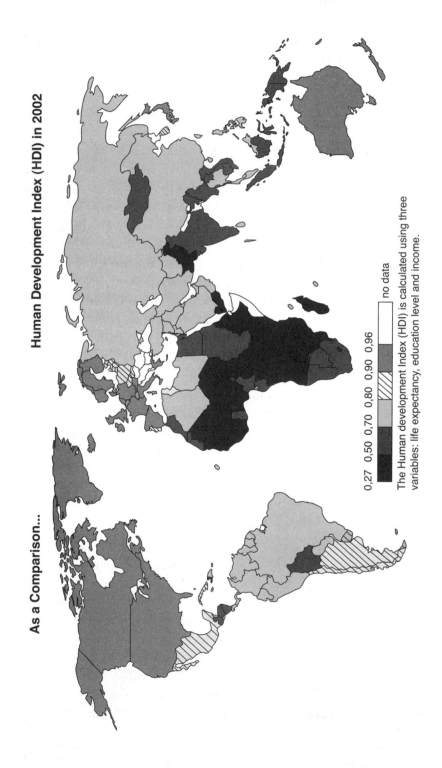

FIGURE 2-1   Human Development Index in 2002

Source: Human Development Index (HDI) in 2002. (2004). In UNEP/GRID-Arendal Maps and Graphics Library. Retrieved 21:15, Philippe Rekacewicz, August 6, 2007 http://maps.grida.no/go/graphic/human-development-index-hdi-i n-2002; Courtesy of UNEP/GRID - Arendal Maps and Graphics Library, http://www.grida.no

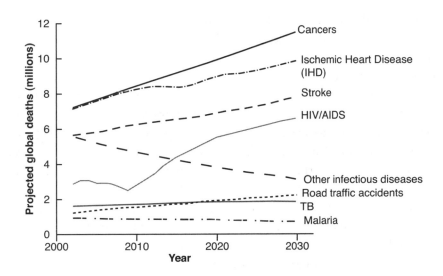

FIGURE 2-2 Projected global deaths for selected causes of death, 2002–2030
Source: Mathers CD and Loncar D. Updated projections of global morality and burden of disease, 2002–2030: data source, methods and results. http://www.who.int/healthinfo/statistics/bodprojectionspaper.pdf

cholesterol levels, high blood pressure, and diabetes mellitus. High blood cholesterol levels can lead to narrowing of the arteries, which may cause blockages, heart attacks, and other complications that can be irreversible.

We also know that genetics and a person's family history are important to health status and that complicated interactions between downstream and fundamental factors determine risk of disease. Although geneticists have not yet found ways to manipulate genes to reduce heart disease, cholesterol, and diabetes, all these conditions are manageable through behavioral, surgical, and pharmaceutical interventions. Lack of availability and lack of affordability of such interventions in this example are tied to fundamental causes, such as poverty and lack of access to preventive health care, which lie even further upstream.

Behavioral factors lie mid-river, between the far upstream fundamental causes (poverty, social marginalization, etc.) and downstream disease diagnosis. These factors include tobacco and alcohol use, poor nutrition, and physical inactivity. In fact, behavioral factors are causally related to elevated cholesterol levels, high blood pressure, and diabetes. But what determines behavioral factors? For example, what determines who smokes and how much they smoke? Surveillance data find different rates of smoking based on age, gender, education, income, occupation, social norms, and geographic location (i.e., where there are differences in tobacco taxes, advertising regulations, and laws regarding who can smoke and where it is acceptable). Behaviors can be influenced directly, such as by raising tobacco taxes; or indirectly, such as by restricting tobacco advertising aimed at children.

Socioeconomic factors such as income, education, and occupation are fundamental causes that influence tobacco use or other behaviors related to heart disease and may be more difficult to influence. According to demographic World Health Surveys from 2003, smoking is most common in the lowest-income households in developing countries. Tobacco-related mortality is also higher where elevated rates of smoking exist in a context with poorer health services and insufficient tobacco cessation programs.[6] These risk factors, along with low literacy or poor working conditions, in places where tobacco regulation does not exist, partly explain the fundamental causes of tobacco use and rates of heart disease in the developing world.

In the developed world, physical inactivity and obesity are most common in poorer socioeconomic classes among people who lack the resources to purchase healthier foods and who live in neighborhoods where fresh vegetables and fruits are not sold, cheap fast food outlets are plentiful, and there is no access to a physical environment conducive to exercise. The people most likely to die prematurely from heart disease are generally least likely to access health screenings or have adequate health insurance coverage and quality health care, and must often pay out of pocket for medications.

Thus, fundamental causes occur at the societal level through social structures that determine the pathways and mechanisms by which health is negatively affected. Returning to the metaphor of disease as a river, fundamental causes occur at the mouth of the river; upstream factors determine the level of risk, and downstream factors become health consequences leading to morbidity or mortality. Although social epidemiologists do not discount that individual choice can affect health and behavior, they recognize that human agency, in the form of choices, alternatives, and resources, is largely determined by the society in which an individual lives and his or her socioeconomic position.

Undoubtedly, categorizing the causes of disease as fundamental is controversial. Identification of fundamental causes challenges the status quo, power bases, and the very way in which societies are organized. Fundamental disparities can expose powerful elites and inequitable decision-making processes that may be partly responsible for deprivation and highlight the lack of rights or equity experienced by vulnerable groups and minorities. Moreover, reform is often undesirable to those who profit from or feel that their needs are satisfactorily met within the existing social hierarchy. Change may deeply conflict with commerce and trade or may require urban renewal, rural development, or more equitable regulation regarding wages, industry, and markets.

PROCESSES IN SOCIETY: HOW DOES SOCIETY ACTUALLY "GET INTO THE BODY"?

Over the lifespan, the human body moves through various processes as it develops. Professor Nancy Krieger of Harvard University describes "bodies in society" as biological species that grow and reproduce.[7] Our bodies begin life in utero and progress into old age, experiencing the constraints or opportunities of our age or stage. Bodies are built to develop and grow physically, intellectually, emotionally, and sexually. We are born with a set of characteristics, such as genetic makeup, physical features, gender, and intellectual aptitude, but we are also biological organisms who evolve as new traits emerge, adaptations occur, or as the body is manipulated. We are able to and do interact with others and with the physical environment.

Our bodies also belong to and are products of the society in which we live. We are born at a certain time or historical period and, as we age, experience life according to our temporal context. Each historical period is marked by its economy, political and legal system, and existing technology. Of course, smaller economies and political systems exist as microcosms within and interacting with larger systems. Thus, we may be overtly excluded from interacting with certain systems (because of social hierarchy or geographic proximity) or choose to boycott certain systems. Still, we cannot divorce our development from the systems into which we are born and interact with or reject during our lifespan and the long history upon which particular contexts are founded.

We are born in a distinct place, but we move across geography, now with greater speed than ever before. Nevertheless, each place or space has advantages and disadvantages, rights and responsibilities, resources, relationships, and institutions.

We are also born, raised, and enter adulthood within a certain social position. We may move up and down the social ladder, but the various ages and stages of our lives are shaped by the social positions we live within and are determined by our class, gender, race/ethnicity, sexual preference, or other divisions based on power or property.[7] As social beings, shaped and developed by the circumstances of our lives and environments, we partake in relationships and processes of production, consumption, and reproduction. As defined by Krieger, social production includes the transactions related to the market economy and culture where goods, services, ideas, and information are produced, shared, traded or sold, and otherwise distributed. We consume ideas, information, advertising, and goods and services that meet our various needs and desires.

Society "enters" the body through our immunologic responses to bacteria, susceptibility to infection, protection from viruses, lifestyle behaviors, knowledge of risks, exposure to harm, attitudes toward health, actions to protect health, and resources for prevention and treatment of disease. We may be exposed to infectious diseases such as malaria, tuberculosis, influenza, HIV/AIDS, hepatitis, schistosomiasis, and other illnesses. We may also develop chronic diseases such as heart disease, arthritis, cancer, diabetes, depression, and drug addiction. Social epidemiologists argue that whether or not we suffer from and survive the infectious or chronic disease is heavily dependent on our place in society.

Social epidemiologists refer to lifecourse theory to help explain the phenomenon by which multiple factors interact to increase susceptibility to disease. For example, there may be disadvantages that accumulate throughout the life cycle so that, by middle age, some populations are highly susceptible to cancer or heart disease. Childhood illness, adverse environmental exposure, accumulated stress, and risky lifestyle behaviors may all interact to cause and worsen heart disease. In the developing world, maternal morbidity and mortality may be largely determined by events that occur throughout the life course. For example, a young girl living in poverty from childhood onward may be more likely to have an early sexual debut leading to an unplanned pregnancy. When childbirth occurs before the reproductive organs are fully formed, there is higher risk of complications, including an obstructed delivery. Persistent deprivation and inadequate nutrition may cause increased mortality among AIDS patients with very low CD4 counts in their first months of receiving antiretroviral treatment in the poorest countries.

Critical periods, during which assaults to the body or exposures destroy or undermine healthy processes or interventions support healthy growth and development, are also important. These critical periods may occur in utero, at birth, during infancy and childhood, at sexual debut, at childbirth, or during other stages and processes. For example, adequate nutrition in early childhood is essential for children to grow to their optimal physical stature, whereas exposure to lead prevents children from reaching their full intellectual potential in adulthood. In addition, prenatal care for mothers affects a child's birth weight, which has long-term health consequences over the lifespan, and exposure to pollution in early years may attack lung function, eventually causing asthma.

SOCIOECONOMIC POSITION

> Life expectancy is shorter and most diseases are more common further down the social ladder in each society. Health policy must tackle the social and economic determinants of health.[8]

Socioeconomic position refers to the indicators that signify a person's status in society. Status is most frequently gained through the ownership of resources, power, and skills that can be used to accumulate wealth or exert influence. In every society, political, cultural, and institutional factors determine the ways in which socioeconomic status influences health, with the steepest gradients found in the most unequal societies and the flattest gradients in the most egalitarian.[9] Although complex patterns of disease distribution exist globally, studies have consistently found that socioeconomic position is robustly related to most health outcomes in nearly all populations.[9] Whereas sociologists seek to explore this social stratification, social epidemiologists aim to explain its influence on health.

As a discipline, social epidemiology is founded on the hypothesis that although the direction and strength of relationships between morbidity and mortality and socioeconomic position vary, the underlying relationship persists. For example, in the United States, socioeconomic status affects low birth weight, injuries, asthma, diabetes, depression, cancer, stroke, and other diseases. In addition, a gradient occurs whereby children from families of lower socioeconomic status have been found to be markedly more likely to suffer from injuries, ear infections, or chronic illness and to be less physically active than children from families of higher socioeconomic status. In fact, children from families in the top third of the socioeconomic status hierarchy have a 50% lower risk of asthma than children from the bottom third. And children in the lowest income quintile are nearly three times as likely to suffer an injury as those from the highest quintile.[9] These socioeconomic influences persist throughout the life course, increasing susceptibility to disease, shaping coping behaviors, and reducing the body's ability to heal itself when confronted by multiple stressors.

MEASUREMENT

Measures of socioeconomic position include indicators of "life chances" such as income, education, and occupation, as well as assets or wealth. In essence, income, education, and occupation are the links between the individual and social stratification that determine life chances as well as market and cultural value.[10] An individual's "value" affects job prospects and opportunities in life. In addition, our income, education, and occupation determine where we live, the groups we belong to and interact with, the resources we can access, the environments in which we live, and the stressors we experience.

Income is a key indicator that captures the resources used to meet basic needs and determines an individual's material conditions, which have direct implications for health. In the United States, for example, a family with high income can afford both health insurance and a physician's copayment and will seek care immediately if a child has an asthma attack. A low-income family without insurance must pay full price for medical attention, which may cause them to delay seeking help until the child is much sicker. Income is often difficult to measure in health research because some people are reluctant to report household income, regarding it as a private matter or a cause of shame.

Education is an easily measured indicator of socioeconomic status that most people freely reveal to health researchers. Education is a marker of socioeconomic status even when individuals are not in the labor force. Education is also rather stable over the lifespan, whereas income may fluctuate based on current employment status. However, indicators of the highest level of achieved education do not capture any information about the quality of schooling, which often determines an individual's value in the marketplace. Educational indicators may also not be sensitive enough to measure inequalities, which are closely linked to the resources used to purchase goods and services. Also, the link between higher levels of education and health is not necessarily obvious, so it is not always clear why education is health promoting or creates protection against illness. Furthermore, the links between health and education can be confusing. For example, research in Nigeria and other developing countries suggests that level of education is positively associated with appropriate prevention and treatment practices for malaria.[11] However, level of education is not consistently associated with patient adherence to medication regimens in either developing or developed country contexts.

Occupation is an important indicator of socioeconomic position because it is the obvious and stable link between individuals and economic processes. Occupation also forms the link between the measures of education and income. Unfortunately, occupational classification systems may not capture important nuances such as formal and informal roles, which may relate directly to benefits and security and the workplace environment. Given the large number of occupations in every society, type of work may also be hard to organize into meaningful categories.

Finally, earned wealth or assets are important indicators of socioeconomic position. Ownership of stocks, real estate, or valuable assets can sustain households and economic activities during unemployment or other household shocks when income declines. Wealth can be readily measured in the developing world, where assets tend to be durable goods (livestock, radios, bicycles, automobiles, indoor plumbing) that are easy to observe (rather than assets such as stocks or investments). Still, it may be difficult to place value on different assets, whose value may decline over time or vary according to culture, geography, and infrastructure.

Researchers seeking to quantify the extent to which socioeconomic factors affect morbidity or explain varying levels of disease in populations must be intentional as they choose the indicators of socioeconomic status. These various measures may have different meanings and levels of sensitivity. For example, a single measure of education used as an indicator of socioeconomic status in a study may not fully capture the differences between populations that would be captured using measures of income or occupational classifications. Social epidemiologists are charged with identifying risk factors for disease, and they must also identify the mechanisms or describe how these factors affect disease. If the occupation of a group of people places them at higher risk of asthma, social epidemiologists must explain how this happens. What occurs within the workplace, or as a result of that occupation, to increase risk of asthma?

INCOME INEQUALITY AND HEALTH

Whereas poverty is an important determinant of health globally, an individual's *relative* position within the social hierarchy is also critical to health outcomes. Evidence from developed countries suggests that unequal access to resources, power, or services appears to affect satisfaction with life, participation in society, and ultimately morbidity and mortality. Although controversial, the evidence suggests that societies with higher levels of inequality have worse measures of health and that income inequality undermines health through various processes and mechanisms. In fact, a 2005 review of 168 analyses of income inequality and population health found that three of four studies associated worse health outcomes with societies with greater inequality, or in which the majority of wealth is heavily concentrated among a small elite.[12] Income inequality in the United States is such that the top 1% of households owns between 40% to 50% of the nation's wealth, whereas the bottom 20% owns just 3.7% of the nation's wealth.[12]

Kawachi argues that inequality leads to underinvestment in human capital, and provides compelling evidence at the state level.[13] For example, he found that states in the United States with greater income inequality devote fewer resources toward education, which results in higher school dropout rates and greater percentages of youth with no high school education and lower reading and math scores.[13] In addition, Kawachi argues that inequality undermines social ties that bind families and community members, compromising social networks during economic or other hardships. He makes the case that strong social ties promote health, but that these bonds are undermined by inequality, leading to mistrust and a focus on the individual over social relationships, although this hypothesis has not been proven.[13]

Finally, Kawachi argues that income inequality undermines health through the psychological effects of relative deprivation, so that those higher up on the economic ladder experience significant and steady advances, while the lower-status groups watch this progression with frustration.[13] The end of apartheid in South Africa has not led to improved socioeconomic conditions for all citizens. Although upward social mobility and wealth are now theoretically available to all, regardless of race or family background, the wide gap between the rich and poor continues. In 2001, 57% of the population lived below the poverty line—unchanged from 1996 (two years after apartheid ended)[14]—and in 2006 the unemployment rate was 25.5%.[15] In this example, frustration or the stressful psychological experience of inequality for 40% of the population who live on less than one U.S. dollar a day actually undermines health.[16]

Income inequalities are further exploited in comparing out-of-pocket expenditures for medicines within and across countries. Inevitably, people living in poorer developing and transitional countries are responsible for paying a great portion of their healthcare and medicine costs compared with those living in transitional and developed countries. In developed countries, social, public, and private insurance protects residents from excessive medicine costs, whereas residents in low-resource countries often encounter catastrophic financial circumstances after encountering unexpected and unaffordable expenditures on medicines.[17] In the Republic of Georgia (formerly part of the Soviet Union), for example, a household study revealed that 19% of respondents had to sell personal property in order to pay for health expenses, and 16% of respondents could not afford to purchase medicines prescribed by doctors.[18]

Social epidemiologists continue to study the ways in which inequality "gets into the body" and undermines population health. The mechanisms and processes most likely operate at various levels, such as through exclusionary laws and policies, the pricing of goods and services, and psychological processes, but more evidence is needed to explain how these processes affect health.

DISCRIMINATION AND HEALTH

The ways in which discrimination is embodied among individuals in society are complex and multifaceted. Anyone who has ever been discriminated against because of age, accent, skin color, gender, sexual preference, or other characteristics can describe the anger or frustration that the experience generates. Beyond anger however, the evidence that discrimination affects health is compelling: in the United States, people of color (including blacks, Latinos, Native Americans, and others) die younger and have higher infant mortality rates and age-adjusted mortality rates.[19] Although women live longer than men, women have higher rates of disability and illness and therefore fewer years of disability-free life. Gay men, bisexuals, and lesbians have higher rates of smoking, suicide, and substance abuse. But how does discrimination harm health?

First, understanding the parameters of discrimination is important. Discrimination can take many forms and occur throughout the life course, determining prenatal care, early childhood education, schooling options, and job prospects. Episodes of discrimination may vary by frequency, intensity, and duration, creating differential impacts on health even with the same population.[19] Discrimination may occur at the individual level, in neighborhoods, states, or countries and can occur in one or more domains, such as at home, in school, or at the workplace. Discrimination may also occur in the marketplace, as people attempt to purchase goods and services such as housing or health care. Public agencies such as police and social workers may discriminate. Discrimination may be overt or covert and be expressed verbally or even through aggressive force. Discrimination is sometimes legislated, allowing individuals and institutions to discriminate against individuals and entire racial/ethnic or other targeted groups. In the United States, the Americans with Disabilities Act of 1990 made barring access to persons with disabilities to public services and employment illegal. In South Africa, apartheid, or the legal discrimination against black South Africans, was not abolished until 1994.

In addition to socioeconomic status and race/ethnicity, societal value is frequently determined by age, gender, and sexuality. Throughout history, the elite in society have often placed a higher value on working-aged adults (who are favored over the very young or old), on men over women, on heterosexuals over homosexuals or bisexuals, and on whites over blacks and others. This value determines life chances and opportunities for work and education and may afford social and economic protection from harm. Thus, discrimination may affect health through economic and social deprivation, increased exposure to hazardous conditions, the often cumulative experience of socially inflicted trauma, targeted marketing, and inadequate health care and resources for health.[7] In healthcare settings, discrimination by physicians may delay patient care or the type of treatment and/or medications prescribed.

Gender roles related to health are complex and varied among different cultures. Gender norms and values influence whether an individual in a household will ultimately seek care, including the purchase and use of medicines, for a given illness or condition. In some regions where gender inequality exists for women, girls and women carry a disproportionate burden of disease and are less likely to seek care and purchase medicines compared with boys and men. In low-resource settings, decisions about whether to seek care for a condition in contexts of gender inequality for women are typically made by men, specifically the husband or father. A community-based study in Benin revealed that decisions regarding use of resources for health services are commonly made without involving women.[20]

Compared with men, Nepalese women delay seeking medical care for the treatment of tuberculosis, instead choosing to seek care from traditional healers prior to seeking treatment from Western medicine practitioners.[21] Other research on household decision making on child health care in Nepal suggests that boys are more likely to be identified as sick than girls, but once deemed sick, there is no difference in care seeking among boys and girls.[22] On the other hand, in areas such as Central Asia, adult men account for less than 25% of all healthcare visits, compared with 50% for adult women.[23] In this region, men assume a much greater burden of disease compared with women. In these examples, a social epidemiologic approach can be used to identify how gender relates to disease distribution and the role gender plays in decision making and care seeking for the treatment of illness, including decisions to purchase and use medicines.

The evidence quantifying racial disparities in health is robust and complex. For example, in the United States, racial and ethnic health disparities, caused in part by discrimination occurring through different mechanisms, are not fully explained by race alone. In fact, a large body of science describes how race, ethnicity, and socioeconomic status combine to undermine health and increase mortality. Consequently, for example, poor black infants have the lowest birth weights in the United States, a condition that sets children up for increased morbidity and mortality throughout the life course. Numerous studies in the United States have revealed disparities in medicine use among African Americans. A study of subjects receiving treatment for schizophrenia revealed that African Americans were less likely to receive newer and more tolerable antipsychotic medicines, such as clozapine and risperidone, than white subjects, but African American subjects were more likely to receive less desirable, deep intramuscular injections of antipsychotic medicines.[24] A study of subjects with elevated serum cholesterol revealed that African Americans and Mexican Americans were less likely than whites to undergo cholesterol screening and less likely to take cholesterol-lowering medicines once diagnosed with elevated cholesterol.[25] In a study evaluating appropriate treatment of asthma, white, non-Hispanic subjects were more likely to have used appropriate inhaled corticosteroid therapy to control asthma compared with minority subjects.[26]

SOCIAL INTEGRATION, SOCIAL NETWORKS, AND SOCIAL SUPPORT AND HEALTH

Social ties and connectedness to family and friends affect all causes of mortality. Studies from many parts of the world have found that people who do not have social ties are at higher risk of dying of heart disease, cancers, and other causes of death.[27]

Thus, the social support gained from relationships is health promoting, and having someone to rely on increases longevity. Support may be financial, informational, emotional, or functional.

Although having someone who can lend a helping hand is important, an individual's social relationships also affect knowledge, behaviors, attitudes, and disease outcomes in both positive and negative ways. For example, a nonsmoking teenager who hangs out with a group of kids who smoke cigarettes may also begin smoking. Parents of a newly diagnosed diabetic child who join a support group might learn how to manage the child's diabetes and insulin shots with ease. Research on adherence to antiretroviral therapy (ART) consistently reveals associations between the need for social support and long-term adherence to ART for the treatment of HIV/AIDS; however, stigma and discrimination within a society may impede the ability of an individual to seek social support concerning treatment for HIV/AIDS. So, whereas an HIV-positive person living in the United States or sub-Saharan Africa may benefit from programs that utilize buddies or community health workers to provide social support to promote ART adherence, an HIV-positive person living in the former Soviet Union may choose nondisclosure of HIV status and forgo such support systems for fear of the discrimination he or she might face if the individual's HIV status were known to his or her community. Social epidemiologists aim to look beyond traditional predictors of adherence such as regimen complexity, pill burden, and side effects to understand the societal factors that prevent or promote adherence to medicines. Social constructs and relationships can also affect acceptability of treatment modality. One U.S. study on depression found that African Americans and Hispanics were less likely to find antidepressant medicine treatment acceptable compared with whites; however, Hispanics were more likely to find counseling methods acceptable than whites.[28]

People belong to social networks at home, in their neighborhoods, at school or work, in communities, at churches, in clubs, and even online. Although these memberships in social organizations may be health or disease promoting, belonging to multiple networks creates complexity in understanding how behaviors are affected by various memberships.

SUMMARY

The great public health challenges of the early 21st century include poverty, malnutrition (food insecurity and obesity), chronic disease (in both developed and developing countries), pandemic infectious diseases (HIV/AIDS, malaria, tuberculosis, influenza), and the threat of drug-resistant "superbugs." The discipline of social epidemiology is founded on the assumption that all of these health outcomes are inextricably tied to social context. This chapter offered two metaphors by which to envision this relationship: the porous human body, absorbing every influence of its external social and physical environment, and the fast-moving river current of fundamental sociocultural influences carrying populations of human bodies downstream from health to disease, through distal risk behaviors, to the accumulating silt of proximal symptoms, eventually ending in disease diagnosis. Whereas clinicians screen, diagnose, and treat individuals, often taking into account socioeconomic background, genetic predisposition, domestic environment, and more, social epidemiologists track complex patterns of morbidity and mortality across populations with the objective of recognizing risk dynamics. Armed with a wealth of details and data about cultural norms, economic determinants, and environmental dangers and protections, social epidemiology is integral to designing, implementing, and evaluating public health interventions to improve access and use of medicines in communities and societies.

REFERENCES

1. Stallones RA. To advance epidemiology. Ann Rev Publ Health 1980;1:69-82.
2. Krieger N. Epidemiology and the web of causation: has anyone seen the spider? Soc Sci Med 1994;39(7):887-903.
3. Engels F. The condition of the working class in England in 1844. New York: J.W. Lovell, 1887:118-9.
4. Allende S. La realidad médico-social Chilena [The structure of national health]. Santiago, Chile: Ministerio de Salubridad, 1939.
5. UNEP/GRID-Arendal Maps and Graphics Library. Human Development Index (HDI) in 2002. 2004. (Accessed August 6, 2007, at http://maps.grida.no/go/graphic/as_a_comparision_human_development_index_hdi_in_2002.)
6. Mathers CD, Loncar D. Updated projections of global morality and burden of disease, 2002–2030: data source, methods and results. Geneva: World Health Organization, 2005. (Accessed at http://www.who.int/healthinfo/statistics/bodprojectionspaper.pdf.)
7. Krieger N. Bodies count and body counts: social epidemiology and embodying inequality. Epidemiol Rev 2004;26:92-103.
8. Marmot M, Wilkinson R, eds. Social determinants of health: the solid facts. 2nd ed. Geneva: World Health Organization, 2003. (Accessed at http://www.euro.who.int/document/e81384.pdf.)
9. Chen E, Matthews KA, Boyce T. Socioeconomic differences in children's health: how and why do these relationships change with age? Psychol Bull 2002;128:295-329.
10. Lynch J, Kaplan G. Socioeconomic position. In: Berkman L, Kawachi I, eds. Social epidemiology. New York: Oxford University Press, 2000:13-35.
11. Dike N, Onwujekwe O, Ojukwu J, et al. Influence of education and knowledge on perception and practices to control malaria in Southeast Nigeria. Soc Sci Med 2006;63(1):103-6.

12. Wilkinson R, Pickett K. Income inequality and population health: a review and explanation of the evidence. Soc Sci Med 2006;62(7):1768-84.

13. Kawachi K. Income inequality and health. In: Berkman L, Kawachi I, eds. Social epidemiology. New York: Oxford University Press, 2000:76-94.

14. Schwabe C. Fact sheet: poverty in South Africa. Human Sciences Research Council, 2004. (Accessed at http://www.sarpn.org.za/documents/d0000990/index.php.)

15. Statistics South Africa. Statistics South Africa, Pretoria. 2007. (Accessed at http://www.statssa.gov.za/PublicationsHTML/P0318July2006/html/P0318July2006.html.)

16. South African Regional Poverty Network. The annual poverty report for the SADC region, 2007. (Accessed at http://www.sarpn.org.za/publications/annual.php.)

17. Xu K, Evans DB, Kawabata K, Zeramdini R, Klavus J, Murray CLJ. Household catastrophic health expenditure: a multicountry analysis. Lancet 2003;362:111-7.

18. Skarbinski J, Walker K, Baker LC, Kobaladze A, Kirtava Z, Raffin TA. The burden of out-of-pocket payments for health care in Tbilisi, Republic of Georgia. JAMA 2002;287:1043-9.

19. Krieger N. Discrimination and health. In: Berkman L, Kawachi I, eds. Social epidemiology. New York: Oxford University Press, 2000:36-75.

20. Ngom P, Wawire S, Gandaho T, et al. Intra-household decision-making on health and resources allocation in Borgou, Benin. Report for United States Agency for International Development. November 2000. (Accessed at http://www.popcouncil.org/pdfs/frontiers/FR_FinalReports/Benin_Decision_Making.pdf.)

21. Yamasaki-Nakagawa M, Ozasa K, Yamada N, et al. Gender difference in delays to diagnosis and health care-seeking behaviour in a rural area of Nepal. Int J Tuberc Lung Dis 2001;51(1):224-31.

22. Pokhrel S, Sauerborn R. Household decision-making on child health care in developing countries—the case of Nepal. Health Policy Planning 2004;19(4):218-33.

23. Cashin CE, Borowitz M, Zuess O. The gender gap in primary health care utilization in Central Asia. Health Policy Planning 2002;17(3):264-72.

24. Kuno E, Rothbard AB. Racial disparities in antipsychotic prescription patterns for patients with schizophrenia. Am J Psychiatry 2002;159(4):567-72.

25. Nelson K, Norris K, Mangione CM. Disparities in the diagnosis and pharmacologic treatment of high serum cholesterol by race and ethnicity. Arch Intern Med 2002;162:929-35.

26. Adams RJ, Fuhlbrigge A, Guilberrt T, Lozano P, Martinez F. Inadequate use of asthma medication in the United States: results of the Asthma in America national population survey. J Allergy Clin Immun 2002;116(1):58-64.

27. Kawachi I, Berkman L. Social cohesion, social capital and health. In: Berkman L, Kawachi I, eds. Social epidemiology. New York: Oxford University Press, 2000:36-75.

28. Cooper LA, Gonzales JJ, Rost KM, et al. The acceptability of treatment for depression among African-American, Hispanic, and white primary care patients. Med Care 2003;41(4):479-89.

Models and Frameworks for Health and Illness Behaviors

CHAPTER 3

Individual and Interpersonal Models of Health and Illness Behavior

Susan J. Blalock, PhD, MPH, Ashley J. Beard, PhD, MPH, and Stacie B. Dusetzina, BA

This chapter focuses on individual and interpersonal theories of health and illness behavior. These theories deal primarily with how the behavior of individuals is influenced by their knowledge, beliefs, attitudes, and emotions and their interactions with others—including their interactions with healthcare providers. Before embarking on this road, however, it is important for readers to recognize that individuals exist within larger social units. Individual behavior is influenced by social and political forces that are not incorporated into most of the individual and interpersonal theories reviewed in this chapter. In a sense, individuals can be thought of as the building blocks for larger social units such as couples, families, social networks, organizations, and communities. As members of these larger social units, individuals have the opportunity to influence policies and regulations that affect health behavior, but their behavior is also influenced by existing policies and regulations. For example, individuals may influence health policy through collective political pressure to increase funding for research in a particular area. However, individual access to new and often expensive therapies is influenced by the rules and regulations regarding use developed by larger social units, such as health insurance organizations.

The social ecological model is a theoretical framework that recognizes this interplay between individuals and the social and physical environments in which they live and function.[1] With its wide-angle lens, the social ecological model provides an excellent framework for understanding factors that affect human health and illness. Individual health behavior must be viewed as the product of individual action, the environment, and the larger social units to which individuals belong. This model identifies domains of variables that may influence health behavior, including individual-level factors, family-level factors, organizational factors, and community factors. Within these domains, however, the ecological framework does not provide guidance on the specific factors that are likely to have the greatest impact on health or illness. Therefore, to fill in the gaps, practitioners and researchers must draw on theories and models that are specific to each domain, remembering that the factors within each domain provide only a limited view of the complex determinants of health and illness behavior.

Theories identify distinct sets of interrelated concepts, define these concepts using precise terminology, specify how the concepts are related to one another, and identify the conditions under which these relationships apply.[2] Theories, by their nature, are abstract and can be applied to a wide variety of behavioral phenomena, helping us understand why people behave in certain ways under specified conditions and how they are likely to respond when those conditions change.

When faced with a health problem, theories can help us design interventions to address the problem by identifying the following:

- *Why* people are experiencing the health problem
- *What* information is needed before developing interventions to address the health problem
- *How* best to develop interventions to address the health problem
- *What* to measure to determine whether the intervention is effective[3]

By providing a systematic way to examine health problems, as well as guidance on developing interventions and assessing their effects, health behavior theories save practitioners from having to reinvent the wheel every time a new problem is faced.

This chapter reviews several contemporary individual and interpersonal theories that are useful in understanding and predicting human health behavior. It starts with value-expectancy theories because they are often a basis for other health behavior theories. Value-expectancy theories are based on the very simple notion that individuals are more likely to engage in a behavior if they believe that performing the behavior is likely to lead to desirable outcomes. When faced with a choice between two or more behavioral options, value-expectancy models posit that individuals will tend to adopt the behavior that maximizes the likelihood of obtaining desired outcomes and avoiding undesired ones. While incorporating the value-expectancy notion, social cognitive theory expands on this notion considerably by emphasizing the interplay between individual and environmental factors.

The chapter then introduces two stage models of health and illness behavior. Stage theories view behavior change as a process and posit that, in the process of moving from inaction to action, people pass through a series of stages—sometimes moving forward toward change, sometimes moving backward away from change, and sometimes remaining in the same stage indefinitely. A central premise that underlies stage theories is that the factors that influence behavior change depend on one's current stage in the behavior change process. Finally, the chapter provides a critique of the theories reviewed, emphasizing issues that they do not consider.

VALUE-EXPECTANCY THEORIES

Rotter's Social Learning Theory

A central notion underlying Rotter's social learning theory is that through the course of their life experiences, people develop expectations concerning the types of outcomes that are most likely to occur if they perform a particular behavior in a particular situation.[4] Consequently, when given an option, people usually choose to perform those behaviors that maximize the perceived likelihood of obtaining desired outcomes and minimize the perceived likelihood of obtaining undesired ones. This is the core tenet underlying all value-expectancy theories.

Rotter summarized this notion in the following formula, where BP stands for *behavior potential*, E for *expectancy*, and RV for *reinforcement value*:

$$BP = f(E, RV)$$

The formula hypothesizes that the likelihood that a person will perform a particular behavior in a particular situation is a function of the person's judgment of how likely the behavior is to lead to a specific outcome and the reinforcement value attached to that outcome.

When using value-expectancy theories, it is important to remember that expectancies and reinforcement values are subjective. Thus, different people will vary in their assessments of the likelihood that a particular behavior will result in a particular outcome. They may also differ in terms of the reinforcement value attached to different outcomes. Even for a single individual, expectancies and the reinforcement value attached to different outcomes will vary across situations, depending on the person's subjective interpretation of the environment. Moreover, expectancies and values may change as individuals gain life experience, including experience with an illness and the medications used to treat it. Thus, behavior is best viewed as a learned response to environmental contingencies.

Most research on health behavior that has used Rotter's social learning theory as a theoretical framework has focused on only one key concept derived from the theory: health locus of control. *Health locus of control* is a generalized expectancy concerning the factors that a person believes influence his or her health. As originally conceptualized by Rotter, these generalized expectancies were viewed as existing on a continuum.[4] At one end of the continuum, individuals believed that health outcomes were totally within their personal control. At the other end of the continuum, individuals believed that health outcomes were totally under the control of factors external to themselves (e.g., powerful others, chance, fate). Thus, this conceptualization did not allow for the possibility that a person could strongly believe that health outcomes are influenced by both internal and external factors.

In the 1970s, this unidimensional conceptualization of health locus of control was replaced by a multidimensional one that recognized that individuals could believe that both internal and external factors influence health outcomes. The Multidimensional Health Locus of Control (MHLC) scales have been widely used to assess this concept.[5] The MHLC assesses perceptions of three different sources of control: internal (e.g., "If I get sick, it is my own behavior that determines how soon I get well again"), powerful others (e.g., "Health professionals keep me healthy"), and chance (e.g., "When I am sick, I just have to let nature run its course"). Studies have examined the relationship between health locus of control and medication adherence in the context of a wide variety of chronic health problems, including cardiovascular illness,[6,7] asthma,[8] renal disease,[9,10] cancer,[11-13] mental health conditions,[14,15] and HIV/AIDS.[16,17] Typically, it has been hypothesized that adherence would be positively associated with beliefs in internal control over health outcomes and negatively associated with beliefs in external control such as powerful others or chance. However, only mixed support has been found for these hypotheses. As noted by others, it seems likely that any effect that locus of control may have on medication adherence will depend on other factors, such as whether individuals believe that they have the ability and resources needed for adherence.[18,19] Thus, research is needed to better understand how locus of control beliefs may interact with other individual beliefs as well as environmental factors to influence medication adherence.

Theory of Reasoned Action and Theory of Planned Behavior

The theory of reasoned action (TRA) was introduced in the 1970s and extended the value-expectancy notion considerably.[20] As shown in Figure 3-1, this theory posits that the best predictor of behavior is *behavioral intention*, which is a person's self-rated likelihood of performing the specified behavior. As we move backward in the model, from right to left, we gain insight into the factors that influence behavior through their effects on behavioral intentions. According to the model, behavioral intentions are influenced by two factors: attitude toward the behavior and subjective norms.

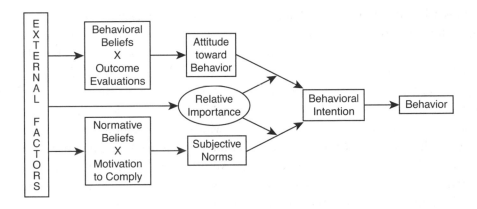

FIGURE 3-1   Various factors at different levels that interact to influence health status

Attitude toward the behavior is an overall judgment of the extent to which a person believes that his or her performance of the behavior is a good or bad idea. Attitude toward the behavior is influenced by a set of salient *behavioral beliefs*, reflecting how likely individuals believe specific outcomes are to occur if they perform the behavior of interest, with each behavioral belief weighted by the value the person attaches to the outcome (i.e., outcome evaluation). For example, a truck driver may believe that taking a particular medication is very likely to cause drowsiness (i.e., a behavioral belief) and that this side effect is very undesirable (i.e., the associated *outcome evaluation*). These factors would have a negative effect on the truck driver's attitude toward using the medication. However, in most cases, attitudes are influenced by multiple salient beliefs. Thus, the same truck driver may also believe that the medication will alleviate bothersome symptoms and that this is more important than the possibility of experiencing drowsiness. Thus, the truck driver may take the medication despite his concerns about experiencing drowsiness.

The second factor that has a direct effect on behavioral intention is *subjective norms*, which reflect the extent to which an individual perceives social pressure to perform the behavior of interest. Subjective norms are influenced by a set of *normative beliefs*, each indexing an individual's perception that a specific other person (or group of people) believes that the individual should perform the behavior, with each normative belief weighted by *motivation to comply* (i.e., the extent to which the individual believes he or she should comply with the wishes of these other people or groups). For example, the truck driver introduced earlier is likely to believe that his doctor thinks he should take the prescribed medication. Assuming that he also believes he should follow his doctor's wishes, his subjective norm will favor taking the medication. However, in the same way that attitude toward the behavior is influenced by multiple salient beliefs, subjective norms are influenced by multiple normative beliefs. Thus, the truck driver may also believe that family members, friends, and coworkers think he either should or should not take the medication. Subjective norms reflect the integration of perceived social pressure from all people (or groups of people) who are important to the individual.

According to the TRA, behavioral intention is influenced directly only by attitude toward the behavior and subjective norms. All other factors (e.g., gender, race, age, education, health status), labeled *external factors* in Figure 3-1, exert their effect on behavioral intention through their effects on attitudes and subjective norms. In some cases, attitudes will have the greatest effect on intention; in other cases, subjective norms will have a greater effect. Thus, it is important to determine, in any particular instance, the extent to which behavior is under attitudinal or normative control.

The theory of planned behavior (TPB) is an extension of the TRA.[21] As shown in Figure 3-2, the TPB identifies a third variable, perceived behavioral control, that can have a direct effect on both behavioral intention and behavior. *Perceived behavioral control* is a person's overall perception of how easy or difficult it is for him or her to perform a behavior. Perceived behavioral control is influenced by a set of salient *control beliefs*, reflecting the presence of factors that either facilitate or interfere with performance of the behavior of interest, with each control belief weighted by the extent to which the person believes the factor makes performing the behavior either easier or more difficult (i.e., *perceived power*). To continue with the earlier example, the truck driver may believe that it is difficult to remember to take the medication multiple times a day. As a result, he may decide not to even try to take the medication as directed—assuming that he would fail. Moreover, to the extent that his belief is accurate (i.e., he really does experience difficulty remembering to take the medication throughout the day), he will be unlikely to take the medication as directed. This suggests that if perceptions of behavioral control are accurate, they may have a direct effect on behavior in addition to the indirect effect that is mediated by behavioral intention.

In practice, individuals who wish to use the TRA or TPB must begin by identifying the salient behavioral, normative, and control beliefs that underlie the behavior of interest. For example, if one is interested in better understanding the factors that predict adherence to a particular medication, members of the target population (i.e., individuals who are either users or potential users of the medication) should be interviewed to assess their behavioral, normative, and control beliefs regarding use of the medication. For those interested in learning more about how to conduct elicitation interviews, Fishbein[20] and Ajzen[22] provide detailed guidelines.

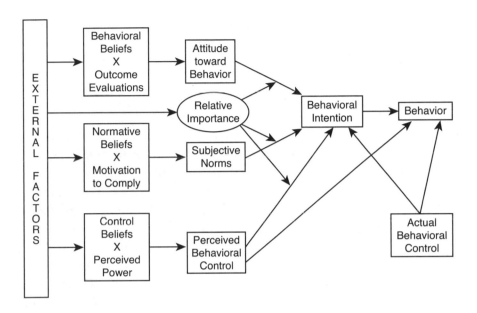

FIGURE 3-2 Theory of Planned Behavior

The TRA and TPB have been used to investigate a number of medication use issues. These include medication adherence,[23-29] duration of benzodiazepine therapy,[30] utilization of postoperative analgesics,[31] utilization of herbal remedies,[32,33] intention to use a medication within the context of a hypothetical scenario,[34] patient–pharmacist communication about antibiotics and antibiotic resistance,[35] pharmacist recommendations concerning the treatment of vaginal candidiasis with nonprescription medications,[36] pharmacist intention to provide Medicare medication therapy management services,[37] and physician use of different sources of drug information.[38,39] For the most part, this research has supported the major tenets of the TRA and TPB. An interesting exception, however, involved a study of analgesia use following orthopedic surgery in which actual analgesia use was not related to patients' presurgery ratings of the amount of analgesia they intended to use (rating scale ranged from 0 = *No medication* to 10 = *The most that I am allowed*).[31] This study is highlighted because it illustrates an important limitation of the TRA and TPB. That is, the link between intention and behavior will be strongest when intentions are based on a good understanding of relevant issues and little new information is subsequently encountered. Obviously, as new information is obtained, intentions may change. In the analgesia study, for example, individuals exhibited a limited understanding of the amount of postsurgical pain they were likely to experience, as evidenced by only a modest correlation between anticipated and actual pain reports. Thus, the lack of a relationship between preoperative intentions and subsequent behavior is understandable.

Health Belief Model

The health belief model (HBM) is one of the most widely recognized individual-level theories of health behavior. It was developed in the 1950s by researchers with the United States Public Health Service to better understand poor rates of participation in a community-based tuberculosis screening program.[40] As shown in Figure 3-3, the model posits that *perceived susceptibility* to a particular health problem and the *perceived severity* of that health problem combine to determine *perceived health threat*. According to the model, a perceived health threat motivates action to prevent the health problem, but it does not determine the specific actions that will be taken. For example, to reduce one's chances of developing complications as a result of having hypertension, one might take medications, lose weight, begin an exercise program, restrict salt intake, or do some combination of these. To determine the specific action or actions to adopt, the model posits that people consider the *perceived benefits* associated with different actions as well as the *perceived barriers* associated with those actions. They then tend to adopt behaviors for which the anticipated benefits outweigh the anticipated barriers. For example, an individual with hypertension may take medications to control her hypertension because she believes that (1) it will reduce the risk of long-term complications and (2) there are few barriers to incorporating medication taking into her daily routine. However, she may not increase her exercise level, despite believing that it would be beneficial to do so, because she believes that exercising on a regular basis is too time-consuming. The HBM also posits that perceived health threat can be increased by exposure to *cues to action*, which can be either internal (e.g., experience of physical symptoms) or external (e.g., exposure to a direct-to-consumer commercial about a medication to reduce disease risk). Finally, in Figure 3-3, the HBM also posits that perceived susceptibility, perceived severity, perceived threat, perceived benefits, and perceived barriers can be influenced by demographic factors (e.g., age, gender, race, ethnicity), psychosocial factors (e.g., personality, peer pressure), and structural factors (e.g., knowledge of the disease, access to resources).[41]

The HBM has been used to better understand the determinants of medication adherence in a variety of different therapeutic areas, including heart failure,[6] malaria chemoprophylaxis,[27,29] hypertension,[42,43] HIV infection,[44,45] mental illness,[46-50] kidney transplant,[51] epilepsy,[52,53] diabetes mellitus,[54] sickle cell disease,[55] a combination of chronic diseases,[56] and following a pediatric emergency room visit.[57] The HBM also

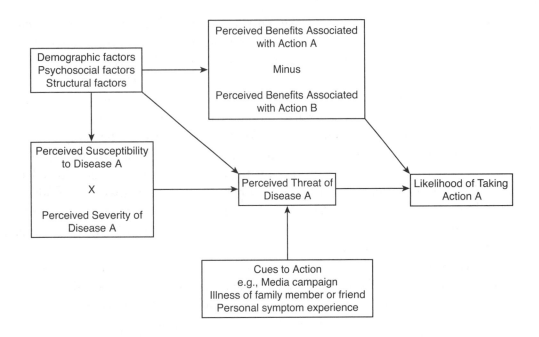

FIGURE 3-3 Health Belief Model

has been used to better understand the determinants of using medications to treat or prevent osteoporosis.[58,59] In general, the findings from these studies provide support for the importance of HBM variables in influencing medication adherence and use. However, the specific factors that emerge as significant vary across studies; the reasons for this variability remain poorly understood.

Bandura's Social Cognitive Theory

Social cognitive theory (SCT) is a dynamic theory addressing both individual and interpersonal factors of human behavior. SCT views behavior as the result of the triadic, reciprocal interaction of personal factors, behavioral patterns, and the environment.[60] *Personal factors* relate to the cognitive, affective, and biological characteristics of the individual. *Environment* refers to objective factors external to the person that affect behavior, including the social environment (family, friends, coworkers) and the physical environment (facilities, temperature, geography). The interaction of person, behavior, and environment is termed *reciprocal determinism*, which implies that the three components are constantly influencing one another, with change in one component effecting change in the other components.

Within SCT, reciprocal determinism provides an overall structure within which other constructs that are important to understanding and changing health behavior operate. Among the critical personal factors are individuals' ability to acquire behavioral competence, learn by observing others, anticipate the outcome of their behavior, develop confidence in performing the behavior of interest (including overcoming performance barriers), self-regulate behavior, and reflect on and evaluate their experiences.[61]

To perform any behavior, a person must know how to perform the behavior and have the required skills. Thus, behavioral competence, or *behavioral capability*, reflects both knowledge and skill. However, even with the requisite knowledge and skills, SCT posits that individuals will not perform a behavior unless (1) they are confident that they can perform the behavior and (2) they believe that performing the behavior will result in valued outcomes. These two types of beliefs are called *self-efficacy* and *outcome expectations*, respectively.

Self-efficacy is perhaps the most powerful SCT construct in predicting and explaining behavioral performance. It reflects the level of confidence individuals have in their ability to perform a specific behavior, including their ability to overcome performance barriers. Results of numerous studies of diverse health behaviors reveal that the effects of behavior change interventions are often mediated, at least in part, by their effects on self-efficacy. The stronger the self-efficacy beliefs that a program instills, the more likely program participants are to initiate behavior change efforts and sustain the effort needed to change detrimental health behaviors.[62]

Self-efficacy has three dimensions: strength, magnitude, and generality. *Strength* reflects how confident individuals are that they can perform a specific behavior. *Magnitude* reflects the level of difficulty associated with performing the behavior. *Generality* reflects the extent to which self-efficacy developed in one situation carries over to other situations. For example, a patient with hypertension and chronic obstructive pulmonary disease may be prescribed both oral tablets and medications delivered via inhalers. The magnitude of difficulty associated with taking the medications prescribed is probably greater for the inhalers than for the oral tablets. Thus, the patient may be very confident that he can take his oral medications correctly when at home, but may be less confident of his ability to use his inhalers correctly in this same situation. In this example, the strength of the patient's self-efficacy beliefs (i.e., level of confidence) varies as a function of the magnitude of task difficulty. The strength of the patient's self-efficacy beliefs may also vary across situations (e.g., taking oral tablets as prescribed when at home versus when on a trip), an issue of generality.

Self-efficacy is influenced by four sources of information: verbal persuasion, vicarious experience, direct experience, and emotional arousal.[63] *Verbal persuasion*, which involves telling a person that he or she has the ability to perform a behavior, is the weakest source of efficacy information. *Vicarious experience*, which is considerably more potent, involves observing others perform the behavior. Through this type of observational learning, individuals can come to better understand how to perform the behavior, the skills that are required for success, and the outcomes that accompany success and failure. Self-efficacy is most likely to be enhanced by observing similar others successfully perform the behavior—the inference being, "If that person can do it, I can too." Many health education interventions include strategies designed to take advantage of learning through vicarious experience. For example, a video on childhood asthma might show a child using his or her inhaler and subsequently experiencing symptom relief. *Direct experience*, which involves performing the behavior oneself, is also often incorporated into health education programs and is the most potent source of information about self-efficacy. Typically, individuals are given an opportunity to practice the behavior in a supportive environment with supervision. In this type of program, complex behaviors might be broken into component steps to facilitate the acquisition of both behavioral capability and self-efficacy. Finally, *emotional arousal* can have either positive or negative effects on self-efficacy. For example, heightened anxiety may undermine self-efficacy, whereas positive affect may enhance it.

The four sources of efficacy information just described also provide information about the outcomes that are most likely to follow performance of a behavior. For example, if an individual experiencing a migraine takes a medication that relieves the migraine, he or she will come to expect that if another migraine is experienced in the future, taking the medication will once again produce relief. Similarly, beliefs concerning the link between behavior and outcomes may be learned by seeing an advertisement on television for a migraine medication that promises symptom relief.

Like Rotter's social learning theory, SCT posits that individuals will tend to engage in behaviors that are likely to result in valued outcomes. In SCT, individuals' beliefs that performance of a specific behavior will lead to given outcomes are called *outcome expectations*, and the values attached to those outcomes are called *outcome expectancies*.[64] These beliefs correspond to the expectations and reinforcement values captured, respectively, in the "E" and "RV" terms in Rotter's social learning theory.

Outcomes that increase the likelihood that a behavior will be repeated are called *reinforcements*. SCT distinguishes between three types of reinforcements: direct reinforcement (e.g., decrease in symptoms after taking a migraine medication), vicarious reinforcement (e.g., observing another person appear to experience symptom relief after taking a migraine medication), and self-reinforcement (e.g., feeling good about oneself after successfully managing a migraine).[64] The mechanisms that underlie self-reinforcement play a central role in SCT because they allow individuals to exercise self-control of behavior. To exercise self-control, individuals must monitor their behavior and its effects, compare their performance to a personal standard or goal, and reward themselves when goals are achieved.[62] Providing people with opportunities for decision making, goal setting, problem solving, and self-reward have all been shown to encourage personal control of behavior.[64]

The final factor that plays an important role in SCT involves *emotional coping responses*. Attempting to learn and enact a new behavior can be emotionally arousing, and negative emotions can inhibit learning and performance of desired behaviors.[61] To be successful, individuals must manage these negative emotions and foster positive ones. Emotional coping responses are the tactics people use to deal with emotional stimuli. In emotionally challenging circumstances, providing people with training and opportunities to practice target behaviors can reduce emotional distress and increase self-efficacy.

SCT has been used to examine adherence to treatment regimens within the context of several chronic diseases. These studies have found high self-efficacy to be associated with greater treatment adherence in diabetes,[65,66] cardiovascular disease,[67,68] HIV/AIDS,[69,70] and rheumatoid arthritis.[71] Interventions using SCT principles have been designed to increase knowledge, expectancies, skills, and environmental support, as well as foster self-regulation, self-monitoring, goal setting, self-incentives, and social support. Results of randomized controlled trials employing SCT constructs have shown marked improvement in outcomes for the intervention group in adherence to treatment for cardiovascular disease[67] and HIV/AIDS.[70]

STAGE THEORIES

Most of the theories that have been reviewed to this point suggest that simple, linear equations can be used to predict behavior and behavior change. For example, Rotter's social learning theory suggests that the likelihood that patients will adopt a recommended behavior can be increased by strengthening their beliefs that valued outcomes will result from adoption of the behavior. Stage theories suggest that it is not that simple. Stage theories view behavior change from a process perspective. These theories suggest that, at any one point in time, individuals will be in one stage of the behavior change process and that, over time, they may move across stages. Moreover, stages theories posit that the factors that influence stage transitions depend on one's current stage in the behavior change process. Stage theorists argue that attempting to apply a simple prediction equation to people in different stages of change is an oversimplification of the behavior change process.[72]

Stage theories include four essential elements:

1. *A classification scheme to define the stages.* Stage theories include rules that allow classification of individuals into different stages of change. These rules must

identify boundaries between stages so that, at any one point in time, an individual can be classified into a specific stage of change and, over time, it is possible to determine when the individual moves to other stages.

2. *An ordering of the stages.* Stages should be ordered in such a way that it is possible to differentiate between people in the early and later stages of change. The earliest stage of change usually includes people who are not considering adopting the target behavior, and the later stages usually include people who are currently performing the behavior. Despite the ordering of stages, progress through the stages is not assumed to be linear, because people may cycle back through stages, skip stages, or remain in one stage indefinitely.

3. *Within stages, assumption of common barriers to change.* Stage theories assume that individuals in the same stage face similar barriers to change. This assumption allows researchers to deliver stage-specific interventions to help people move across stages.

4. *Across stages, assumption of different barriers to change.* Stage theories assume that individuals in different stages face different barriers to change. Thus, different types of interventions are needed by people in different stages to help them progress through the behavior change process.[72]

Completely specified stage theories identify both the criteria that define stages and the stage-specific barriers to change. Although the stage definitions will apply across diverse behaviors, the barriers to change may be behavior specific. For example, barriers relevant to adherence to asthma medications delivered via inhalers probably differ from the barriers relevant to adherence to oral asthma medications. Further, barriers associated with different oral medications may vary depending on their side effect profiles.

Two of the most widely used stage models are the transtheoretical model of change and the precaution adoption process model. These models are described next.

The Transtheoretical Model of Change

The transtheoretical model of change (TTMC) was developed in the 1970s, within the context of addictive disorders, in an effort to produce a comprehensive model of behavior change.[73] Developers of the TTMC drew on concepts from over 300 leading theories of psychotherapy to support one overarching idea—that behavioral change occurs in stages.[74]

As shown in Table 3-1, the TTMC identifies five stages of change: precontemplation, contemplation, preparation, action, and maintenance. A final stage, termination, has been proposed but is not generally emphasized because it is difficult (if not impossible) to achieve.[74]

TABLE 3-1 Stages of Change from the Transtheoretical Model of Change	
Stages of Change	**Description**
Precontemplation	Have no intention to act within the next 6 months. May be uninformed about or unaware of the consequences of their behavior.
Contemplation	Plan to change within the next 6 months. Aware of the pros and cons of their behavior. Some may reach a point of "behavioral procrastination" (not ready for action) and could be stuck in this stage for prolonged periods.
Preparation	Intend to act in the immediate future (next month). Have taken some significant action in the previous year. Have a plan and would be good candidates for an action-oriented program/intervention.
Action	Overt lifestyle change in the past 6 months. Sometimes could be considered behavioral change.
Maintenance	Active relapse prevention and relapse temptation reduction. Individuals have increasing confidence in their ability to continue changes.

In addition to the stages of change, the TTMC emphasizes three key constructs that play critical roles in the behavior change process: decisional balance, self-efficacy, and the processes of change.[74] *Decisional balance* is based on the value-expectancy framework and concerns how individuals weigh the pros and cons of changing.[75] As suggested by value-expectancy theories, individuals are more likely to engage in behaviors if they believe that the pros associated with the behavior outweigh the cons. Moreover, in the behavior change process, research suggests that increases in the perceived pros associated with a target behavior prompt individuals to contemplate behavior change, but that actual behavior change is unlikely to occur as long as perceived cons remain high.[73] In the TTMC, *self-efficacy*, drawn from Bandura's SCT, plays a critical role in predicting relapse following behavior change—especially when dealing with addictive behaviors such as alcohol abuse or smoking.[76] Lower self-efficacy is generally associated with a greater risk of relapse. Finally, the TTMC identifies ten *processes of change*. As shown in Table 3-2, these processes can be aggregated into two higher-order factors: cognitive-affective processes and behavioral processes.[77,78] The processes of change reflect the strategies that people use during the behavior change process. Research suggests that people tend to use cognitive-affective strategies early in the behavioral change process and behavioral strategies in later stages.[79]

TABLE 3-2   Processes of Change from the Transtheoretical Model of Change

Processes of Change	Description
Cognitive-Affective	
Consciousness raising	Gathering information about the behavior
Self-reevaluation	Evaluating the personal consequences for continuing or stopping the behavior
Dramatic relief	Expressing and experiencing emotional arousal related to the behavior
Environmental reevaluation	Evaluating the consequences on others for continuing or stopping the behavior
Social liberation	Evaluating the social norms related to the behavior
Behavioral	
Counter-conditioning	Replacing undesirable behaviors with desirable ones
Stimulus control	Replacing environmental cues to encourage resisting the behavior
Reinforcement management	Introducing rewards for resisting the undesirable behavior
Helping relationships	Using social support to reinforce behavioral change
Self-liberation	Committing to permanent behavioral change

Ficke and Farris reviewed papers published from 1995 to 2004 that used the TTMC to study medication use issues.[80] Two of these papers focused on developing psychometrically sound measures of the stages of change concept.[81,82] The remaining studies used the model to examine adherence to oral contraceptives,[83] discontinuation of therapy with interferon beta-1a,[84] and pharmacists' readiness to provide pharmaceutical care.[85] In addition to these empirical papers, Ficke and Farris identified six conceptual papers that used the TTMC to discuss medication management issues in the context of diabetes,[86] hypertension,[87,88] HIV/AIDS,[89] organ transplant,[90] and pharmaceutical policy.[91] More recently, Berger and colleagues reported positive findings for a TTMC-based intervention designed to decrease discontinuation of therapy with interferon beta-1a.[92] The TTMC also guided a study that involved training pharmacists and pharmacy technicians to identify a pharmacy customer's stage of change for smoking cessation in an attempt to improve counseling and nicotine replacement therapy use.[93] Although smoking cessation rates did not differ between the intervention and control groups, TTMC-trained pharmacists were more likely than untrained pharmacists to talk with their customers about smoking cessation. Thus, the limited evidence available suggests that the TTMC provides a useful framework for studying medication use issues. More work is needed, however, to determine the extent to which interventions based on the TTMC are more effective than non-stage-based interventions in prompting and sustaining behavior change efforts.

Precaution Adoption Process Model

The precaution adoption process model (PAPM) was introduced in 1988 to better describe the processes through which individuals adopt behaviors recommended to reduce the risk associated with potential health threats. The model is similar to the TTMC in many respects; however, a major difference between the two models is the definition of the early stages of change. In the TTMC, all individuals who are not currently either thinking about adopting a recommended behavior or actively involved in the behavior change process are classified together as *precontemplators*. In contrast, the PAPM essentially subdivides the TTMC precontemplation stage into three distinct stages. Thus, as shown in Figure 3-4, in PAPM stage 1, individuals have never heard of the health threat of interest or of precautions recommended to reduce risks associated with the threat. In PAPM stage 2, individuals have heard of the threat, but have never considered adopting the precaution(s) recommended to reduce risk. In PAPM stage 3, individuals have thought about adopting the precaution(s), but have decided against it. The value of distinguishing among people in these three different early PAPM stages is probably greatest in situations where information concerning the health threat or available precautions is actively evolving. For example, the PAPM may be particularly appropriate to study the behavior change process in relation to vaccination against human papilloma virus. Because this vaccine has only become available fairly recently, many women may be unaware that the vaccine exists or have had little opportunity to consider obtaining it. The PAPM also suggests that individuals who have decided against adopting a particular precaution may be especially difficult to engage in behavior change efforts. Research suggests that individuals in this stage (i.e., stage 3) can be quite well informed[94] and that they will tend to reject information that is inconsistent with their decision.[95]

The PAPM has been used to study receipt of hepatitis B vaccination[96] and has been used in a series of studies to examine adoption of precautions recommended to prevent osteoporosis.[94,97-99] In general, this research supports the basic stage model assumption that individuals in different stages face different barriers to change. However, it is too early to determine whether interventions based on the PAPM are superior to non-stage-based interventions in terms of facilitating behavior change efforts.

Stage 1 Not aware of the issue	Stage 2 Unengaged by the issue	Stage 3 Deciding about acting	Stage 5 Deciding to act	Stage 6 Acting	Stage 7 Maintaining behavior change
		Stage 4 Deciding not to act			

FIGURE 3-4 Precaution Adoption Process Model.

LIMITATIONS OF THE THEORIES REVIEWED

The theories reviewed in this chapter provide considerable insight into individual and interpersonal factors that influence health and illness behavior. However, several limitations of the theories should also be noted. First, most of the theories assume that behavior is volitional. Thus, individuals are viewed as consciously deciding whether or not to engage in different behaviors. Because of the heavy emphasis placed on individual perceptions (e.g., perceived benefits, perceived barriers, subjective norms), most of the theories reviewed pay little attention to the effects that objective social and political factors may have on health behavior. Although the theory of planned behavior acknowledges the possible direct effect of environmental constraints (i.e., actual behavioral control) on individual behavior, only Bandura's social cognitive theory explicitly recognizes the reciprocal influences of individual and environmental factors.

Second, the theories reviewed tend to assume that individuals consciously consider the advantages and disadvantages associated with different courses of action and choose to enact behaviors that optimize their outcomes. However, behavior often appears less deliberate than this conceptualization would suggest. For example, while picking up a prescription at a pharmacy, a person might notice an attractive display of vitamin and mineral preparations and be prompted to make a purchase with little consideration of the advantages and disadvantages. In the health belief model, this type of store display would be considered a cue to action. However, none of the other theories reviewed recognize the important role that such environmental cues may have on behavior. In addition, recent work in the area of judgment and decision making suggests that adults often make decisions based on intuitive principles, rather than a careful balancing of the advantages and disadvantages of different courses of action.[100] Additional research is needed to fully understand the practical implications of these findings.

Finally, the theories reviewed in this chapter are primarily cognitive in that they emphasize the effects of beliefs and attitudes on behavior. Although emotional arousal is considered in several of the theories (e.g., Bandura's social cognitive theory, the transtheoretical model of change, and the health belief model), it tends to receive less attention than the cognitive variables. Yet, emotion often has profound effects on health and illness behavior. For example, fear of needles may prevent individuals from obtaining immunizations that they know they need.[101] As another example, depression may interfere with individuals engaging in a broad range of self-care activities, including adhering to prescribed medications.[102] Emotion plays a more integral role in two other theories that were not reviewed in this chapter due to space limitations. These are the dual process model of self-regulation, developed by Leventhal and colleagues,[103] and the transactional model of stress and coping, developed by Lazarus and colleagues.[104,105] Interested readers may refer to the references provided for additional information about these models.

SUMMARY

This chapter reviewed several individual and interpersonal theories of health and illness behavior. It also noted that these models address only a relatively small number of factors that influence health behavior. Other chapters in this book address factors at other levels of the social ecological framework. The chapter also discussed limitations of the various models reviewed. As new findings emerge, current theories are likely to be adapted or replaced by newer theories.

A major weakness of the literature on medication use and pharmacy practice is that often investigators do not use any theoretical framework to guide their work. Given that most of the theories reviewed in this chapter have been widely used to guide research on other health behaviors, it is surprising that they have not been used more often to study issues related to medication use and pharmacy practice. As described in the introduction to this chapter, theories provide a vehicle for summarizing and communicating empirical findings. They provide a mechanism through which the knowledge base in a particular area can be built and organized. As a consequence of the relative dearth of theoretically informed research in pharmacy practice, it is often difficult to synthesize empirical findings across studies in a meaningful way. Pharmacy practitioners developing interventions to improve adherence and treatment outcomes often do so with little consideration given to the existing theoretical literature. Thus, they often end up reinventing the wheel with each new intervention. It is hoped that the information provided in this chapter will increase awareness of the theoretical frameworks that can be used to guide intervention efforts and will stimulate interest in the development of interventions that are both theoretically informed and evidence based.

REFERENCES

1. Cohen DA, Scribner RA, Farley TA. A structural model of health behavior: a pragmatic approach to explain and influence health behaviors at the population level. Prev Med 2000;30(2):146-54.
2. Kerlinger FN. Foundations of behavioral research. 3rd ed. New York: Holt, Rinehart and Winston, 1986.
3. Glanz K, Rimer BK, Lewis FM, eds. Health behavior and health education: theory, research, and practice. 3rd ed. San Francisco: Jossey-Bass, 2002.
4. Rotter JB. Generalized expectancies for internal versus external control of reinforcement. Psychol Monogr 1966;80(1):1-28.
5. Wallston KA, Wallston BS, DeVellis RF. Development of the Multidimensional Health Locus of Control scales (MHLC). Health Educ Monogr 1978;6:160-70.
6. George J, Shalansky SJ. Predictors of refill non-adherence in patients with heart failure. Br J Clin Pharmacol 2007;63(4):488-93.
7. Bane C, Hughes CM, McElnay JC. The impact of depressive symptoms and psychosocial factors on medication adherence in cardiovascular disease. Patient Educ Couns 2006;60(2):187-93.
8. Apter AJ, Reisine ST, Affleck G, Barrows E, ZuWallack RL. Adherence with twice-daily dosing of inhaled steroids. Socioeconomic and health-belief differences. Am J Respir Crit Care Med 1998;157(6 pt 1):1810-7.
9. Weng FL, Israni AK, Joffe MM, et al. Race and electronically measured adherence to immunosuppressive medications after deceased donor renal transplantation. J Am Soc Nephrol 2005;16(6):1839-48.
10. Frazier PA, Davis-Ali SH, Dahl KE. Correlates of noncompliance among renal transplant recipients. Clin Transplant 1994;8(6):550-7.
11. Tamaroff MH, Festa RS, Adesman AR, Walco GA. Therapeutic adherence to oral medication regimens by adolescents with cancer. II. Clinical and psychologic correlates. J Pediatr 1992;120(5):812-7.
12. Atkins L, Fallowfield L. Intentional and non-intentional non-adherence to medication amongst breast cancer patients. Eur J Cancer 2006;42(14):2271-6.
13. McDonough EM, Boyd JH, Varvares MA, Maves MD. Relationship between psychological status and compliance in a sample of patients treated for cancer of the head and neck. Head Neck 1996;18(3):269-76.
14. Haley CJ, Drake RJ, Bentall RP, Lewis SW. Health beliefs link to duration of untreated psychosis and attitudes to later treatment in early psychosis. Soc Psychiatry Psychiatr Epidemiol 2003;38(6):311-6.
15. Budd RJ, Hughes IC, Smith JA. Health beliefs and compliance with antipsychotic medication. Br J Clin Psychol 1996;35(pt 3):393-7.

16. Molassiotis A, Nahas-Lopez V, Chung WY, Lam SW, Li CK, Lau TF. Factors associated with adherence to antiretroviral medication in HIV-infected patients. Int J STD AIDS 2002; 13(5):301-10.

17. Altice FL, Mostashari F, Friedland GH. Trust and the acceptance of and adherence to anti-retroviral therapy. J Acquir Immune Defic Syndr 2001;28(1):47-58.

18. Wallston KA. Hocus-pocus, the focus isn't strictly on locus: Rotter's social learning theory modified for health. Cogn Ther Res 1992;16(2):183-99.

19. Oberle K. A decade of research in locus of control: what have we learned? J Adv Nurs 1991;16(7):800-6.

20. Fishbein M, Ajzen I. Belief, attitude, intention and behavior: an introduction to theory and research. Boston: Addison-Wesley, 1975.

21. Ajzen I. From intentions to actions: a theory of planned behavior. In: Kuhl J, Beckman J, eds. Action-control: from cognition to behavior. Heidelberg: Springer, 1985:11-39.

22. Ajzen I. Constructing a TPB questionnaire: conceptual and methodological considerations. January 2006. (Accessed April 2, 2007, at http://www-unix.oit.umass.edu/~aizen/pdf/tpb.measurement.pdf.)

23. Ried LD, Christensen DB. A psychosocial perspective in the explanation of patients' drug-taking behavior. Soc Sci Med 1988;27(3):277-85.

24. Austin JK. Predicting parental anticonvulsant medication compliance using the theory of reasoned action. J Pediatr Nurs 1989;4(2):88-95.

25. Jackson C. Promoting adherence to antibiotics: a test of implementation intentions. Patient Educ Couns 2006;61(2):212-8.

26. de Bruin M, Hospers HJ, van den Borne HW, Kok G, Prins JM. Theory- and evidence-based intervention to improve adherence to antiretroviral therapy among HIV-infected patients in the Netherlands: a pilot study. AIDS Patient Care STDS 2005;19(6):384-94.

27. Abraham C, Clift S, Grabowski P. Cognitive predictors of adherence to malaria prophylaxis regimens on return from a malarious region: a prospective study. Soc Sci Med 1999;48(11): 1641-54.

28. Miller P, Wikoff R, Hiatt A. Fishbein's model of reasoned action and compliance behavior of hypertensive patients. Nurs Res 1992;41(2):104-9.

29. Farquharson L, Noble LM, Barker C, Behrens RH. Health beliefs and communication in the travel clinic consultation as predictors of adherence to malaria chemoprophylaxis. Br J Health Psychol 2004;9(pt 2):201-17.

30. van Hulten R, Bakker AB, Lodder AC, Teeuw KB, Bakker A, Leufkens HG. The impact of attitudes and beliefs on length of benzodiazepine use: a study among inexperienced and experienced benzodiazepine users. Soc Sci Med 2003;56(6):1345-54.

31. Pellino TA. Relationships between patient attitudes, subjective norms, perceived control, and analgesic use following elective orthopedic surgery. Res Nurs Health 1997;20(2):97-105.

32. Gupchup GV, Abhyankar UL, Worley MM, Raisch DW, Marfatia AA, Namdar R. Relationships between Hispanic ethnicity and attitudes and beliefs toward herbal medicine use among older adults. Res Social Adm Pharm 2006;2(2):266-79.

33. Bharucha DX, Morling BA, Niesenbaum RA. Use and definition of herbal medicines differ by ethnicity. Ann Pharmacother 2003;37(10):1409-13.

34. Bersellini E, Berry D. The benefits of providing benefit information: examining the effectiveness of provision of simple benefit statements on people's judgments about a medicine. Psychol Health 2007;22(1):61-82.

35. Coleman CL. Examining influences of pharmacists' communication with consumers about antibiotics. Health Commun 2003;15(1):79-99.

36. Walker A, Watson M, Grimshar J, Bond C. Applying the theory of planned behavior to pharmacists' beliefs and intentions about the treatment of vaginal candidiasis with non-prescription medicines. Fam Pract 2004;21(6):670-6.

37. Herbert KE, Urmie JM, Newland BA, Farris KB. Prediction of pharmacist intention to provide Medicare medication therapy management services using the theory of planned behavior. Res Social Adm Pharm 2006;2(3):299-314.

38. Gaither CA, Bagozzi RP, Ascione FJ, Kirking DM. A reasoned action approach to physicians' utilization of drug information sources. Pharm Res 1996;13(9):1291-8.

39. Gaither CA, Bagozzi RP, Ascione FJ, Kirking DM. The determinants of physician attitudes and subjective norms toward drug information sources: modification and test of the theory of reasoned action. Pharm Res 1997;14(10):1298-308.

40. Hochbaum GM. Public participation in medical screening programs: a socio-psychological study. Washington: U.S. Department of Health, Education, and Welfare, Public Health Service, Bureau of State Services, Division of Special Health Services, Tuberculosis Program, 1958.

41. Janz NK, Becker MH. The health belief model: a decade later. Health Educ Q 1984;11(1):1-47.

42. Hershey JC, Morton BG, Davis JB, Reichgott MJ. Patient compliance with antihypertensive medication. Am J Public Health 1980;70(10):1081-9.

43. Brown CM, Segal R. The effects of health and treatment perceptions on the use of prescribed medication and home remedies among African American and white American hypertensives. Soc Sci Med 1996;43(6):903-17.

44. Wutoh AK, Brown CM, Dutta AP, Kumoji EK, Clarke-Tasker V, Xue Z. Treatment perceptions and attitudes of older human immunodeficiency virus-infected adults. Res Social Adm Pharm 2005;1(1):60-76.

45. Muma RD, Ross MW, Parcel GS, Pollard RB. Zidovudine adherence among individuals with HIV infection. AIDS Care 1995;7(4):439-47.

46. Kelly GR, Mamon JA, Scott JE. Utility of the health belief model in examining medication compliance among psychiatric outpatients. Soc Sci Med 1987;25(11):1205-11.

47. Adams J, Scott J. Predicting medication adherence in severe mental disorders. Acta Psychiatr Scand 2000;101(2):119-24.

48. Mulaik JS. Noncompliance with medication regimens in severely and persistently mentally ill schizophrenic patients. Issues Ment Health Nurs 1992;13(3):219-37.

49. Seo MA, Min SK. Development of a structural model explaining medication compliance of persons with schizophrenia. Yonsei Med J 2005;46(3):331-40.

50. Nageotte C, Sullivan G, Duan N, Camp PL. Medication compliance among the seriously mentally ill in a public mental health system. Soc Psychiatry Psychiatr Epidemiol 1997;32(2):49-56.

51. Kiley DJ, Lam CS, Pollak R. A study of treatment compliance following kidney transplantation. Transplantation 1993;55(1):51-6.

52. Shope JT. Compliance in children and adults: review of studies. Epilepsy Res Suppl 1988;1:23-47.

53. Al-Faris EA, Abdulghani HM, Mahdi AH, Salih MA, Al-Kordi AG. Compliance with appoint-
    ments and medications in a pediatric neurology clinic at a university hospital in Riyadh, Saudi
    Arabia. Saudi Med J 2002;23(8):969-74.

54. Polly RK. Diabetes health beliefs, self-care behaviors, and glycemic control among older adults
    with non-insulin-dependent diabetes mellitus. Diabetes Educ 1992;18(4):321-7.

55. Elliott V, Morgan S, Day S, Mollerup LS, Wang W. Parental health beliefs and compliance
    with prophylactic penicillin administration in children with sickle cell disease. J Pediatr
    Hematol Oncol 2001;23(2):112-6.

56. Nagy VT, Wolfe GR. Cognitive predictors of compliance in chronic disease patients. Med
    Care 1984;22(10):912-21.

57. Soliday E, Hoeksel R. Health beliefs and pediatric emergency department after-care adher-
    ence. Ann Behav Med 2000;22(4):299-306.

58. Unson CG, Fortinsky R, Prestwood K, Reisine S. Osteoporosis medications used by older
    African American women: effects of socioeconomic status and psychosocial factors. J
    Community Health 2005;30(4):281-97.

59. Cline RR, Farley JF, Hansen RA, Schommer JC. Osteoporosis beliefs and antiresorptive med-
    ication use. Maturitas 2005;50(3):196-208.

60. Bandura A. Social cognitive theory: an agentic perspective. Asian J Social Psychol 1999;2(1):21-41.

61. Bandura A. Self-efficacy: toward a unifying theory of behavioral change. Psychol Rev 1977;
    84(2):191-215.

62. Bandura A. Social cognitive theory and exercise of control over HIV infection. In: DiClemente
    CC, Peterson JL, eds. Preventing AIDS: theories and methods of behavioral interventions.
    New York: Plenum Press, 1994:336.

63. Bandura A. Social foundations of thought and action: a social cognitive theory. Englewood
    Cliffs, NJ: Prentice-Hall, 1986.

64. Baranowski T, Perry CL, Parcel GS. How individuals, environments, and health behavior
    interact. In: Glanz K, Rimer BK, Lewis FM, eds. Health behavior and health education: theory,
    research, and practice. 3rd ed. San Francisco: Jossey-Bass, 2002:165-84.

65. Kavanagh DJ, Gooley S, Wilson PH. Prediction of adherence and control in diabetes. J Behav
    Med 1993;16(5):509-22.

66. McCaul KD, Glasgow RE, Schafer LC. Diabetes regimen behaviors. Predicting adherence.
    Med Care 1987;25(9):868-81.

67. DeBusk RF, Miller NH, Superko HR, et al. A case-management system for coronary risk factor
    modification after acute myocardial infarction. Ann Intern Med 1994;120(9):721-9.

68. Haskell WL, Alderman EL, Fair JM, et al. Effects of intensive multiple risk factor reduction
    on coronary atherosclerosis and clinical cardiac events in men and women with coronary artery
    disease. The Stanford Coronary Risk Intervention Project (SCRIP). Circulation 1994;89(3):
    975-90.

69. Gifford AL, Bormann JE, Shively MJ, Wright BC, Richman DD, Bozzette SA. Predictors of
    self-reported adherence and plasma HIV concentrations in patients on multidrug antiretroviral
    regimens. J Acquir Immune Defic Syndr 2000;23(5):386-95.

70. Smith SR, Rublein JC, Marcus C, Brock TP, Chesney MA. A medication self-management
    program to improve adherence to HIV therapy regimens. Patient Educ Couns 2003;50(2):
    187-99.

71. Taal E, Rasker JJ, Seydel ER, Wiegman O. Health status, adherence with health recommendations, self-efficacy and social support in patients with rheumatoid arthritis. Patient Educ Couns 1993;20(2-3):63-76.

72. Weinstein ND, Sutton SR, Rothman AJ. Stage theories of health behavior: conceptual and methodological issues. Health Psychol 1998;17(3):290-9.

73. Prochaska JO, Velicer WF, Rossi JS, et al. Stages of change and decisional balance for 12 problem behaviors. Health Psychol 1994;13(1):39-46.

74. Prochaska JO, Redding CA, Evers KE. The transtheoretical model and stages of change. In: Glanz K, Rimer BK, Lewis FM, eds. Health behavior and health education: theory, research, and practice. 3rd ed. San Francisco: Jossey-Bass, 2002:99-116.

75. Janis I, Mann L. Decision making: a psychological analysis of conflict, choice and commitment. New York: Free Press, 1977.

76. DiClemente CC, Fairhurst SK, Piotrowski NA. The role of self-efficacy in the addictive behaviors. In: Maddux J, ed. Self-efficacy, adaptation and adjustment: theory, research and application. New York: Plenum, 1995:109-41.

77. Prochaska JO, DiClemente CC. Transtheoretical therapy: toward a more integrative model of change. Psychother Theory Res Practice 1982;19:276-88.

78. Rosen CS. Is the sequencing of change processes by stage consistent across health problems? A meta-analysis. Health Psychol 2000;19(6):593-604.

79. Prochaska JO, DiClemente CC, Norcross JC. In search of how people change: applications to addictive behaviors. Am Psychol 1992;47(9):1102-14.

80. Ficke DL, Farris KB. Use of the transtheoretical model in the medication use process. Ann Pharmacother 2005;39(7-8):1325-30.

81. Cook CL, Perri M 3rd. Single-item vs multiple-item measures of stage of change in compliance with prescribed medications. Psychol Rep 2004;94(1):115-24.

82. Willey C, Redding C, Stafford J, et al. Stages of change for adherence with medication regimens for chronic disease: development and validation of a measure. Clin Ther 2000;22(7):858-71.

83. Johnson SS, Grimley DM, Prochaska JO. Prediction of adherence using the transtheoretical model: implications for pharmacy care practice. J Social Adm Pharm 1998;15:135-48.

84. Berger BA, Hudmon KS, Liang H. Predicting treatment discontinuation among patients with multiple sclerosis: application of the transtheoretical model of change. J Am Pharm Assoc (Wash) 2004;44(4):445-54.

85. Berger BA, Grimley D. Pharmacists' readiness for rendering pharmaceutical care. J Am Pharm Assoc (Wash) 1997;NS37(5):535-42.

86. Corelli RL, Hudmon KS. Promoting treatment adherence in diabetes: a practical strategy for pharmacists. Calif J Health Syst Pharm 1999;Sept/Oct:6.

87. Sher TG, Bellg AJ, Braun L, Domas A, Rosenson R, Canar WJ. Partners for life: a theoretical approach to developing an intervention for cardiac risk reduction. Health Educ Res 2002;17(5):597-605.

88. Willey C. Behavior-changing methods for improving adherence to medication. Curr Hypertension Rep 1999;1(6):477-81.

89. Tuldra A, Wu AW. Interventions to improve adherence to antiretroviral therapy. J Acquir Immune Defic Syndr 2002;31(suppl 3):S154-7.

90. Robbins ML. Medication adherence and the transplant recipient: helping patients at each stage of change. Transplant Proc 1999;31(4A):29S-30S.

91. Roughead EE, Gilbert AL, Primrose JG. Improving drug use: a case study of events which led to changes in use of flucloxacillin in Australia. Soc Sci Med 1999;48(6):845-53.

92. Berger BA, Liang H, Hudmon KS. Evaluation of software-based telephone counseling to enhance medication persistency among patients with multiple sclerosis. J Am Pharm Assoc (Wash) 2005;45(4):466-72.

93. Sinclair HK, Bond CM, Lennox AS, et al. Training pharmacists and pharmacy assistants in the stage-of-change model of smoking cessation: a randomised controlled trial in Scotland. Tobacco Control 1998;7(3):253-61.

94. Blalock SJ, DeVellis RF, Giorgino KB, et al. Osteoporosis prevention in premenopausal women: using a stage model approach to examine the predictors of behavior. Health Psychol 1996;15:84-93.

95. Weinstein ND, Sandman PM. A model of the precaution adoption process: evidence from home radon testing. Health Psychol 1992;11(3):170-80.

96. Hammer GP. Hepatitis b vaccine acceptance among nursing home workers [Doctoral dissertation]. 1997.

97. Blalock SJ. Predictors of calcium intake patterns: a longitudinal analysis. Health Psychol 2007;26(3):251-8.

98. Blalock SJ, Currey SS, DeVellis RF, et al. Effects of educational materials concerning osteoporosis on women's knowledge, beliefs, and behavior. Am J Health Promot 2000;14:161-9.

99. Blalock SJ, DeVellis BM, Patterson CC, Campbell MK, Orenstein DR, Dooley MA. Effects of osteoporosis prevention program incorporating tailored educational materials. Am J Health Promot 2002;16:146-56.

100. Reyna VF, Lloyd FJ, Brainerd CJ. Memory development, and rationality: an integrative theory of judgment and decision making. In: Schneider SL, Shanteau J, eds. Emerging perspectives on judgment and decision research. Cambridge, England: Cambridge University Press, 2003.

101. Crockett M, Keystone J. "I hate needles" and other factors impacting on travel vaccine uptake. J Travel Med 2005;12(suppl 1):S41-6.

102. Rubin RR. Adherence to pharmacologic therapy in patients with type 2 diabetes mellitus. Am J Med 2005;118(suppl 5A):27S-34S.

103. Leventhal H, Leventhal EA, Cameron LD. Representations, procedures, and affect in illness self-regulation: a perceptual-cognitive model. In: Baum A, Revenson TA, Singer JE, eds. Handbook of health psychology. Mahwah, NJ: Erlbaum, 2001:19-47.

104. Lazarus RS, Folkman S. Stress, appraisal, and coping. New York: Springer Publishing, 1984.

105. Lazarus RS. Fifty years of research and theory by R.S. Lazarus: an analysis of historical and perennial issues. Mahwah, NJ: Lawrence Erlbaum Associates, 1998.

CHAPTER 4

Health Disparities: International Perspectives

Janine Morgall Traulsen, PhD, and Paul Bissell, PhD

This chapter outlines some of the ways in which sociologists have sought to understand how social systems (or societies) operate to produce health disparities. As readers will be aware, this is a vast area of social science inquiry; the aim in this chapter is to introduce and discuss key areas of sociological thinking in relation to health disparities. The extent, causes, and consequences of inequalities in health remain one of the most heavily researched and hotly debated areas in social epidemiology and medical sociology. However, there are differences concerning how various disciplines approach health disparities; for example, whereas social epidemiology is primarily concerned with identifying and quantifying the factors that might explain the socioeconomic gradient in health (mainly from within a neopositivist paradigm), sociology is more concerned with understanding and developing theories that better explain how disparities in health have arisen. This chapter summarizes the extent of health disparities and provides an overview of the types of explanations that have been posited, focusing particularly on the newer neomaterialist and psychosocial arguments. Many of these explanations offer important insights into how the social system shapes (some would say determines) our experiences of health and illness.

HEALTH DISPARITIES

Research in the field of health inequality includes the following: measurement of the extent of health disparities; social group inequalities in health; health disparities as a reflection of the effects of poverty; the role of material deprivation and psychosocial mechanisms as they affect health; the effect of relative income on health; and how the life course contributes to health inequalities.[1] This chapter will not attempt to address all of these issues; rather, it introduces the reader to the sociological understanding of the causes and consequences of health disparities and macro sociological concerns. It begins with socioeconomic inequalities, changing demographics, and their links to health and disease, and then discusses measurements of and explanations of disparities.

Let us start by considering the extent of global inequality in income. Studies show that at the beginning of the 21st century, the richest 5% of people received one third of total global income—as much as is shared by the poorest 80%. Although a few poorer countries are catching up with rich parts of the world, economists point out that the differences between the richest and poorest individuals around the globe are growing.[2] A recent study on per capita wealth in different countries found that average wealth amounted to $144,000 per person in the United States in the year 2000, and $181,000 in Japan.[3] In contrast, India was found to have per capita assets of $1,100 and Indonesia $1,400.[3]

Richer countries have generally grown faster than poorer countries, and according to the World Bank, inequality between nations is increasing. At the same time, the two most populous nations on earth—China and India—have experienced dramatic rates of economic growth, but this has been accompanied by growing inequalities in domestic wealth that have increased over the past two decades.[2] Not only are there dramatic and continuing inequalities in wealth, but also a less dramatic but widening inequality in personal and household income, that is, the growing inequality of earnings.

Like wealth, health and disease are not distributed equally. A growing body of evidence shows persistent differences in health status both within countries as well as between countries. At the beginning of the 21st century, inequalities among the world's individuals are staggering, and we continue to find links between poverty, material deprivation, social class, and ill-health.[4] In reviewing the evidence, we find that whichever indicator of socioeconomic status is used—income, class, housing, deprivation, or education—those who are worse off socioeconomically also have the worst health.[5]

In both national and international literature, *health inequalities*, *health inequality*, and *health disparities* are used interchangeably. However, these terms can hold different meanings for different people. For some policy makers, health disparities refers to the fact that individuals do not have the same health status—that is, within any given society, some are ill and some are not. Yet health disparities are most widely understood as the differences between social groups rather than the individual variations between people. Within the field of sociology, health disparities often refers to differences in health that arise because of other social inequalities experienced by subgroups in the population. To put this slightly differently, there are systematic differences in health, disease, and mortality associated with the positions in society of people or groups in the population. This concept links the health of individuals to the structures producing social inequalities that shape people's lives.[6]

Various organizations such as the World Health Organization (WHO) and the World Bank have studied inequalities as they relate to and influence health, and have pointed to the fact that wealth provides access to economic resources and thereby more freedom of choice.[7] Economic resources mitigate the impact of unexpected expenses or income losses—for example, as a result of unemployment or work injuries. Wealthy nations (as well as individuals) have the possibility to reduce work hours, providing time for holidays and recreation, and, most important, they can afford health insurance and health services. However, the lack of economic resources makes these options less likely, and in the case of abject poverty, even impossible. For example, natural disasters on the scale of the tsunami in the Indian Ocean in 2004 and Hurricane Katrina in the United States in 2005 focused attention on the susceptibility of poor and vulnerable populations to such catastrophes.

Global demographic changes appear to further exacerbate inequalities in wealth and health. Aging and the increase in chronic conditions, including diabetes and cardiovascular disorders, are just a few examples of the emerging demographic patterns affecting health, and are more pronounced in certain population groups and socioeconomic categories. In addition to these examples, in today's global world we find an ever-increasing movement of people as labor migrants, soldiers, and refugees. Seen from this perspective, the link between social and economic factors, changing demographics, and health is more visible than ever. This constant and increasing movement of people facilitates the spread of communicable diseases such as tuberculosis and HIV/AIDS. Migrants and refugees—in most cases with few economic resources—have little or no access to health care in host countries, and their ability to use services is increasingly becoming a pressing issue.

Various social as well as economic factors contribute to the persistent patterns of health disparities, including changing demographics. For example, many low- and middle-income countries are now facing the so-called double burden of disease: while continuing to deal with the problems of infectious disease and undernutrition, they are also experiencing a rapid upsurge in chronic disease risk factors such as obesity, particularly in urban settings. It is not uncommon to find undernutrition and obesity existing side by side within the same country, the same community, and even within the same household. According to WHO, the double burden is caused by inadequate prenatal, infant, and young child nutrition followed by exposure to high-fat, energy-dense, micronutrient-poor foods and lack of physical activity.[8]

Measuring Health Disparities

Historically, measurements of health have focused largely on the prevalence of disease. By the mid-20th century, however, the health picture had changed—the populations living in the West were not disease ridden, and ideas about what has been referred to as *positive health* emerged. This approach led to the widespread adoption of the seminal WHO definition of health as "physical, mental and social well-being, not merely the absence of disease or infirmity," a definition that has been subsequently revised and enhanced.[9] In this tradition, health status is measured by variables such as life expectancy, mortality, morbidity, and disability.

In the West, mortality rates have fallen dramatically over time, beginning in the 18th century in a few countries, and they continue to fall in most countries today. However, when looking at life expectancy at birth, we find a range of almost 50 years between rich and poor countries: 33 years in Swaziland, compared with 81.9 years in Japan.[10] We find also that the probability of a man dying between ages 15 and 60 is 8.3% in Sweden, 46.4% in Russia, and 90.2% in Lesotho.[11] Life expectancy in several sub-Saharan African states is little more than 40 years (Malawi, Uganda, and Zambia) and slightly more than 45 in Botswana, compared with over 75 in the United Kingdom and 77 in the United States.[10] By any index, Africa is the poorest continent in the world.

Differences within countries can be just as startling. One study carried out in Bangladesh looked at the relationship between household wealth inequality and chronic childhood undernutrition and found that children in the poorest 20% of households were more than three times as likely to suffer from adverse growth-rate stunting as children from the wealthiest 20% of households.[12] Another example is Indonesia, where under-five mortality is nearly four times higher in the poorest fifth of the population than in the richest fifth.[13] However, perhaps the most shocking and tragic statistics are from those countries where life expectancy has been spiraling downward. For example, in 1995 the life expectancy at birth in Zimbabwe was 55.6 years, and by 2005 it had plummeted to 37.2, most likely due to a combination of HIV/AIDS, poverty, and the socioeconomic crises that have occurred in the last decade.[10]

Inequalities within countries are not confined to poorer countries. In the United States, there is a 20-year gap in life expectancy between the least and most advantaged.[14] The post-neonatal (28 days to 11 months) death rate for Native Americans and Alaska Native people is almost double that of white Americans.[15] Similar patterns in health disparities can also be found in the United Kingdom, where life expectancy at birth for boys is about 5 years less in the two lowest social classes than in the two highest, at 70 and 75 years, respectively. Men between 20 and 64 years from the bottom social class are three times more likely to die from coronary heart disease and stroke than those in the top social class.[6]

A widely referenced WHO-commissioned report from 2003 entitled *The Solid Facts* reviewed evidence from Europe aimed at reducing inequalities in health within countries and found that poor social and economic circumstances affect health throughout life, and that those persons further down the social ladder usually run at least twice the risk of serious illness and premature death as those near the top.[16] It is important to remember that the effects of socioeconomic differences are not confined to the poor alone. The so-called social gradient in health refers to the fact that this pattern tends to be evident across the society. This means that people in each socio-economic category have worse health than those above them in the hierarchy, so that even among middle-class office workers, lower-ranking staff suffer much more disease and earlier death than higher-ranking staff.[16]

According to Marmot, the social gradient in health is influenced by such factors as social position, relative versus absolute deprivation, control, and social participation.[17] In seeking to understand causes for the social gradient, Marmot made two observations. First, the social gradient applies to nonhuman primates and other social animals as well as humans (that is, the lower the status, the higher the disease risk and the shorter the lifespan). Second, it applies to many societies and at different time periods. This pattern has been confirmed by data from the United States and elsewhere.[17] One should not see this as a cause for despair, because it is possible for the health of everyone to improve and for the gap between rich and poor to shift toward more equal distribution; in other words, the slope of the social gradient in mortality is not fixed.

The factors that are believed to contribute to these differences in morbidity and mortality are both material and psychosocial, and their effects extend to most diseases and causes of death. When we speak of disadvantaged people and populations, we speak of disadvantages as both absolute or relative and as encompassing a multiple set of factors, including having few family assets, having poor education, having insecure employment, becoming stuck in a hazardous or dead-end job, living in poor housing, trying to bring up a family in difficult circumstances, and living on an inadequate retirement pension. *The Solid Facts* points out that these disadvantages tend to concentrate among the same people and that their effects on health accumulate during life. In other words, the research indicates that the longer people experience stressful economic or social circumstances, the greater the physiologic problems they suffer and the less likely they are to enjoy life into old age.[16]

In summary, the key messages on the social determinants of health from *The Solid Facts* include the following:[16]

- *The social gradient:* Poor social and economic circumstances affect health throughout life.
- *Stress:* Continuous anxiety, insecurity, low self-esteem, social isolation, and lack of control over work and home life all have stressful effects on health.
- *Early life:* Foundations of adult health are laid in childhood; for example, poor nutrition, maternal smoking, drinking, or drug use, and maternal stress all contribute to a poor foundation of adult health.
- *Social exclusion:* Social exclusion (racism, stigmatization, discrimination, etc.) often implies denied access to decent housing, education, and transport, all of which affect health.
- *Work:* Employment is better for health than unemployment, and jobs that couple high demand and low control carry special risk for stress that contributes to sickness absence, social status difference in health, and premature death.
- *Unemployment:* Unemployment puts health at risk, and risk is higher in regions where unemployment is widespread.
- *Social support:* Social support and good social relations contribute to good health.
- *Addiction:* Drug use, alcoholism, and eating disorders have adverse effects on health.
- *Food:* Nutrition and food safety are important to health.
- *Transportation:* Healthy transport means less driving and more walking and cycling.

This section explored the links between health and social, economic, and demographic factors. The focus now shifts to sociological explanations for health disparities.

EXPLAINING HEALTH DISPARITIES

Explanations for health disparities have become more nuanced over time, moving from biological factors to social and environmental factors; however, attempts to understand and explain health disparities are varied. Scambler points out that much of the epidemiologic research has been atheoretical to date and takes a largely positivist view of health and illness, by which he means it simply looks for relationships between variables rather than attempting to develop theory to explain the data.[18]

Scambler points out that in the United Kingdom there has been a strong commitment to social class analysis among quantitative researchers using a measurement that sorts occupations into five groups ranging from professional to unskilled—the so-called Registrar Generals Social Scale (RGS).[18] For example, the impressive and influential Black Report published in 1980 attempted to link social class—based on the RGS—to health and illness. The Black Report showed that while there continued to be an improvement in health across all the classes (during the first 35 years of the British National Health Service), there was still a correlation between social class and infant mortality rates, life expectancy, and inequalities in the use of medical services. This seminal report was fundamental in demonstrating that although overall health had improved since the introduction of the welfare state, there were still widespread health disparities. For example, the death rate for men in social class V (unskilled manual workers) was twice that for men in social class I (professional and managerial), and the gap between the two was increasing rather than decreasing as expected. The report also argued that the main cause of these inequalities was poverty, and that to attack these inequalities, the gap between upper-class and lower-class peoples must be narrowed. More recent studies, such as the Whitehead Report published in 1987 and the Acheson Report published in 1998, came to the same conclusions as the Black Report.[18] Just why these inequalities have been so persistent has been a matter of continuing debate.

A number of explanations for these health disparities have been offered. One argument points out that the gradient of class differences in health will depend to some extent on how class and health are measured.[19] Another is that there is evidence of "social drift," in which people with poor health suffer a decline in socioeconomic position, whereas the opposite argument posits that the healthy rising in class is less likely, because many health problems emerge only in adulthood, once career choices have been made. There is also evidence that risk behaviors are unevenly distributed between the classes and that this contributes to the health gradient. Poverty is demonstrably bad for health, yet material explanations are not sufficient on their own to explain class differences in health. Other factors, such as gender, race, and ethnicity, have been shown to play a significant part in health.

One approach to explaining these discrepancies is that of *social ecology*. In his book *The Impact of Inequality: How to Make Sick Societies Healthier*, Richard Wilkinson compares the United States with other market democracies, and one state with another.[20] He presents evidence that unequal societies create poor health, more social conflict, and more violence. According to Wilkinson, despite their material success, modern societies are social failures, largely because of the social inequalities that characterize them, particularly inequalities in relation to wealth and status. He uses various examples to explain how and why inequality has such devastating effects on the quality and length of our lives. In what has become known as Wilkinson's social ecology argument, he shows that inequality leads to stress, that stress creates sickness on the individual and mass level, and that overall society suffers widespread unhappiness and high levels of violence, depression, and mistrust across the social spectrum. His conclusion is simple: social, economic, and political equality is essential for improving life for everyone. Wilkinson argues that even small reductions in income inequality can make an important difference to the health of a population; for example, he calculates that a difference of only 7% of the share of income going to the bottom 50% of the population would result in a two-year increase in life expectancy.[21]

Others have been more critical of such arguments. Scambler has developed a hypothesis based on greed wherein he argues that it is quite plausible to regard health disparities (for example, in the United Kingdom) "as the (largely unintended) consequences of the ever-adaptive behavior of members of its (weakly globalized) power elite, informed by its (strongly globalized) capitalist-executive."[18] In other words, the rich have managed to grab more and more slices of the cake in conjunction with largely controlling the executive functions of government. This can be observed in the intersection between the experiences of ill health (lifeworld narratives) and how these are perceived and processed in healthcare systems (expert culture). Examples of this can be found in attempts to mix preventive medicine with individual and community empowerment—thus abstracting individuals from the social relations of which they are a part and assuming that their choices about lifestyle and health are both individual and rational.

Gender, Race, and Ethnicity

Although social determinants of mortality and morbidity have long been utilized in health planning and in developing health services, it is only more recently that the importance of gender, race, and ethnicity has become internationally recognized and accepted in healthcare planning and politics.

Whereas gender affects the health of both men and women, it is widely recognized that women's health is especially affected as a result of gender. Powerful barriers that include poverty, unequal power relationships between men and women, and lack of education prevent millions of women worldwide from having access to health care and from attaining—and maintaining—the best possible health.

Although worldwide fertility rates have declined in most countries thanks to effective family planning programs, childbirth is still recognized as a major factor affecting women's overall health. In the developing world as a whole, the total fertility rate, or the average number of births per woman, had fallen from 5.7 births per woman in 1970 to 3.5 by 2000, excluding China.[22] Still, one third of births (32%) in the developing world are ill timed or unwanted, as documented in the Demographic and Health Surveys estimates for 51 developing countries.[22]

Unintended pregnancies affect the well-being of women, children, and families. In fact, some health experts believe that unintended pregnancies carried to term are more likely to involve complications.[23] Women with unintended pregnancies may be subject to increased physical abuse by their partners during pregnancy.[24] Moreover, many unintended pregnancies end in abortion. In 2000, of the 46 million pregnancies that were terminated each year around the world, it was estimated that 19 million were carried out under unsafe conditions. According to WHO, every year 68,000 women die of complications from abortions performed by unqualified people or under unhygienic conditions or both; many suffer serious, often permanent, disabilities.[25] Unintended pregnancy is the result of many factors, among them lack of access to contraception. About 114 million women—more than one in six—in the developing world have an unmet need for contraception, often because of lack of access to a choice of modern methods.

Reproduction is only one part of the picture. The WHO Gender and Women's Health Program places emphasis on the health consequences of the discrimination against women that exists in nearly every culture, as well as the need to understand not just absolute levels of health but how it varies within populations. Gender is an important determinant of health that interacts with many factors, including material and cultural resources. Therefore, understanding the relationship between gender and health requires analysis of the distribution of power and economic resources among men and women.[26]

A quarter of a century ago, race and ethnicity did not figure prominently in the work of health services researchers, medical sociologists, or public health researchers. The experiences of ethnic minority groups were either absent or confined to specialist texts. In the final quarter of the 20th century, the relationship between race, ethnicity, and health began to figure more prominently in mainstream medical and social science journals. Today it is widely recognized that there is an urgent need to identify and research the experiences of ethnic minority client groups in relation to their use of community and hospital pharmacy. There is also considerable scope for adding to the research on ethnic minority groups' use of medicines and their self-care activities.

Changing Demographics

One issue to be considered when looking at the relationship between race, ethnicity, and health is the constant change in demographics. Migration is one of the important demographic trends in many parts of the world today. Migration patterns in the European Union (EU) and the increase in so-called mobile patients are proving a serious challenge to national healthcare and pharmacy services in Europe. The migration patterns can be seen as follows:

- East to west: The influx of non-Westerners into the EU
- South to north: The influx of Africans into the EU
- North to south: The influx of retirees from northern to southern Europe

There are many reasons for migration. War, unstable governments, poverty, and unemployment have driven thousands of political refugees from their homes in search of a better life. This pertains mostly to east-to-west and south-to-north migration.

Increasing migration is often fueled by war and poverty, and the consequences for large groups of immigrants or refugees who come to live as "guests" in host countries can be devastating. Migration and racial discrimination may in itself provide the basis for ill health. Migrants may suffer from victimization, stress, and personal injury, as well as physical and emotional distress. Refugees from war-torn areas bring health problems to host countries, such as the long-term physical and mental effects of deprivation, torture, and post-traumatic stress. Excluded groups, often refugees and immigrants, tend to undertake more risky physical labor that has low status and therefore higher levels of injury and occupational disease and ill health.

Newcomers are not the only ones to experience exclusion and discrimination, and although differences in health due to race and ethnicity are often linked to economic disadvantages, socioeconomic status as a health variable cannot stand alone. There is also evidence that nonsocioeconomic causes of racial/ethnic differences in health, in addition to income, may depend on wealth, education, occupation, neighborhood socioeconomic characteristics, or past socioeconomic experiences.[27]

A British study on ethnic inequalities in health suggests a link between the different forms of social disadvantage experienced by ethnic minority groups and the various ways in which racism itself can affect physical and mental health.[28] The study suggests that racism and its accompanying social disadvantage are important aspects of the lives of people from ethnic minority groups, and that this must be incorporated into strategies to address ethnic inequalities in health.

A more recent form of migration, which has only recently received attention, is the increase of economically well-off adults—primarily retired EU citizens—moving from the north (e.g., from the United Kingdom and the Nordic countries) to southern Europe (mostly Spain, Portugal, and France). The reason for this—the milder climate in the south—is similar to the north-to-south migration of elderly persons also found in the United States. However, the problems in Europe are much more complex than those found in the United States. As a rule, these retirees—with above-average medicine needs—move to host countries where they neither speak nor understand the language and where they do not understand the structure and legalities of the healthcare system and health services.

SUMMARY

This chapter has shown how sociology provides different perspectives on how the system operates at the structural level to produce health disparities. In summary, we would like to point out that the policy implications of the health disparities discussed in this chapter are tremendous. If policy fails to address the links between social inequality and health, it not only ignores the most powerful determinants of health standards in modern societies but also ignores one of the most important social justice issues facing modern societies.[16]

REFERENCES

1. Kawachi I, Subramanian S, Almeida-Filho N. A glossary for health inequalities. J Epidemiol Community Health 2002;56(9):647-52.
2. Milanovic B. Worlds apart: measuring international and global inequality. Princeton, NJ: Princeton University Press, 2005.
3. Davies J, Shorrocks A, Sandstrom S, Wolff E. The world distribution of household wealth. Helsinki: World Institute for Development Economics Research of the United Nations University, 2006.
4. Whitehead M, Bird P. Breaking the poor health-poverty link in the 21st century: do health systems help or hinder? Ann Trop Med Parasitol 2006;100(5-6):389-99.
5. Shaw M, Dorling D, Davey-Smith G. Poverty, social exclusion and minorities. In: Marmot M, Wilkinson R, eds. Social determinants of health. Oxford, England: Oxford University Press, 1999:220-41.
6. Graham H. Tackling inequalities in health in England: remedying health disadvantages, narrowing health gaps or reducing health gradients? J Soc Policy 2004;33(1):115-31.

7. Morissette R, Zhang X. Revisiting wealth inequality. Perspectives, December 2006. Statistics Canada Catalogue no. 75-001-XIE. (Accessed April 17, 2007, at http://www.statcan.ca/english/freepub/75-001-XIE/11206/art-1.pdf.)

8. World Health Organization. Obesity and overweight. September 2006. (Accessed April 17, 2007, at http://www.who.int/mediacentre/factsheets/fs311/en/print.html.)

9. Preamble to the Constitution of the World Health Organization as adopted by the International Health Conference, New York, 19 June–22 July 1946; signed on 22 July 1946 by the representatives of 61 States (Official Records of the World Health Organization, no. 2, p. 100) and entered into force on 7 April 1948. (Accessed at http://www.who.int/suggestions/faq/en/.)

10. United Nations Development Programme. Human development report: beyond scarcity—power, poverty and the global water crisis. New York: United Nations Development Programme, 2006.

11. World Health Organization. World health report 2003: shaping the future. Geneva: World Health Organization, 2003.

12. Hong R, Banta JE, Betacourt JA. Relationship between household wealth inequality and chronic childhood under-nutrition in Bangladesh. Int J Equity Health 2006;5:15. (Accessed April 17, 2007, at http://www.pubmedcentral.nih.gov/articlerender.fcgi?artid=1702347.)

13. Victora CG, Wagstaff A, Schellenberg JA, Gwatkin D, Claeson M, Habicht JP. Applying an equity lens to child health and mortality: more of the same is not enough. Lancet 2003; 362:233-41.

14. Murray CJL, Michaud CM, McKenna MT, Marks JS. U.S. patterns of mortality by county and race: 1965–94. Cambridge, MA: Harvard Center for Population and Development Studies, 1998.

15. National Center for Health Statistics. Health, United States, 2004, with chartbook on trends in the health of Americans. Hyattsville, MD: U.S. Department of Health and Human Services, 2004.

16. Wilkinson R, Marmot M. The solid facts. Copenhagen: World Health Organization, 2003.

17. Marmot MG. Understanding social inequalities in health. Perspect Biol Med 2003; 46(3 suppl):9-23.

18. Scambler G. Health and social change: a critical theory. Philadelphia: Open University Press, 2002.

19. Macintyre S. The Black Report and beyond: what are the issues? Soc Sci Med 1997;44(6):723-45.

20. Wilkinson R. The impact of inequality: how to make sick societies healthier. New York: New Press, 2006.

21. Wilkinson R. Unhealthy societies: the afflictions of inequality. London: Routledge, 1996.

22. Westoff CF. Unmet need at the end of the century. Calverton, MD: Macro International, 2001. (Demographic and Health Surveys Comparative Reports no. 1.)

23. Institute of Medicine. Prenatal care: reaching mothers, reaching infants. Washington, DC: National Academy Press, 1988.

24. Goodwin MM, Gazmararian JA, Johnson CH, Gilbert BC, Saltzman LE, PRAMS working group. Pregnancy intendedness and physical abuse around the time of pregnancy: findings from the Pregnancy Risk Assessment Monitoring System, 1996–1997. Matern Child Health J 2000;4(2):85-92.

25. World Health Organization. Unsafe abortion: global and regional estimates of incidence of unsafe abortion and associated mortality in 2000. Geneva: World Health Organization, 2004.

26. Wamala S, Ågren G. Gender inequity and public health—getting down to real issues . Eur J Public Health 2002;12:163-5.

27. Braverman PA, Cubbin C, Egeter S, et al. Socioeconomic status in health research—one size does not fit all. JAMA 2005;294(22):2879.

28. Nazroo JY, Karlsen S. Ethnic inequalities in health: social class, racism and identity. Lancaster, England: Lancaster University, Health Variations Programme, September 2001. (Research Findings no. 10.) (Accessed April 19, 2007, at http://www.lancs.ac.uk/fss/apsocsci/hvp/pdf/fd10.pdf.)

Ecological Models for Change in Health and Illness Behaviors

CHAPTER 5

Health Promotion: Program Planning and Evaluation

Health Promotion: Program Planning and Evaluation

Karen S. Hudmon, DrPH

Perhaps the most challenging aspect of health promotion is *effective integration of theory and models* in the conceptualization, development, implementation, and evaluation of our interventions. It is not enough to understand a given theory—it is necessary to understand numerous theories, their applicability to specific behaviors, and their relevance to specific populations. Theory, if applied appropriately, should be intricately woven throughout the entire process. As such, systematic application of theory, from the point of conceptualization of an intervention through the analysis of program evaluation results and dissemination, requires robust comprehension of the theoretical constructs as well as the measurement and analysis of these constructs. Evaluation is, in many ways, both an art and a science.

Program planning and evaluation together constitute an ongoing, cyclical process whereby planning informs evaluation and evaluation informs subsequent planning (Fig. 5-1). Although much of the remaining content of this chapter focuses on the specifics of health promotion planning, it is important to understand the science and importance of program evaluation. Evaluation can be defined as "the systematic assessment of the worth or merit of some object."[1] Two key categories of evaluation are formative and summative.[1]

- *Formative evaluation:* Strengthens or improves a program by examining its delivery, the quality of its implementation, or the organizational/environmental context of the program in which the program is delivered. Examples of questions addressed via formative evaluation include the following.
  (a) What is the definition and scope of the problem?
  (b) Where does the problem occur—for example, in what location(s), in what population(s)? How pervasive and how serious is the problem?

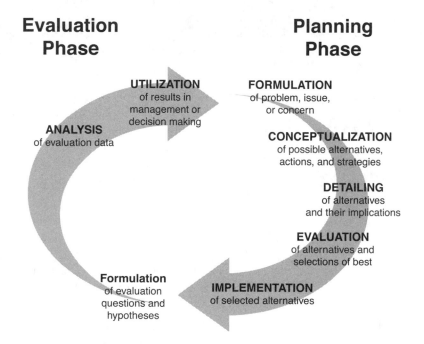

FIGURE 5-1   The Planning Evaluation Cycle
Source: From W.M.K. Trochim. The Research Methods Knowledge Base, 2nd edition © 2001 Custom Solutions, a part of Cengage Learning, Inc. All rights reserved. Reproduced by permission. No further reproduction permitted without prior written permission of the publisher. www.cengage.com/permissions

    (c) How should a program be delivered to address the problem?

    (d) To what extent is a program concept being implemented?

- *Summative evaluation:* Examines the effects or outcomes of programs, estimating the overall impact and/or estimating associated costs. Examples of questions addressed via summative evaluation include the following.

    (a) What is the efficacy or effectiveness of the program on relevant health outcomes?

    (b) Is the program cost-effective?

Most health promotion programs undergo some level of evaluation at either the formative or summative level (see Table 5-1 for examples); however, the approach is often unsystematic or desultory. Commonly, evaluation procedures are designed *after* a program has already been developed and implemented. Although this information can be useful in informing future changes, often the results reveal major changes that are needed, which can be costly to implement.

TABLE 5-1   Evaluation: Types and Examples

Formative Evaluation

Needs assessment: To (1) identify the target population for a program, (2) estimate the extent of need for the program, or (3) delineate what type of program might meet the needs of a target population

Feasibility assessment: To determine whether an evaluation is feasible to conduct

Implementation or process evaluation: To monitor the extent to which a program complies with the implementation protocol

Summative Evaluation

Outcome evaluation: To investigate the effect(s) of a program on defined target outcomes

Impact evaluation: To assess the overall effects (intended or unintended) of a program

Cost effectiveness and cost-benefit analysis: To estimate efficiency by standardizing outcomes in terms of their costs and values

Secondary analysis: To utilize existing data to examine new questions or to apply methods not previously employed

Meta-analysis: To combine the results of multiple studies, creating a summary judgment on an evaluation question

Adapted from Trochim WMK. The research methods knowledge base. 2nd ed. Cincinnati, OH: Atomic Dog Publishing, 2001.

The pages that follow describe several different frameworks for program planning and evaluation. Finally, the chapter concludes with comments about the importance of these frameworks within the broader context of public health and health promotion.

PROGRAM PLANNING

Planning and evaluation are crucial to health promotion. Too often, institutions or organizations identify a problem and concoct a short-sighted quick fix without taking time to gain an in-depth understanding of the problem and its determinants. The planning process must operationalize program components and the target population, but it also must address factors associated with adoption and implementation. And all of this should be evaluated, on an ongoing basis, to gauge the appropriateness of programs and to make amendments as needed.

Several relevant frameworks have been presented in the literature over the past several decades. This chapter presents three options that are commonly used to facilitate program development and evaluation:

1. PRECEDE-PROCEED
2. Intervention mapping
3. RE-AIM

The *PRECEDE-PROCEED model* offers a stepwise method for program planners to work in tandem with communities throughout the planning, implementation, and evaluation process.[2] A strength of PRECEDE-PROCEED, if applied effectively, is that the approach necessitates a systematic and comprehensive examination of the public health problem and the environment in which it occurs and considers a wide range of potential outcome determinants at the needs assessment stage before the program is developed. *Intervention mapping*, developed in the 1980s and 1990s, draws from PRECEDE-PROCEED by emulating the needs assessment process but, in contrast, applies a more heavy emphasis on the intervention development process and its interrelatedness with behavioral theory.[3] *RE-AIM*, which was introduced more recently (in the late 1990s), similarly offers a systematic approach for evaluating health behavior interventions, with particular attention to five elements (described later in this chapter) that the creators describe as being equally important.[4,5]

Each of these frameworks has many strengths, and with the exception of the need for time and labor allocations for more complete characterization of constructs, there are no major drawbacks. To date, the three frameworks have not undergone comparative analysis in a research setting. Notably, all three frameworks apply an ecological approach to health promotion and evaluation, whereby the "health" of an individual or group is examined within the context of the environment (e.g., impact of family, social networks, community, organization, and policy).

THE PRECEDE-PROCEED PLANNING MODEL

The PRECEDE framework (Fig. 5-2), developed in the 1970s by Green and colleagues, is perhaps the most widely used model for health promotion program planning.[2] PRECEDE stands for predisposing, reinforcing, and enabling constructs in educational/ecological diagnosis and evaluation. Phases 1 to 4, which focus on formative evaluation comprise PRECEDE. In 1991, the model was expanded to include PROCEED (policy, regulatory, and organizational constructs in educational and environmental development). This addition highlights the importance of environmental factors and their influence on health behavior and health outcomes. Phases 5 to 8,

PRECEDE

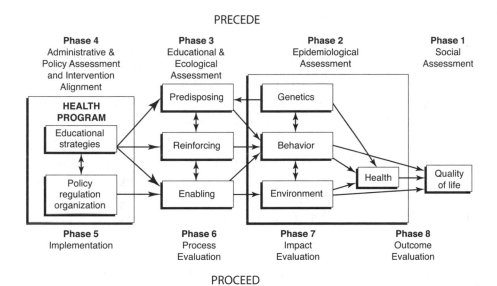

PROCEED

FIGURE 5-2 PRECEDE-PROCEED planning model for health education planning and evaluation
Source: L. Green, M. Kreuter. Health Promotion Planning: An Educational and Ecological Approach, 4th edition, The McGraw-Hill Companies, 2005. Reproduced with permission of the McGraw-Hill Companies.

which focus on development, comprise PROCEED. This stage follows the PRECEDE stage and marks the beginning of the program implementation and evaluation process.

The PRECEDE-PROCEED model emphasizes community participation so as to foster community ownership in the process, the proposed solution, and the implementation of the resulting programmatic intervention. This approach is congruent with the principles of *community-based participatory research* (CBPR). As defined by the Agency for Healthcare Research and Quality, CBPR is a "collaborative process of research involving researchers and community representatives; it engages community members, employs local knowledge in the understanding of health problems and the design of interventions, and invests community members in the processes and products of research. In addition, community members are invested in the dissemination and use of research findings and ultimately in the reduction of health disparities."[6]

The PRECEDE-PROCEED model necessitates careful assessment of the social environment, the epidemiology of the problem, the behavior or behaviors that are affecting the health problem in question, educational and ecological factors, and administrative and policy factors. As delineated in Figure 5-2, each of these is important to the planning process and informs intervention development. The following sections detail each component as described by Green and Kreuter.[2,7]

Phase 1: Social Assessment

The social assessment phase focuses on characterizing a population's perceived needs and quality of life, as opposed to simply assessing the disease-related outcomes. There are many ways to assess different aspects of quality of life, but in general all of these assessments attempt to ascribe a number or set of numbers to quantify "the perception of individuals or groups that their needs are being satisfied and that they are not being denied opportunities to pursue happiness and fulfillment."[7] Methodology can include objective social indicators (e.g., unemployment rates, air quality, healthcare insurance coverage) or subjective assessments of perceptions, provided by community members. These assessments are important because quality of life and health are closely connected—quality of life impacts health, and health affects quality of life. If a health program aims to meet patient needs, one must first understand what those needs are. One must also gain a clear understanding of the capacity of the population—what are their strengths and weaknesses, and how will these affect their receptivity to an intervention?

Immersion in the community, through varied data collection efforts, fosters an enhanced understanding of the problem. Specifically, planners should observe the population, conduct in-depth interviews with key informants (e.g., community leaders, opinion leaders), conduct focus groups, host community forums, and/or administer surveys to representative members of the broader community population. The goal in this phase is to gain a complete understanding of quality of life concerns from the community's perspective.

Phase 2: Epidemiologic Assessment

The epidemiologic assessment phase aims to (a) identify all health-related factors that contribute to, or interact with the societal problems defined in phase 1, and (b) identify etiological factors or determinants of health such as genetics (genes, as well as gene-environment interactions), patterns of behavior, and environment. Specifically, the phase 2 assessment attempts to obtain objective measures that pinpoint which health-related conditions are important and to identify the various factors contributing to the incidence of those conditions.

Epidemiologic data are available through national databases maintained by the National Center for Health Statistics, the Centers for Disease Control and Prevention, the Department of Health and Human Services, the Census Bureau, and state and local health departments. Typically, an epidemiologic assessment examines morbidity, mortality, and disability in a population. Statistics can include prevalence (the *proportion* of a population that possesses the characteristic at a given point in time) or incidence (the *rate* at which members of a population convert status from nondiseased to diseased, creating new cases).

Phase 3: Behavioral and Environmental Assessment

This phase also aims to assess the myriad factors that are known or hypothesized contributors to the negative health outcome under investigation. *Behavioral factors* are the specific behaviors and lifestyle choices that manifest in the target population and contribute to incidence or severity. In contrast, *environmental factors* include social and physical forces that are external to an individual and often not under his or her control. Ideally, many of these factors will be modifiable through intervention. Factors that are not modifiable, such as genetic predisposition, might be useful in identifying specific subgroups of a population that are at an elevated risk.

A series of steps constitutes the *behavioral assessment:*

1. *List potential behavioral risks for the health problem.* This involves refining the list of behavioral factors to specify preventive behaviors (e.g., smoking cessation, regular exercise, mammography screening, stress reduction) versus associated actions or treatment/interventions (e.g., adherence with medical regimens, smoking cessation, weight reduction). Note that some behaviors might be classified in both categories. For example, smoking cessation is a preventive behavior (e.g., in an adolescent patient) but it also might be a treatment (e.g., in a patient with emphysema).

2. *Rate the behaviors based on importance.* Any behavior that is closely correlated with the outcome of interest is considered important. In this step, the goal is to reduce the list of behaviors to include only those that are most important, where importance is gauged by the behavior's frequency and level of relatedness to the health problem.

3. *Rate the behaviors based on extent of changeability.* Behaviors that are closely associated with the outcome of interest but offer little opportunity for change typically are not ideal targets for program planning. In estimating changeability, it is important to consider anticipated time lines for change—how long will it take for the change to occur? High changeability typically is more likely when behaviors are in the developmental stages or have recently been established (e.g., smoking initiation among adolescents or young adults) than when the behavior

is well established. Behaviors with high relapse rates tend to be more difficult to change and often require more intensive interventions.

4. *Choose behavioral targets.* Based on information gathered and processed in steps 1 through 3, the focus of the intervention is chosen.

5. *State behavioral objectives.* The conclusion of the behavioral assessment process requires careful specification of behavioral objectives. Objectives should state and address the following: Who is the target population? What is the desired change to be achieved? How much of the condition or outcome is to be achieved? In what time frame is the change expected to occur?

The *environmental assessment* follows the same methodology, with a focus on environmental influences. If the scope of environmental factors becomes unmanageable, consider limiting the list to environmental aspects that are more social than physical (e.g., organizational and economic factors), are interactive with behavior in its impact on health, and have the potential to be changed through social action or health policy.[7]

Green and Kreuter provide guidelines to assist planners in setting priorities for health programs:[2]

1. Which health problem has the greatest impact (e.g., death, disease, disability, absenteeism, cost)?
2. Are any subpopulations (e.g., children, mothers, racial/ethnic groups) at an elevated risk?
3. Which problems would be most susceptible to an intervention?
4. Which problems are not being addressed by other agencies or programs?
5. Which problems have the greatest potential for achieving a significant intervention impact?
6. Are any of the health problems ranked high at the national or local level?
7. To what extent does the problem(s) constitute a disproportionately high burden compared to other areas or communities?

After these seven questions have been answered and priorities are aligned, objectives must be delineated. This is achieved by asking four questions:[2]

1. Who will receive the program?
2. What health benefit should the population receive?
3. How much of that benefit should be achieved?
4. By when should it be achieved, and for how long will the program run?

These objectives must be carefully operationalized—for example, "the prevalence of smoking in African American women in Los Angeles will be reduced by five percentage points in the next 12 months, and by an additional three percentage points in the following 24 months." Defining measurable program objectives enables evaluators to gauge the overall success of a program and facilitates associated resource allocation.

Three categories of factors affect individual or group behavior and are targeted in phase 3 of PRECEDE:

- *Predisposing factors:* Antecedents to behavior that provide the rationale or motivation for the behavior. Examples: knowledge, awareness, attitudes, beliefs, perceived needs, self-efficacy, and existing skills.
- *Enabling factors:* Factors that facilitate the performance or enactment of a behavior. Examples: availability, accessibility or convenience, affordability, new skills, and environmental conditions. Some enabling factors might exert a negative impact on change.
- *Reinforcing factors:* Consequences of action that provide either positive or negative feedback for the action. Examples: physical response, reactions of peers or coworkers, social support, advice from a clinician.

Phase 3 is the assessment step for which behavioral theory tends to be most relevant. This step focuses on the delineation of factors that affect behavioral and environmental factors. Constructs from existing behavioral theories, such as the health belief model,[8-11] the transtheoretical model of change,[12,13] the theory of reasoned action or planned behavior,[14,15] or social cognitive theory,[16] can help us to understand the target behavior.

Selecting factors to be targeted and setting priorities is achieved by identifying all the causal factors and categorizing them based on whether they exhibit predisposing, enabling, or reinforcing properties. Among the three categories, the constituent factors should be prioritized. Finally, the planners must determine which factors in each category are to be targeted first. Characteristics to consider are importance (frequency and extent of relatedness to the outcome of interest) and changeability. As a final step in the PRECEDE component of the model, one must write learning and resource objectives that (1) define the predisposing factors and skills that will be targeted by the new intervention, (2) provide measurable criteria by which the program can be evaluated, and (3) specify what resources or conditions will be present at the conclusion of the program.

Phase 4: Administrative and Policy Assessment

Phase 4 involves the delineation of intervention strategies and outlines the logistics of program implementation. A planner must clarify the resources needed for program implementation, any organizational barriers and facilitators for implementation, and any policies that are relevant to the success of the program. This information is used to establish project time lines, allocate resources, and develop a working budget.

Administrative Assessment

Administrative assessment encompasses the following:

1. *Assessment of necessary resources.* What resources are needed to implement the proposed program? Items to consider include time, personnel, and budget.
2. *Assessment of available resources.* What resources does the planning team have available to support the program? A primary focus here is on identifying personnel to accept responsibility for the various duties. Are new employees needed, or can existing employees be retrained? What level of funding is available, and what are the budgetary constraints? Lack of funding might necessitate modifications to the program's components or its reach.
3. *Assessment of factors influencing implementation.* Investigation of potential factors influencing program implementation might reveal barriers that can be circumvented up front or might identify positive facilitators, such as program champions that might otherwise have gone unnoticed. At this step, planners should assess staff commitment and attitudes, revisit the programmatic goals (and adjust as necessary), consider the anticipated rate of change (for example, it might be prudent to take smaller, more manageable steps), promote familiarity of the new procedures among staff through training, attempt to reduce complexity where possible, ensure that appropriate space is available, and anticipate resistance that might be encountered from community members. Also at this step, planners should make certain that program personnel have received adequate training and that a plan for ongoing supervision is in place. This promotes quality assurance.

Policy Assessment

Does your proposed program fit within the existing polices, regulations, and organizational structure and values? Are there any political forces that must be reconciled before the program is launched? Several approaches exist for examining the policy environment within an organization or system. The interested reader is referred to Green and Kreuter for a more detailed discussion.[2]

Phases 5 to 8: Implementation and Evaluation

Moving from the PRECEDE (assessment and diagnostic steps) to the PROCEED component of the model, phase 5 is where the program is actually developed and implemented. All necessary resources are in place, and the program launch is imminent. In phase 6, the team conducts an ongoing assessment of the program processes to estimate the extent to which the program was implemented according to plan. This *process evaluation* is a necessary component of all program evaluations because it enables the team to more fully interpret the results from the impact and outcome evaluations (phases 7 and 8). According to the model, *impact measures* capture changes in the behavioral and environmental factors as well as the predisposing, enabling, and reinforcing factors. *Outcome measures* estimate the effect of the program on health and quality of life.

In summary, the PRECEDE component begins with analysis of quality of life; health, behavioral, and environmental factors; and predisposing, enabling, and reinforcing determinants of the health problem under investigation and its associated environmental factors. In the PROCEED component, a health promotion program is developed, implemented in the defined setting, and evaluated using process, impact, and outcome measures. This comprehensive approach is achieved through collaboration between planners and the target community. The PRECEDE-PROCEED model has been used as an intervention framework in nearly 1,000 published studies and is an integral component of training for public health advocates.[17] Its underlying principles are germane to the next framework that we present, intervention mapping.

INTERVENTION MAPPING

Intervention mapping, developed by Bartholomew and colleagues, provides a protocol for the development of theory-based health promotion programs.[3] The six-step protocol (Fig. 5-3) enables the effective translation of knowledge about behavioral determinants into specific change goals, and subsequently into theory-based intervention methods and strategies. It has been applied to a variety of health behaviors and settings.[3,18-26]

Intervention mapping builds on the work achieved in a PRECEDE-PROCEED phase and facilitates the development of proximal program objectives, the selection of theory-based intervention methods and practical strategies to promote change, the delineation of program components, the anticipation of program dissemination and adoption, and the anticipation of process and outcome evaluations. This process is assisted by the creation of intervention matrices—the matrices collectively create an "intervention map" that guides the translation of objectives to change strategies and intervention activities. The approach, which builds on existing frameworks and applies behavioral theories in the planning process, is a tool that "maps the path from recognition of a need or problem to the identification of a solution."[22(p87)]

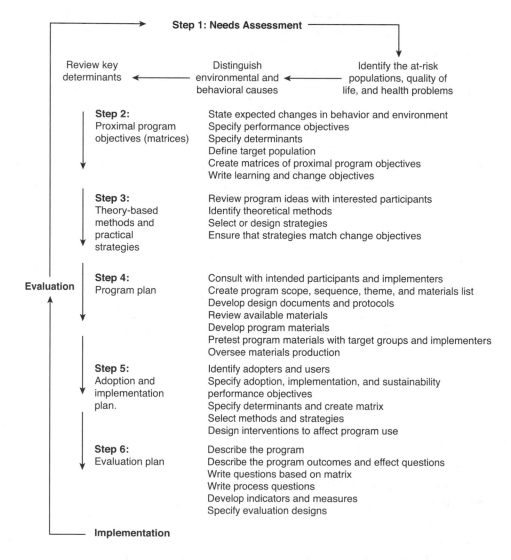

FIGURE 5-3   Intervention Mapping: A 6-step protocol for health promotion programs
Source: L.K. Bartholomew, G.S. Parcel, G. Kok, N.H. Gottlieb. Planning Health Promotion Programs: An Intervention Mapping Approach, John Wiley & Sons, Inc., 2006. Adapted with permission of John Wiley & Sons, Inc.

Although intervention mapping is presented as a series of steps, the planning process is more iterative and cumulative than linear.[3] Several core processes are integral to intervention mapping (Table 5-2); these are applied through group process, with interactive discussion. The mapping process, which operationalizes the theory-based intervention, begins after the needs assessment (e.g., the PRECEDE-PROCEED component, step 1) has been completed. The mapping process is labor intensive, but is comprehensive in approach. This section provides a summary of the steps (see also Fig. 5-3). The interested reader is referred to the intervention mapping website (www.interventionmapping.nl) and also to the textbook by Bartholomew and coauthors that describes the approach in great detail.

In step 2 (Fig. 5-3), planners specify *who* and *what* will be the target of the intervention. Toward this goal, a set of matrices is created for each of the relevant ecological levels (e.g., individual, group, organization, societal), which integrates performance objectives for each ecological level with behavioral determinants to produce change objectives. In step 3, the team identifies evidence-based theories and methods and strategies that are hypothesized to be effective in promoting change at the relevant ecological levels. The end products of step 4 include a defined scope and sequence of the intervention components, a complete set of program materials, and carefully operationalized program implementation protocols. All materials and protocols should have undergone pilot testing with the personnel who are responsible for implementing the program as well as the recipients of the program. The emphasis in step 5 is program adoption, implementation, and maintenance of implementation over time. In step 6, the

TABLE 5-2   Core Processes for Intervention Mapping
Process
Pose questions
Brainstorm provisional answers
Search the literature for empirical findings
Evaluate the relevance and strength of evidence
Access and apply theory
Identify and address needs for new data

Adapted from Bartholomew LK, Parcel GS, Kok G, Gottlieb NH. Intervention mapping: designing theory- and evidence-based health promotion programs. New York: McGraw-Hill, 2001. Reproduced with permission from McGraw-Hill Companies.

team finalizes an evaluation plan that is designed to parallel the intervention map. The focus is on both process and impact/outcome measures, as described earlier.

In summary, intervention mapping is a tool to aid health planners in applying behavioral science theories to program development and evaluation. It is a practical approach, and although it does not offer new theories or strategies per se, it increases the likelihood that new interventions are theoretically solid and are directly linked to the programmatic objectives.

RE-AIM

The RE-AIM framework was designed in response to an identified need to expand the number of "dimensions of quality" that are addressed in the evaluation of health promotion programs. This section describes the RE-AIM model and its comprehensive approach toward emphasizing the reach and representativeness of the target populations and settings for health promotion programs.

According to the RE-AIM framework, the impact of a health promotion program is a function of five key factors, each of which can be expressed on a scale that ranges from zero to one (or, as a percentage, from 0% to 100%). The factors, summarized in Table 5-3, are described in greater detail in the following subsections. Online tools for computing these percentages are available at www.re-aim.org/2003/calculations.html.

Reach

The *reach* of a program describes the proportion of at-risk persons who are exposed to the impact of a policy or program. Careful consideration is given to defining both the numerator and the denominator composing the proportion. Examples of denominators could include the total number of patients serviced at a specific inpatient or outpatient clinic, the number of employees at a specific worksite, or census data. In estimating the extent to which a program is reaching its intended target population, it is important to define the target population and to identify both overinclusion (did some individuals who received the program not need it?) and underinclusion (were there individuals in need who did not receive the program?). Whereas underinclusion can lead to increased healthcare costs, overinclusion can result in wasted resources.

Efficacy or Effectiveness

In evaluating the *efficacy* or *effectiveness* of a new medication, one would want to identify the positive therapeutic benefits as well as the adverse events. One would expect

Dimension	Level	Definition
Reach	Individual	The absolute number, proportion, and representativeness of individuals who are willing to participate in a given initiative.
Efficacy or effectiveness	Individual	The impact of an intervention on important outcomes, including potential negative effects, quality of life, and economic outcomes.
Adoption	Organizational	The absolute number, proportion, and representativeness of settings and intervention agents who are willing to initiate a program.
Implementation	Organizational	At the setting level, implementation refers to the intervention agents' fidelity to the various elements of an intervention's protocol. This includes consistency of delivery as intended and the time and cost of the intervention.
Maintenance	Individual and organizational	Setting level: The extent to which a program or policy becomes institutionalized or part of the routine organizational practices and policies.

Individual level: The long-term effects of a program on outcomes (6 or more months after the most recent intervention contact). |

TABLE 5-3   RE-AIM Evaluation Framework

Adapted from Kaiser Permanente. RE-AIM. 2006. (Accessed October 15, 2007 at http://www.re-aim.org/.)

the same approach when evaluating a health promotion program—it is important to capture both positive and negative outcomes of the program. In addition, evaluators should assess changes in clinical outcomes, behavioral outcomes, and quality of life. The impact of the intervention should be estimated using sound study designs that are able to capture changes over time. Prospective designs are best in most cases, and these should include baseline measures and either a control group or a comparison group so as to protect the internal validity of study results.

Adoption

The third component of the RE-AIM model is *adoption*, which answers the question, what is the proportion and representativeness of settings that adopt the program? Whereas some programs might target only one setting, others are designed for more broadscale dissemination. Some change agents or sites will be early adopters, some will be late adopters, and some will not adopt at all. It is important to examine a representative sample of all persons or settings, regardless of adoption status. Sometimes the most useful information comes from those that do not choose to adopt. Extent of adoption can be assessed through direct observation, interviews, or surveys.

Implementation

The *implementation* factor is essential in understanding the extent to which the program adhered to the specified protocol. Was the program delivered as intended? If not, how did it deviate? Deviations can occur at the individual and the setting level. At the individual level, some patients might not have participated fully in the program—for example, some might have attended only three of five scheduled group sessions, or some might not have taken their medication as prescribed. At the setting level, some staff might have implemented the intervention with 100% of patients who met the inclusion criteria, whereas other staff members might have applied the intervention intermittently when time was limited. Implementation is assessed by computing the percentage of process objectives that were achieved—for example, the proportion of brochures that were distributed, how many of the planned training sessions were taught, or what proportion of the prescribed medication was consumed. Other process measures that are important and can inform future work includes costs of staff time and other resources expended during implementation.

Maintenance

Many program evaluations examine adoption but fail to examine ongoing maintenance of the program. At the individual level, program evaluators might want to assess relapse (e.g., recidivism to smoking, for a cessation program). At the setting level, once a program has been disseminated, one might assess the predictors of ongoing institutionalization.

In summary, the RE-AIM model provides a structure for conducting program evaluation. It also has been used in designing interventions.[27] Each of the five elements is critical for evaluations of programs that are designed for broadscale dissemination. RE-AIM draws on previous work in several areas, including Rogers's diffusion of innovations theory[28] and the PRECEDE-PROCEED approach.[2] RE-AIM differs from existing models in that it was designed to facilitate translation of research into practice, places equal emphasis on internal and external validity and emphasizes the representativeness of individuals as well as settings, and outlines standard methods to guide assessment of key factors involved in evaluating potential for public health impact and dissemination.

SUMMARY

Healthcare resources are limited, and therefore one cannot overstate the need for effective program planning and evaluation in our public health efforts. Although behavioral theories such as those presented in Chapter 3 offer guidance, theory contributes to but is not an effective substitute for program planning or evaluation. The three frameworks presented here each offer a systematic approach for the successful development, implementation, and evaluation of health programs. PRECEDE-PROCEED has been in existence the longest, and intervention mapping and RE-AIM both build from its strong foundation for conducting baseline needs assessments. PRECEDE-PROCEED and intervention mapping tend to be used for both planning and evaluation; RE-AIM, which also is applicable to planning, has mostly been applied for program evaluation efforts. One of RE-AIM's strengths is that it is particularly relevant to programs that are intended for broadscale dissemination.

As stated at the beginning of this chapter, evaluation is both an art and a science. The frameworks presented here should be used in tandem with sound research designs, psychometrically solid study measures, and carefully operationalized protocols for program implementation, data collection, data management, and data analysis. Book chapters and class lectures can present methodologies; however, there is no substitute for practical experience. The real world of program planning and evaluation is challenging, but also rewarding. There is no doubt that successful programs have the potential to substantially alter the landscape of public health.

REFERENCES

1. Trochim WMK. The research methods knowledge base. 2nd ed. Cincinnati, OH: Atomic Dog Publishing, 2001.
2. Green LW, Kreuter MW. Health program planning: an educational and ecological approach. New York: McGraw-Hill, 2005.
3. Bartholomew LK, Parcel GS, Kok G, Gottlieb NH. Intervention mapping: designing theory- and evidence-based health promotion programs. New York: McGraw-Hill, 2001.
4. Glasgow RE, Vogt TM, Boles SM. Evaluating the public health impact of health promotion interventions: the RE-AIM framework. Am J Public Health 1999;89(9):1322-7.
5. Kaiser Permanente. Re-AIM. 2006. (Accessed October 15, 2007, at http://www.re-aim.org/.)

6. Agency for Healthcare Research and Quality. Community-based participatory research. (Accessed at http://www.ahrq.gov/about/cpcr/cbpr/cbpr1.htm.)

7. Green LW, Kreuter MW. Health promotion planning: an educational and ecological approach. 3rd ed. Mountain View, CA: Mayfield Publishing, 1999.

8. Becker MH, Maiman LA. Sociobehavioral determinants of compliance with health and medical care recommendations. Med Care 1975;13:10-24.

9. Becker MH, Maiman LA, Kirscht JP, Haefner DP, Drachman RH, Taylor DW. Patient perceptions and compliance: recent studies of the health belief model. In: Haynes RB, Taylor DW, Sackett DL, eds. Compliance in health care. Baltimore: Johns Hopkins University Press, 1979:78-109.

10. Janz NK, Becker MH. The health belief model: a decade later. Health Educ Q 1984;11:1-47.

11. Rosenstock IM. The health belief model and preventive health behavior. Health Educ Monogr 1974;2:354-86.

12. Prochaska JO. Systems of psychotherapy: a transtheoretical approach. Homewood, IL: Dorsey Press, 1979.

13. Prochaska JO, DiClemente CC. The transtheoretical approach: crossing traditional boundaries of therapy. Homewood, IL: Dow Jones-Irwin, 1984.

14. Ajzen I, Fishbein M. Understanding attitudes and predicting social behavior. Englewood Cliffs, NJ: Prentice-Hall, 1980.

15. Ajzen I. The theory of planned behavior. Organizational Behav Human Decision Processes 1991;50:179-211.

16. Bandura A. Social foundations of thought and action. Englewood Cliffs, NJ: Prentice Hall, 1986.

17. Precede-Proceed. (Accessed at http://www.lgreen.net/precede.htm.)

18. Abbema EA, Van Assema P, Kok GJ, De Leeuw E, De Vries NK. Effect of evaluation of a comprehensive community intervention aimed at reducing socioeconomic health inequalities in the Netherlands. Health Promot Int 2004;19(2):141-56.

19. Bartholomew LK, Parcel GS, Kok G. Intervention mapping: a process for developing theory- and evidence-based health education programs. Health Educ Behav 1998;25(5):545-63.

20. Fernandez ME, Gonzales A, Tortolero-Luna G, Partida S, Bartholomew LK. Using intervention mapping to develop a breast and cervical cancer screening program for Hispanic farmworkers: Cultivando La Salud. Health Promot Pract 2005;6(4):394-404.

21. Heinen MM, Bartholomew LK, Wensing M, van de Kerkhof P, van Achterberg T. Supporting adherence and healthy lifestyles in leg ulcer patients: systematic development of the Lively Legs program for dermatology outpatient clinics. Patient Educ Couns 2006;61(2):279-91.

22. Kok G, Schaalma H, Ruiter RA, van Empelen P, Brug J. Intervention mapping: protocol for applying health psychology theory to prevention programmes. J Health Psychol 2004;9(1):85-98.

23. Kwak L, Kremers SP, Werkman A, Visscher TL, van Baak MA, Brug J. The NHF-NRG In Balance-project: the application of intervention mapping in the development, implementation and evaluation of weight gain prevention at the worksite. Obes Rev 2007;8(4):347-61.

24. van Empelen P, Kok G, Schaalma HP, Bartholomew LK. An AIDS risk reduction program for Dutch drug users: an intervention mapping approach to planning. Health Promot Pract 2003;4(4):402-12.

25. Van Kesteren NM, Kok G, Hospers HJ, Schippers J, De Wildt W. Systematic development of a self-help and motivational enhancement intervention to promote sexual health in HIV-positive men who have sex with men. AIDS Patient Care STDS 2006;20(12):858-75.

26. van Oostrom SH, Anema JR, Terluin B, Venema A, de Vet HC, van Mechelen W. Development of a workplace intervention for sick-listed employees with stress-related mental disorders: intervention mapping as a useful tool. BMC Health Serv Res 2007;7:127.

27. Glasgow RE, Toobert DJ, Hampson SE, Strycker LA. Implementation, generalization and long-term results of the "choosing well" diabetes self-management intervention. Patient Educ Couns 2002;48(2):115-22.

28. Rogers EM. Diffusion of innovations. 5th ed. New York: Free Press, 2003.

PART II

Approaches to Resolve Health Problems

The first part of this textbook discussed the overall context of health and illness and how individuals and social systems respond to change. The second part of the book explores more specifically the different alternatives and experiences that individuals and social systems use when engaging in treatment options. This set of seven chapters begins with a description and history of the evolution of behavioral medicine (Chapter 6) and pharmacy practice (Chapter 7) as two distinct approaches to treatment. Given the understanding of the historical aspects of how pharmacists have become socialized to engage in greater clinical services in Chapter 7, the book delves deeper in Chapter 8 to identify how these changes in the professional socialization of pharmacists stimulate pharmacies and pharmacy organizations toward change in providing even greater services to patients receiving drug therapy. It is also important to know what factors affect the type of drug therapy provided to patients (Chapter 9), patient receptivity to and participation in that treatment process (Chapter 10), how pharmacist–patient communication influences patient participation in treatment (Chapter 11), and how the integration of the roles of caregivers can modify the pharmaceutical care received by patients (Chapter 12).

Chapters 13 to 15 focus on the processes that affect patient use of drug therapies. Chapter 13 explores the psychosocial aspects of patient adherence to drug therapies. Chapter 14 examines approaches that can be used by pharmacists to help patients engage in more consistent adherence to treatment. Although improving medication use can be an end in itself, clinicians and researchers often desire to know how medication use leads to improved patient outcomes. For this reason, this second part of the textbook ends with Chapter 15, which presents a discussion of different ways in which to measure patient-reported outcomes of their treatment.

In the spirit of Donabedian's framework for understanding how systems behave, Part I of the book presented the structure of health and illness behaviors related to medication use, and Part II focuses both on the processes that affect those behaviors and the outcomes of those processes.

SECTION A

Behavioral Medicine

CHAPTER 6
Behavioral Medicine

Behavioral Medicine

John M. Lonie, EdD, and John Pappan, MA, MS

Over the past three decades, the behavioral sciences have become a well-recognized resource for healthcare professionals. Today, few healthcare professionals can argue against the role that the mind (and its impact on behavior) plays in health and illness. Dolinsky,[1] using Shunichi's[2] definition of behavioral medicine, noted that "behavioral medicine is an interdisciplinary applied science concerned with the development and integration of behavioral and biomedical science, knowledge and techniques related to health and illness, and the application of this knowledge and these techniques to prevention, diagnosis, treatment and rehabilitation."

This chapter focuses on the primary areas in which contributions from the behavioral sciences have affected the health professions, based on empirical evidence. The chapter is organized by four major topic areas: an overview of the theoretical basis of behavioral medicine, the mind–body connection to behavioral medicine, the human stress response, and the placebo response.

As mentioned, behavioral medicine is an adaptation and application of many concepts, principles, and theories from a number of scientific disciplines. These include psychology, sociology, and anthropology as well as medicine, nursing, and pharmacy. Research shows that social psychology, health psychology, and cognitive psychology have greatly contributed to the development of behavioral medicine treatments. This chapter begins with a focus on the theories within each of these disciplines that were used to advance the understanding of how behavioral medicine has affected patient care.

THE THEORETICAL BASIS OF BEHAVIORAL MEDICINE

The theoretical basis of behavioral medicine spans a number of disciplines; however, a question that often arises in pharmacy practice and education is whether students (and pharmacists) are able and motivated to apply theories from other disciplines (e.g., psychology, sociology) to real-life professional practice problems. In seeking an answer to this problem, Sleath sought to determine whether pharmacy students would be able to apply social psychological theories to the solution of real-life pharmacy practice situations.[3] She found that students were able to make connections and apply these theories in order to solve patient care problems. However, just what are these theories, and which may be used with the greatest practicality by pharmacists?

The discipline of health psychology is an area that traditionally has guided theory in behavioral medicine. Health psychology is primarily concerned with the understanding, prevention, and treatment of illnesses using a psychosocial framework. This understanding, prevention, and treatment occur from within the biopsychosocial model of health and illness.[1] That is, health psychologists operate from the framework that physical illness can best be explained and treated if the illness is viewed from its biological, psychological, and sociological components.[1]

Health Belief Model

Within the field of health psychology, the health belief model (HBM) is one of the most widely used theories in behavioral medicine. As noted in Chapter 3, the purpose of the HBM is to explain and predict why people make specific health-related decisions.[3] The HBM is predicated on several key assumptions: individuals will take or not take action based upon (1) their perceived susceptibility to a particular illness, (2) the perceived severity of the illness, (3) the perceived costs (barriers) of taking action, and (4) the perceived benefits of taking action. The HBM has been successfully used in a number of areas, including predicting and explaining adherence to medical regimens.[4] For example, a patient visits his physician, and it is determined that the patient has elevated cholesterol levels. The physician prescribes a modification in the patient's diet as well as an exercise program for the patient to follow. According to the HBM, the patient will or will not follow the advice of his physician based on the assumptions of the HBM. The patient may ask himself, "How susceptible am I to the medical effects of having high cholesterol? How severe are these effects? What are the costs versus the benefits of me adhering to my physician's advice? Will I have to substantially change my lifestyle? How important is it for me to change my lifestyle?" How the patient decides to answer these questions (i.e., cognition) will determine adherence or nonadherence to his physician's advice (i.e., behavior).

Recent research using the HBM on issues related to the profession of pharmacy include defining the cognitive predictors of adherence to malaria prophylaxis regimens,[5] studying the impact of attitudes and beliefs on the length of benzodiazepine use,[6] and predicting noncompliance among warfarin therapy outpatients.[7]

Learning Theories and Health Behavior

Learning theorists believe that behavior change is not only based on the decisions an individual makes, but also on the external environment in which the decision is made. In addition, learning theorists place a great deal of importance on the consequences that decisions have on the individual (i.e., rewards, punishments, etc.).[8] This section examines the following learning theories as they relate to health behavior change: operant conditioning, observational learning, and self-efficacy.

Operant Conditioning

Operant conditioning is based on the premise that positive behavioral responses will occur if the person is rewarded for his or her behavior.[9] Essentially, the reward feels good to the individual, and people tend to repeat behaviors that make them feel good. An aspect of the principle of operant conditioning that has important implications for health behaviors is the gradient of reinforcement, which implies that immediate rewards are more effective than delayed rewards.[10] For example, if a patient smokes cigarettes and attempts to begin an exercise program, she may become discouraged if she is short of breath after a small amount of exercise. If that same patient stops smoking and sees an immediate increase in her exercise tolerance, she might decide to continue not to smoke. An example of recent research utilizing operant conditioning as a theoretical approach was conducted by Heapy, who studied diabetic patients' adherence to treatment regimens using the inherent consequences model (ICM).[11] This model is based on operant conditioning principles. Heapy found that the ICM has significant predictive power and may be useful in determining adherence issues.

Observational Learning

As defined by Bandura, observational learning is any learning that occurs through observing the behavior of others.[12] The learning can manifest in a number of ways, including the imitation of the learned behaviors. Research also supports the notion that individuals who operate at various cognitive developmental levels respond differently to observed events than they would respond to verbal or written instructions.[12] For example, a graphic television commercial highlighting the negative health effects of smoking may be a more powerful stimulus to stop smoking for some individuals than would verbal advice from a physician. It appears that for some individuals, the act of observing is a powerful cognitive influence. This has important implications for individuals practicing any form of behavioral modification. If cognitive developmental levels are assessed appropriately, the desired behavioral modification can be delivered more efficiently.

Self-Efficacy

Perhaps more influential than his theory of observational learning was Bandura's theory of self-efficacy.[12] Bandura noted that people regularly monitor (self-regulate) their actions in line with predetermined goals. Central to the self-efficacy theory is the idea that people's beliefs about the successful attainment of those goals will influence their ability to attain those goals. For example, if an individual wants to lose 20 pounds, his level of self-efficacy (the belief that he can lose 20 pounds) will be affected by the magnitude of the goal itself as well as his ability to self-regulate his behavior (i.e., exercise) in order to meet that goal.[12,13]

Self-efficacy theory has been used in a myriad of health-related research projects, including the development of an intervention to improve nurses' knowledge, self-efficacy, and ability to perform a specific nursing ability,[13] applying social learning theory to alleviate children's dental anxiety,[14] and using social learning theory to help achieve behavior modification in a nonliterate patient population.[15] As noted, various aspects of behavioral medicine have contributed greatly to the improvement of health outcomes. The next section describes the mind–body relationship from a behavioral medicine perspective.

THE MIND–BODY CONNECTION

The belief that the mind and body are connected goes back to ancient times. Although different cultures have had various understandings of the mind–body connection, most considered the mind and body as one element.[16] The ancient Greek and Chinese societies first conceptualized health and disease as being due to natural (as opposed to supernatural) causes. Although both of these cultures developed a more sophisticated understanding of illness, the idea that the mind and body were intimately connected was still viable. During this time it was understood that physical illness might be caused by a malady within the blood or nervous system, but it was also understood and accepted that the person's mental state played a key role in the outcome of the illness.[16] However, throughout the Middle Ages there was an emphasis on the view that health and illness were solely spiritually mediated. This was due more to the influence and control of the Catholic Church than to a widespread change in core belief systems.

It was not until the Renaissance and the Scientific Revolution that a systematic theory of health and illness took hold. The biomedical model became the commonly used theory that guided thinking regarding the determinants of health and illness. As useful as this concept has been, it has also received some criticism. For example, the biomedical model breaks all physical illness down into its component parts. By doing so it does not take into account the myriad of psychological and social factors that contribute to health and illness. Therefore, a biopsychosocial approach to health and illness emerged. As the name suggests, the biopsychosocial approach takes into account the biomedical, psychological, and social factors that contribute to health and illness.

Research has shown that the mind can influence the perception of many different physical and psychological illnesses. A large percentage of patient visits to primary healthcare providers are the result of psychological issues.[17] Researchers have examined the role that family practitioners and primary care physicians have in treating patients with psychosomatic complaints. They determined that over half of all patient visits to these healthcare practitioners were the result of psychosocial problems that presented as somatic complaints.[17] Psychological stress may be the most common inducer of psychosomatic complaints.[18]

Mind–body treatments have been used with varying success in many physical and psychological disorders. The most well known mind–body treatments used in behavioral medicine have been meditation, relaxation, mindful breathing techniques, massage, biofeedback, hypnosis, prayer, and yoga. Some of these mind–body approaches to health have been used in the treatment of respiratory disorders,[18] as an adjunct to help dieters lose weight,[19] and in the management of diabetes mellitus.[20]

THE HUMAN STRESS RESPONSE

Stress results when an organism is required to change or adapt to its environment.[21] According to this definition, stress can result from anything. For example, just getting up from a seated position can be stressful because of the physical demand that gravity exerts on the body. Stress can be either useful or damaging to both the physical body and an individual's psychological state. Stress that is helpful to individuals is known as *eustress*.[22] Examples of eustress can be seen when an individual has a small amount of anxiety before speaking in public, or when an athlete is about to take the field in a big game. In both of these instances, the stress experienced is not debilitating and can actually lead to better performances by the speaker and the athlete. Stress becomes a problem when it leads to some form of debilitation or alteration of normal activities in an individual.

Stress can be acute (short term) or chronic (long term). Acute stress is the response to an abrupt threat and often manifests physiologically as the fight-or-flight response. The threat can be any situation that is interpreted consciously or unconsciously as possibly causing harm to the individual. Common acute stressors include noise, pollution, crowded settings, sudden danger, and certain illnesses.[21] Common forms of chronic stressors are prolonged tensions in work environments, problems in interpersonal relationships, and various social, economic, and cultural adaptations.[21]

Stress and Human Physiology

A number of biochemical and neurochemical changes occur in response to stress. The hypothalamic-pituitary-adrenal (HPA) system becomes activated in the brain. The HPA system activates the production and release of the steroid hormones and neurotransmitters.[23] A wide range of biological functions within the human body, including the immune system, integumentary system, and metabolic system, are affected. Both the cardiovascular and respiratory systems respond to stress by means of adaptation. For example, the heart rate and blood pressure increase in response to perceived threats. Prolonged elevation of heart rate and blood pressure has detrimental effects on the body.[22,23] Prolonged and severe stress can alter the individual's neurophysiology, causing depression and anxiety.[22,23] Research has shown that two thirds of participants who experienced a stressful situation had nearly six times the risk of developing depression within the same month.[23(p2)] Additional findings suggest that the repeated release of cortisol produces hyperactivity in the HPA axis, which disrupts the normal levels of serotonin, a neurotransmitter that is responsible for feelings of well-being.[23(pp1-2)] Prolonged psychological stress has been shown to cause injury to the inner lining of blood vessels, leading to hypertension.[23(pp2-3)] There is also evidence that stress contributes to changes in the immune system. Chronic stress hinders the immune response and poses a greater risk for infections.[24] Patients with chronic stress often present with below-normal levels of white blood cells, making these patients more susceptible to cold and flu viruses.[23(pp2-3)] Research has shown that HIV-positive men who experience prolonged high levels of stress have a greater incidence of developing AIDS.[23(pp2-3)]

Evidence exists for relationships between various types of headaches, muscular and joint pain, and stress.[23(pp2-3)] Other studies relate stress to a vast number of other conditions, including insomnia, external pollutants that cause allergies, skin disorders, hair loss, premature teeth loss, gum disease, sexual and reproductive dysfunction, premenstrual syndrome, fertility, and pregnancy conditions leading to miscarriages and premature births.[23,24]

Stress also impairs memory, concentration, and learning. Research focusing on the effects of acute stress on short-term memory found that increased cortisol levels impaired the ability of participants to memorize. Enduring chronic stress, such as post-traumatic stress, has been shown to shrink the hippocampus region of the brain.[23(pp2-3)] Although more research is being conducted to confirm the negative effects of stress on psychological and biological systems, one is able to draw preliminary relationships between the negative effects of stress and the imbalance of biochemical responses of the human anatomy and physiology.[14,23(pp2-3)]

Impact of Stress on Pharmacists

Stress is a common phenomenon among pharmacists and other healthcare professionals. A study examining community pharmacists' job satisfaction found that, among other factors, the routine stressors of pharmacy practice led in some cases to negative evaluations of their job satisfaction.[25]

A study showed that prolonged stress can be a causative factor in many medication errors.[26] Recently, investigators have begun incorporating theory from the cognitive sciences to better understand the effect of stress on behavior. For example, research using the cognitive system model examined how stress contributes to medication errors among pharmacists.[27]

Gaither conducted a cross-sectional mail survey of 1,088 licensed pharmacists in the United States practicing in chain, independent, or hospital pharmacies to determine whether career commitment mediates the effects of job stress on pharmacists.[28] The research examined the effects of job stress, career commitment, met expectations, job satisfaction, and organizational commitment on job turnover intention. The results indicated that more than 65% of the respondents were satisfied with their present job, and 50% indicated that they would choose pharmacy again as a career. Seventy percent of pharmacists indicated that their work was creative and important. The results suggested that career commitment and other factors can mediate the effects of job stress. The author suggested that strategies should be developed to increase the career commitment of pharmacists through career planning and the use of mentors.

In another study, researchers investigated the levels of job satisfaction and job stress among consulting and community pharmacists. The results of this study showed that the majority of pharmacists surveyed would choose to be pharmacists again despite the stressors that they experienced.[29] Among the pharmacists in this study, the most common stressors included personal obligations that were difficult to carry out because of long hours at work, overload of work as a result of short staffing, and the lack of opportunities for job advancement. The most common stressor, experienced by one third of respondents, was the fear of making a mistake when filling a prescription.[29]

Stress is a natural phenomenon that in moderate levels can be motivating. However, in high levels and under prolonged conditions, stress can be debilitating and lead to physical and psychological damage. The practice of pharmacy is stressful; this stress can be mediated through the various factors discussed in this section.

THE PLACEBO EFFECT

A *placebo* is a substance with no medicinal properties used to treat a physical or psychological condition.[30] A placebo used in research is an inactive substance or procedure used as a control in an experiment.[30] The clinical use of the placebo effect began among physicians who intended to please their patients with medicines that instilled the hope of a speedy recovery when in reality the medicinal substance had no therapeutic significance to the medical condition. Placebos that are administered through ingestion, injection, or incision often are considered more powerful than noninvasive placebos.[31]

When administered by healthcare providers, placebos can have beneficial effects on various physical and psychological disease processes. These beneficial effects are a result of the beliefs and expectations of the person receiving the placebo treatment. Whether or not a placebo will work depends a great deal on the amount of faith the patient has in the treatment itself and in the practitioner administering the placebo. It is understood that the more a patient believes in the benefits of treatment, the more likely it is that the patient will experience a positive medical benefit from the placebo treatment.[32] Research has shown that as many as one third of patients feel better in response to treatments with placebos.[32]

As noted previously, there is a powerful connection between the mind and the body. *Suggestion* is the term used to describe the process by which a physical or mental state is created by a thought or idea.[33] Placebo effects frequently demonstrate an influence of suggestion, or how the body is influenced by the mind. A person's psychological state when influenced by suggestion can trigger neurochemical releases that then can affect that person's physiology.[34] Research conducted on patients with illnesses ranging from arthritis to depression showed a 30% to 60% substantial improvement in their symptoms after receiving placebo treatments.[35]

Other examples of the effects of placebo treatment include a study conducted by the Coronary Drug Project in which researchers set out to find the safety and effectiveness of drugs used for long-term treatment of men with coronary heart disease. The results showed that those who were adherent to the placebo treatment demonstrated nearly half the mortality rate of those who were not.[36] Placebo treatments have been used to alter immune responses in cancer patients and in patients suffering from rheumatoid arthritis.[35] Placebos have also been used with success in treating patients with depression.[37]

BEHAVIORAL MEDICINE INTERVENTIONS

There are many different forms of behavioral medicine interventions. This chapter briefly discusses two common behavioral medicine interventions: relaxation and meditation.

Relaxation

Relaxation techniques have been used with great success in combating various physical and psychological disorders. Relaxation techniques have been used to treat hypertension, migraine headaches, and stress disorders.[38] In traditional medical practices, relaxation techniques have been used to combat stress and anxiety. Various forms of relaxation can be used for this purpose. Examples include the tense-release method and deep breathing.[39]

The tense-release relaxation method involves tensing different muscle groups in the body and then releasing them completely and relaxing. This technique usually requires individuals to begin at the feet and then systematically move through the body. This method can be performed several times per day and is popular because it can be done in 2 to 3 minutes.

The deep breathing technique is also a popular relaxation technique because it can be done in a relatively short time in almost any space. Deep breathing is thought to reduce stress through both physiological and psychological mechanisms. The act of taking in oxygen at a slow rate, gently holding the breath, and then slowly releasing the breath has positive effects on the central nervous system, cardiovascular system, and gastrointestinal system.[38]

Meditation

Meditation has been used for centuries by many different cultures and religions as a means of centering the mind and body. It is difficult to precisely define what meditation is because there are many different forms. It is perhaps better to discuss the benefits of meditation as described by its practitioners. One of the most popular forms of meditation is called *mindfulness meditation*, which involves focusing the consciousness on what one is doing in the present moment. This involves gently pushing aside random thoughts and ideas that may creep into one's consciousness while meditating. For many people, this is a difficult process to learn. However, proponents of various meditative practices claim that a steady practice of meditation can increase self-awareness, self-trust, and self-acceptance. Many claim that meditation enhances appreciation of life and provides serenity. There is also evidence that meditation provides long-term decreases in stress-related physical and psychological health problems.[40]

SUMMARY

Behavioral medicine became widely recognized as a discipline in the 1970s. Since then, the field of behavioral medicine has gained a number of proponents as well as skeptics. The two areas where behavioral medicine has experienced its greatest successes are cardiovascular disease and cancer. Research in these areas now focuses on modifiable risk factors associated with these diseases. However, despite some advances in behavioral medicine, there are still challenges that exist in the field that hinder its full integration into mainstream medical practice. Such hindrances include concerns about the validity and reliability of behavioral medicine research. Some scientists dispute the quality of the data that support the efficacy of various interventions. Healthcare decision makers also question how best to integrate theory and concepts of behavioral medicine into the healthcare system as it exists today. Despite these limitations, research in behavioral medicine will continue to grow well into the twenty-first century.

REFERENCES

1. Dolinsky D. Recent developments in behavioral medicine. In: Smith MC, Wertheimer AI, eds. Social and behavioral aspects of pharmaceutical care. Binghamton, NY: Haworth Press, 1996.
2. Shunichi A, ed. An integrated behavioral approach to health and illness. Amsterdam: Elsevier, 1992.
3. Sleath B. Teaching pharmacy students how to use social psychological theories when monitoring chronic disease patients. J Soc Adm Pharmacy 1997;14(1):16-25.
4. Wallston BS, Wallston KA. Social psychological models of health behavior: an examination and integration. In: Baum A, Taylor SE, Singer JE, eds. Handbook of psychology and health. Hillsdale, NJ: Erlbaum, 1984.
5. Abraham C, Clift S, Grabowski P. Cognitive predictors of adherence to malaria prophylaxis regimens on return from a malarias region: protective study. Soc Sci Med 1999;48(11):1641-54.
6. Van Hulten R, Bakker AB, Lodder AC, et al. The impact of attitudes and beliefs on length of benzodiazepine use: a study among inexperienced and experienced benzodiazepine users. Soc Sci Med 2003;56(6):1345-54.
7. Orensky IA, Holdford DA. Predictors of noncompliance with warfarin therapy in an outpatient anticoagulation clinic. Pharmacotherapy 2005;25(12):1801-8.
8. Lonie JM. From counting and pouring to caring: the empathic developmental process of community pharmacists. Res Soc Adm Pharm 2006;2(4):439-57.
9. Chesney MA. Behavior modification and health enhancement. In: Matarazzo JD, Weiss SM, Herd JA, Miller NE, eds. Behavioral health: a handbook of health enhancement and disease prevention. New York: Wiley, 1984.
10. Miller NE. Behavioral medicine: symbiosis between laboratory and clinic. Ann Rev Psychology 1984;34:1-31.
11. Heapy AA. The inherent consequences and prediction of diabetic regimen adherence [Dissertation]. Purdue University, 2004.
12. Bandura A. Self efficacy: toward a unifying theory of behavioral change. Psychol Rev 1977;84: 191-215.
13. Ngo A, Murphy S. A theory based intervention to improve nurses' knowledge, self-efficacy, and skills to reduce PICC occlusion. J Infusion Nurs 2005;28(3):173-81.
14. Do C. Applying social learning theory to children with dental anxiety. J Contemp Dental Practice 2004;5(1):126-35.
15. Ngoh L, Shepherd M. Design, development and evaluation of visual aids for communicating prescription drug instructions to nonliterate patients in rural Cameroon. Patient Educ Couns 1997;30(3):257-70.
16. Kaplan HI. Current psychodynamic concepts in psychosomatic medicine. In: Pasnau RO, ed. Consultation-liaison psychiatry. New York: Grune & Stratton, 1975.
17. Wickramasekera I, Davies TE, Davies SM. Applied psychophysiology: a bridge between the biomedical model and the biopsychosocial model in family medicine. Professional Psychology Res Pract 1996;27:221-33.

18. Braun L. The use of complementary and alternative medicine in respiratory diseases. Austr J Pharmacy 2002;83:682-6.

19. Eaton J. Safe dieting. Part 3. Natural Pharmacy 1999;3:18-20.

20. Kligler B, Lynch D. An integrative approach to type 2 diabetes mellitus. Altern Ther Health Med 2003:9(6):24-32.

21. American Heritage Dictionary of the English Language, 4th ed. Stressor. (Accessed November 6, 2006, at http://www.answers.com/topic/stressor.)

22. LeFevre M, Kolt GS, Matheny J. Eustress, distress and their interpretation in primary and secondary occupational stress management interventions: which way first? J Managerial Psychology 2006;21(6):547.

23. Simon H. Stress. October 10, 2005. (Well-Connected Report no. 31.) (Accessed November 20, 2006, at http://www.wellconnected.com/report.cgi/pdf/000031.pdf.)

24. Padgett DA, Glaser R. How stress influences the immune response. Trends Immunol 2003; 24(8):444-8.

25. Longshaw RN, Asghar MN. Where the grass is not greener. Pharmacy Practice (England) 1999;9:276.

26. Wick JY, Zanni GR. Stress in the pharmacy: changing the experience. J Am Pharm Assoc 2002; 42(1):16-20.

27. Buckley J. Daily life stresses of pharmacists can contribute to medication errors. Pharmacy Practice News 2002;29(7):21-2.

28. Gaither CA. Career commitment: a mediator of the effects of job stress on pharmacists' work-related attitudes. J Am Pharm Assoc 1999;39(3):353-61.

29. Lapane KL, Hughes CM. Baseline job satisfaction and stress among pharmacists and pharmacy technicians participating in the Fleetwood phase III study. Consulting Pharmacist 2004;19(11):1029-37.

30. Wolman B, ed. Placebo. Dictionary of Behavioral Science. New York: Van Nostrand Reinhold, 1973.

31. Leslie A. Ethics and practice of placebo therapy. Am J Med 1956;16(6):854-62.

32. Nordenberg T. The healing power of placebos. FDA Consumer 2000;34(1). (Accessed at http://www.fda.gov/fdac/features/2000/100_heal.html.)

33. Henderson CE. Hypnosis suggestion formulation and application part 1. Hypnotica December 8, 2003. (Accessed at http://www.bcx.net/hypnosis/suggest.htm.)

34. Hyland ME. Using the placebo response in clinical practice. Clin Med 2003;3(4):349.

35. University of California Neuropsychiatric Institute. Placebo research at the UCLA Neuropsychiatric Institute. (Accessed at http://www.placebo.ucla.edu/.)

36. Influence of adherence to treatment and response of cholesterol on mortality in the Coronary Drug Project. New Engl J Med 1980;303(18):1038-41.

37. Dworkin RH, Katz J, Gitlin MJ. Placebo response in clinical trials of depression and its implications for research on chronic neuropathic pain. Neurology 2005;65:S7-S19.

38. Hart JA, 2007 was reviewed on: 4/17/2007 by Patrika Tsai, M.D., M.P.H., Assistant Clinical Professor, Pediatric Gastroenterology, Hepatology and Nutrition, University of California, San Francisco, San Francisco, CA. Review provided by VeriMed Healthcare Network. (Accessed at http://adam.about.com/care/weightloss/weight_drhart.htmls.)

39. Benson H, Dusek JA, et al. Study of the Therapeutic Effects of Intercessory Prayer (STEP) in cardiac bypass patients: a multicenter randomized trial of uncertainty and certainty of receiving intercessory prayer. Am Heart J 2006;151(4):762-4.

40. WholeHealthMD.com. Meditation. 2006. (Accessed at http://wholehealthmd.com/ME2/dirmod.asp?sid=17E09E7CFFF640448FFB0B4FC1B7FEF0&nm=Reference+Library&type=AWHN_Therapies&mod=Therapies&mid=&id=7936709D16B94C8F9960E53BCF52C6E7&tier=2.)

CHAPTER 7

Professional Socialization of Pharmacists

Gregory J. Higby, PhD

How does one become a pharmacist? At first glance, the answer to this question appears simple and straightforward: a person attends pharmacy school, gains the requisite amount of education and training, passes a qualifying examination, obtains a license, and finds a job. Actually, that is how someone attains the qualifications to practice as a licensed pharmacist. To *become* a pharmacist, a man or woman also must be socialized.[1] Robert Merton defined socialization as "the process by which people selectively acquire the values and attitudes, the interests, skills and knowledge—in short, the culture—current in the groups of which they are, or seek to become, a member. It refers to the learning of social roles."[2] All functioning members of a society undergo a process of primary socialization whereby individuals learn their major identifying roles within a culture, such as gender, ethnicity, and religious beliefs. These identities are inculcated primarily within the family. Secondary socialization occurs when people join a group after their identities have been formed through earlier primary socialization. When someone takes a new job, he or she quickly learns the mores of the new work culture and how to function in this adult role.

In the case of most pharmacists today who practice in the community setting, their role is one that mixes two distinct identities, professional and commercial.[3] One hundred years ago, these two identities were compatible, but during the last 40 years they have diverged as pharmacy practice and the healthcare marketplace have evolved.[4] New pharmacists entering the workforce, especially in community settings, often discover an environment that contradicts the ideals of professional practice taught in pharmacy school, leading to disillusionment or "realistic disenchantment."[3,5] Moreover, the hopes of educators and leaders that lengthened education (PharmD degree) and innovative practice models (pharmaceutical care) would expand the societal role of pharmacists and elevate their stature have failed to be realized fully. As a result, the subject of professional socialization (professionalization) in pharmacy has attracted increased attention in recent years. This chapter explores this topic with a focus on the historical roots of its development.

PHARMACY AS A PROFESSION

Merton's definition of socialization is generally accepted, but the same cannot be said about the meanings of the word *profession*. The *Oxford English Dictionary* retains a traditional view of the term: "The occupation which one professes to be skilled in and to follow a vocation in which a professed knowledge of some department of learning or science is used in its application to the affairs of others or in the practice of an art founded upon it. This applies specifically to the three learned professions of divinity, law, and medicine; also to the military profession."[6] Historically, an individual made a claim or "profession" to have the requisite abilities to fulfill a socially accepted and understood role such as *pharmacist*. Fully established in American society by the middle of the 1800s, pharmacists were retailers of medicines, spices, oils, flavorings, sponges, cosmetics, and sundry other "drugstore items." Their professional claim rested on their specialized skill in preparing drugs and compounding medicines upon a physician's prescription order. In the late 1800s the American public began to value paper credentials (school diplomas and governmental licenses) as indicators of professional competency as much as personal reputation. Pharmacy, with its dual cultures, however, has clung to both individualistic (drugstore proprietor) and collective (licensed graduate) approaches to pursuing societal recognition.[7]

Definitions of *profession* and *professionalism* abound, and scholars have struggled to find ones that fit pharmacy well.[8] Throughout the 20th century, authors did not include pharmacists as full professionals, classifying them as semiprofessionals or "incomplete professionals."[9-12] They observed that most pharmacists spent their days selling packaged goods in a commercialized retail setting. Moreover, even in their "professional" practice—filling prescriptions—pharmacists lacked autonomy; they were just following the orders of physicians.[9-12] For this reason, Supreme Court Justice Warren Burger deemed pharmacists no more professional than store clerks selling law books.[13]

Pharmacy historian Glenn Sonnedecker, building on Carr-Saunders and Thorner, put forward a useful set of "essentials" or traits that result in an occupation attaining professional status:

A relatively specific, socially necessary function upon the regular performance of which the practitioner depends for his livelihood and social status; a special technique, competence in which is demanded, resting upon a body of knowledge embracing generalized principles, the mastery of which requires theoretic study; a traditional and generally accepted ethic subordinating its adherents' immediate private interests to the most effective performance of the function; and a formal association fostering the ethic and improvement of performance.[14]

For pharmacy in the count-and-pour era of the 1950s, Sonnedecker's traits were an ambitious target. The "socially necessary function" of the pharmacist in 1960 was to dispense medicines according to a physician's order. Compounding, the crux of community pharmacy's professional claim from the 1870s through the 1940s, had all but disappeared. Mass manufacturers made almost all end dosage forms. Laws prohibited generic substitution and limited refills. Pharmacists were not allowed to discuss the content or actions of drugs with their patients. In fact, to protect patients, pharmacists did not put the name of the medicine on the prescription container. Pharmacists were often called "the most over-educated professionals" because they possessed a large "body of knowledge" in the chemical sciences but their "special technique" was little demanded.[15]

The pharmacy profession, represented by the American Pharmaceutical Association (APhA), did possess a "generally accepted ethic," put forward in the APhA Code of Ethics. This code, like those of other occupations, was "a detailed, explicit, operational blue-print of norms of professional conduct, a public recital of desirable and undesirable actions having an impact upon the character of a professional and its functional reliability."[16(pp39-40)] The APhA had revised its code periodically since the founding of the organization in 1852. A few excerpts from the 1952 version illustrate the restricted role of the pharmacist in the count-and-pour era:

> The primary obligation of pharmacy is the service it can render to the public in safeguarding the preparation, compounding, and dispensing of drugs and the storage and handling of drugs and medical supplies. . . .
>
> The pharmacist holds the health and safety of his patrons to be of first consideration; he makes no attempt to prescribe for or to treat disease or to offer for sale any drugs or medical device merely for profit. . . .
>
> The pharmacist willingly makes available his expert knowledge of drugs to the other health professions. . . .
>
> The pharmacist does not discuss the therapeutic effect or composition of a prescription with a patient. When such questions are asked, he suggests that the qualified practitioner [i.e., the physician] is the proper person with whom such matters should be discussed.[16(pp155-6)]

Despite the high-sounding tone of the code, readers should remember that in the early 1950s the vast majority of pharmacists worked in small, independent shops that prospered by the sale of over-the-counter medicines, tobacco products, candy, magazines, greeting cards, and other similar merchandise. Prescription sales brought in less than 25% of the average community pharmacy's income.[17] Most of the young men who entered pharmacy aspired to be drugstore owners, and to achieve this goal they first had to become pharmacists. Generally, they had experience as stock boys, soda jerks, or store clerks, and had already been socialized into the "drug business," not unlike the apprentice apothecaries of the 1800s.

CLINICAL PHARMACY

In the middle of the 1960s, a major paradigm shift in the profession occurred with the rise of the *clinical pharmacy* movement. Innovative pharmacists, mainly in hospital settings, actively sought to expand their practice roles through the staffing of drug information centers, adoption of unit dose distribution methods, and other ideas that pushed daily practice beyond mundane counting and pouring, licking and sticking. In the late 1960s and early 1970s, pharmacy educators embraced the new model of pharmacists as drug information specialists and medication counselors. Biology, physiology, and therapeutics courses were added to the chemistry and physical pharmacy subjects that dominated curricula in the 1950s and early 1960s. Rotations in hospitals and clinics exposed pharmacy students to collaborative practices. In turn, pharmacy students were encouraged to look forward to careers as clinical pharmacists.[18] Graduates in the 1970s often sought placement in hospital settings with prospects for advanced practice, but soon discovered that most open positions were to be found in community pharmacies. There the opportunities for clinical pharmacy were few and far between. Most pharmacists continued to spend their days dispensing prescriptions without providing additional services. The result was frustration and disappointment among young practitioners.

A number of pharmacy scholars in the mid-1970s noticed this trend among beginning pharmacists, which educator Robert Buerki had earlier called "realistic disenchantment."[5] Henri Manasse, in his dissertation and a series of articles that followed it, explored this phenomenon with an eye toward the important role of socialization.[19] In a classic article published in 1975, Manasse, Stewart, and Hall argued that the underlying cause was a pattern of "inconsistent socialization," that is, "the process by which the individual develops or acquires incompatible or conflicting behaviors, beliefs and values from formal or informal sources due to the absence of uniformity or agreement within the idealized group model into which he is being socialized."[20(p616)] In the case of pharmacy, the environment in which a student completed his or her practical experience was key. If that environment contradicted the ideals inculcated within the classroom, "role conflict" resulted.[20(p658)]

During the clinical pharmacy era (1965–1990), pharmacy educators attempted to rectify the inconsistent-socialization problem through lengthening and altering the experiential learning portions of the curriculum. Studies done on the professionalism of students as they progressed through school, clerkships, and early work experiences, however, revealed no improvement or even a decline in their social and occupational attitudes.[21-23] Cynicism and anxiety increased.[24] Negative experiences with supervisors or physicians tended to push students into passivity and discouragement.[25] And those graduates who worked in community pharmacy found an environment as commercialized and professionally discouraging as in the 1950s.[26,27]

PHARMACEUTICAL CARE

The *pharmaceutical care* concept introduced by Hepler and Strand in the late 1980s seemed to offer pharmacy something it had lacked for full growth as a profession: a set of universal shared values within the occupation. In addition to their traditional roles of filling prescriptions with due diligence, pharmacists were to accept full responsibility for drug therapy outcomes. They would actively care for patients and be their therapeutic advocates. When Douglas Hepler spoke at the Pharmacy in the 21st Century Conference in 1989, the gathered group of American pharmacy leaders endorsed pharmaceutical care as the future of the profession's direction.[28] During this same time period, the American Council on Pharmaceutical Education announced its intent to only accredit after 2001 those programs that led to the doctor of pharmacy degree. The Omnibus Budget Reconciliation Act of 1990 (OBRA '90) included provisions calling for pharmacists to utilize their expertise to promote rational drug outcomes.[29] The scene was set for major professional advancement through dual paradigm shifts in education and in the practice model.[30]

The 1990s, initially heralded as the "pharmaceutical care era," witnessed huge growth in the prescription drug sector of health care, with subsequent efforts to control exploding costs through a group of methods euphemistically called "managed care." Caught between a burgeoning number of prescriptions to fill and time spent wrangling with pharmacy benefits managers over coverage issues, most community pharmacists had no real time to "care." When the first generation of students educated within the pharmaceutical care paradigm entered the hectic and restrictive realm of community pharmacy, they expressed disappointment and disillusionment, just like their predecessors a generation before.

In 1995, a special American Association of Colleges of Pharmacy (AACP) committee looked at the situation and made this stark observation:

> It has been argued that students are presented the ideal, patient-oriented perspective by pharmacy educators, only to have those levels of expectations unsupported and unmet as they progress through the curriculum, gain experience in the real world, and enter practice. If students are unclear about what should be expected of them, as a result of mixed, inconsistent messages during socialization, they might experience role ambiguity where they are unsure exactly what their role should be. Their behaviors could be significantly swayed by the opinions of powerful others (e.g., employers, physicians, patients). The difference in role expectations (by some pharmacists) in current practice may not be consistent with the role expectations of recent graduates (they are trained at a higher level to pursue expanded roles) culminating in role stress/strain and a dissatisfaction with practice.[3(p85)]

The committee recommended "continuing efforts within AACP to encourage faculty to give comparable attention to professional socialization as to optimizing the traditional academic components. These two educational (professional socialization and academic learning) processes should be planned as mutually dependent and mutually reinforcing contributions to student growth in achieving the overall educational goals adopted by the faculty."[3(p87)]

Since the mid-1990s, a large number of studies, task force reports, and white papers have been generated on the subject of pharmacy student professionalism and professionalization. Of special value is the "White Paper on Pharmacy Student Professionalism," the product of a joint task force of members from the American Pharmaceutical Association's Academy of Students of Pharmacy and the AACP Council of Deans.[31] It returned to first principles, providing valuable contemporary definitions of key concepts:

> *Profession*: An occupation whose members share ten common characteristics:
> 1. Prolonged specialized training in a body of abstract knowledge
> 2. A service orientation
> 3. An ideology based on the original faith professed by members
> 4. An ethic that is binding on the practitioners
> 5. A body of knowledge unique to the members
> 6. A guild of those entitled to practice the profession
> 7. A set of skills that form the technique of the profession
> 8. Authority granted by society in the form of licensure or certification
> 9. A recognized setting where the profession is practiced
> 10. A theory of societal benefits derived from the ideology

Professional: A member of a profession who displayed the following ten traits:

1. Knowledge and skills of a profession
2. Commitment to self-improvement of skills and knowledge
3. Service orientation
4. Pride in the profession
5. Covenantal relationship with the client
6. Creativity and innovation
7. Conscience and trustworthiness
8. Accountability for his/her work
9. Ethically sound decision making
10. Leadership

Professionalism: The active demonstration of the traits of a professional.

Professional socialization (*professionalization*): The process of inculcating a profession's attitudes, values, and behaviors in a professional. The goal of professional socialization is to develop professionalism, as defined by the ten character traits above.[31]

The recommendations of the APhA-AACP task force continue to resonate today. First of all, the task force contended that "students have a significant role in advancing the process of professional socialization" and that the concepts of professionalism should be introduced to students on their first day in school. Students should take on two parallel tasks from that day: learning how to assume more responsibility for patient care and more responsibility for their own professional development. (This last assignment could be documented through a professional portfolio.) Second, the task force recommended that schools of pharmacy create structured programs to facilitate "the development of professional attitudes, behaviors, and identity." The task force gave advice concerning recruitment, admissions, educational programs, and experiential learning. Finally, the task force recognized that practicing pharmacists had a "critical role in professional socialization." It insisted that practitioners avoid situations that reinforce inconsistent socialization. Instead, they were to serve "as professional mentors and role models to recent pharmacy graduates and pharmacy students."[31]

Rather than depend completely upon clerkships and other experiential learning to inculcate professional values, schools of pharmacy in the 21st century have accepted the challenge to socialize students. As one group of authors put it, "Schools of pharmacy exist to develop professionally mature pharmacy practitioners who can render pharmaceutical care."[8] This is a far cry from the educational *raison d'être* of the Philadelphia College of Pharmacy in 1821, which was to provide a night finishing school for those learning pharmacy (and being socialized) during the day through apprenticeship in a shop, wholesaler, or factory. Students today are encouraged to take on the persona of what they imagine a professional pharmacist might be. This process of "anticipatory socialization" can include behaviors such as wearing more professional dress, acting more mature and responsible, and relating with faculty more as peers. In addition, students and faculty work together on counseling competitions and other activities through which students emulate idealized practitioners.

And yet, for all the white coat ceremonies and other professionalizing activities, progress has been slow. In 2006, Marilyn Speedie, president of AACP, made these observations:

> I find that our students are often frustrated by the distance between what they are being taught as the ideal practice of pharmacy, i.e., pharmaceutical care (or medication therapy management) and what they actually see in practice. This frustration leads to cynicism in some and a curbing of practice ambitions in others. Some will maintain their optimism and idealism throughout the curriculum only to emerge from the program into a practice setting without the skills to create the changes in that setting so they can serve patients the way they want to. There are not enough patient-care-providing practices available to accommodate all our students in experiential education, much less to hire all of our graduates. Clearly our students and our graduates must be part of a practice change and practice improvement process if we have any hope of meeting the needs of society for medication therapy management.[27]

Twenty years before Speedie's editorial, Broadhead and Facchinetti had made the then-controversial accusation that some educators possessed a "hidden agenda" to expand pharmacy practice by making students "agents of social and occupational change."[25(p231)] Nothing is hidden today as schools adopt wide-ranging professionalization programs from orientation courses through clerkships to inculcate values and change the culture of pharmacy.[8,32] And after years of philosophizing about professional socialization in pharmacy, faculty members have suggested some concrete assessments of professionalism to facilitate evaluation of student advancement. Although these "professionalism criteria" center on seemingly trivial outward manifestations of professional attitudes (appearance, attire, timeliness, and good manners), they are a beginning.[33]

Is there a professionalism crisis in 21st-century pharmaceutical education? A number of pharmacy educators advocating for "more professionalism" have lamented the "erosion of values and civility" and a general "demoralization of society."[33,34] Despite the importance of pharmacy schools in the development of the pharmacist, we should remember what Manasse, Kabat, and Wertheimer observed in 1976:

> The focus of the professional socialization process is on how professional aspirants exchange their lay views and imagery of a profession for those the profession ascribes

to itself. In this layman-to-professional exchange, students acquire a self-image within the context of their professional role and, at the same time, begin to adjust to professional demands and uncertainties. The major feature of professional socialization is that the process occurs under strictly defined conditions and is administered by the "gate-keeping" professional group. What cannot be controlled in professional socialization are those behaviors of the "socializee" which are exhibited outside the sphere of professional practice.[35]

SUMMARY

From the colonial period up to the start of the 20th century, American pharmacy was an apprenticeship-based trade whose leadership sought to transform it into a modern, credentialed profession. Despite the development of much more rigorous educational requirements from the 1920s to the 1990s—from two-year PhG courses to six-year PharmD programs—pharmacy continues to struggle for full professional recognition. Socialization, once simply regarded as the means through which a newcomer adopted the culture of the pharmacy workplace, has recently gained the attention of educators and leaders hoping to utilize this process consciously to inculcate values of caring and professionalism in pharmacy students.

In 1996, William Zellmer put forward a simple mission for American pharmacists: "Let's dedicate ourselves to remaking this occupation of ours into a profession that gives people what they want and need. This is not an agenda that we can assign to someone else. Each of us must take personal responsibility for making this happen."[36] Rather than laying the responsibility for change upon pharmacy students and graduates, let us work to understand more fully the subculture that is pharmacy and accept the strengths of its dual identity. Rather than forcing abstract (and unreachable) ideals of *professionalism* upon the young, it might be better for all pharmacists to rededicate themselves to the traditional values of *pharmacy:* expertise, accuracy, diligence, and integrity.

REFERENCES

1. Schwirian PM, Facchinetti NJ. Professional socialization and disillusionment: the case of pharmacy. Am J Pharm Educ 1975;39:18.
2. Merton RK, Reader GG, Kendall PL. The student-physician. Cambridge, MA: Harvard University Press, 1957:40–41. For a further discussion of the cultural concept in pharmacy, see Zellmer WA. The culture and subcultures of pharmacy. Am J Hosp Pharm 1992;49:841.
3. Chalmers RK, Adler DS, Haddad AM, et al. The essential linkage of professional socialization and pharmaceutical care. Am J Pharm Educ 1995;59:85-90.

4. For two differing opinions on this divergence, see Parks LM. What price professionalism. Am J Pharm Educ 1961;25:527-34 and Francke DE. Let's separate pharmacies and drug stores. Am J Pharm 1969;141:161-76.

5. The term *realistic disenchantment* was coined by Robert Buerki in the mid-1960s; see Buerki RA. Pharmacist Smyth and druggist Smith—a study in professional aspirations. Am J Pharm Educ 1977;41:28-33.

6. Oxford English Dictionary. Profession. Oxford, England: Oxford University Press, 1933; 6:1427.

7. Higby GJ. Professionalism and the nineteenth-century American pharmacist. Pharm History 1986;28:115-24.

8. Hammer DP, Berger BA, Beardsley RS, Easton MR. Student professionalism. Am J Pharm Educ 2003;67:96.

9. Flexner JA. A vanishing profession. Atlantic Monthly 1931;98:16-25.

10. McCormack TH. The druggists' dilemma: problems of a marginal occupation. Am J Sociol 1956;61:308-15.

11. Wilensky HL. The professionalization of everyone? Am J Sociol 1964;60:141.

12. Denzin NK, Mettlin CJ. Incomplete professionalization: the case of pharmacy. Social Forces 1968;46:375-81.

13. Flannery MA, Buerki RA, Higby G. 150 years of American pharmacy as reflected in its trade press. Drug Topics 2007;151(May):58; The professionalism issue. Drug Topics 1976;120(June):10.

14. Sonnedecker GA. To be or not to be—professional. Am J Pharm 1961;133:243-54.

15. Tom Rowe, quoted in Francke DE. Let's separate pharmacies and drug stores. Am J Pharm 1969;141:165.

16. Buerki RA, Vottero LD. Ethical responsibility in pharmacy practice. Madison: American Institute of the History of Pharmacy, 1994:39-40.

17. Jackson RA, Worthen DB, Garner DD. Total income for pharmacy owners at record highs. America's Pharmacist 2003;125:29-31.

18. Parascandola J, Brodie DC, Benson RA, Francke DE, Whitney HA, Rodowskas CA. Clinical pharmacy in historical perspective. Drug Intell Clin Pharm 1976;10:505-28.

19. Manasse HR. The states and process of socialization in the profession of pharmacy [PhD dissertation]. University of Minnesota, 1974.

20. Manasse HR, Stewart JE, Hall RH. Inconsistent socialization in pharmacy—a pattern in need of change. J Am Pharm Assoc 1975;15:616-21, 658.

21. Manasse HR, Kabat HF, Wertheimer AI. Professional socialization in pharmacy: a cross-sectional analysis of dominant value characteristics of agents and objects of socialization. Soc Sci Med 1977;11:653-9.

22. Speranza KA, McCook WM. The effects of an institutional clinical experience on pharmacy student professional status perceptions. Am J Pharm Educ 1978;42:11-4.

23. Hatoum HT, Smith MC. Identifying patterns of professional socialization for pharmacists during pharmacy schooling and after one year in practice. Am J Pharm Educ 1987;51:7-17.

24. Hatoum H, Smith MC, Sharpe TR. Attitudes of pharmacy students towards psychosocial factors in health care. Soc Sci Med 1982;16:1240-1.

25. Broadhead RS, Facchinetti NJ. Clinical clerkships in professional education: a study in pharmacy and other ancillary professions. Soc Sci Med 1985;20:231-40.

26. Anderson RD. The peril of deprofessionalization. Am J Hosp Pharm 1977;34:133-9.

27. Speedie M. Introductory experiential education: a means for introducing concepts of health-care improvement. Am J Pharm Educ 2006;70:145.

28. Conference on Pharmacy in the 21st Century, October 11–14, 1989, Williamsburg, VA. Am J Pharm Educ 1989;53(suppl):1S-78S.

29. Brushwood DB, Catizone CA, Coster JM. OBRA 90: what it means to your practice. US Pharmacist 1992;17:64-72.

30. Higby GJ. American pharmacy in the twentieth century. Am J Health-System Pharm 1997; 54:1814.

31. APhA-AACP Task Force on Professionalism. White paper on pharmacy student professionalism. J Am Pharm Assoc 2000;40:96-102.

32. Berger BA, Butler SL, Duncan-Hewitt W, et al. Changing the culture: an institution-wide approach to instilling professional values. Am J Pharm Educ 2004;68:22.

33. Boyle CJ, Beardsley RS, Morgan JA, de Bittner MR. Professionalism: a determining factor in experiential learning. Am J Pharm Educ 2007;71:31.

34. Hammer D. Improving student professionalism during experiential learning. Am J Pharm Educ 2006;70.59.

35. Manasse HR, Kabat HF, Wertheimer AI. Professional socialization in pharmacy I: a cross-sectional analysis of personality characteristics of agents and objects of socialization. Drugs Health Care 1976;3(3):4.

36. Zellmer WA. Searching for the soul of pharmacy. Am J Health Syst Pharm 1996;53:1911-6.

CHAPTER 8

Organizational Change

Salisa Westrick, PhD

QUEST FOR CHANGE: FROM A PRODUCT FOCUS TO A PATIENT FOCUS

A 2007 report, published in a *Health Affairs* online edition, reveals that the overall cost of health care is estimated to double over the next 10 years.[1] By the year 2016, nearly 20 cents of every dollar earned in the U.S. economy will be spent on health care, compared with the expenditure of 16 cents of every dollar earned in 2006. This report further suggests that prescription drug spending will show an accelerated growth of an annual average of 8.6%.[1] It is estimated that, in the next 10 years, prescription drug expenditures will also double the 2006 amount. As a result of rising healthcare costs, third-party payers have put forth efforts to control the costs of health care while improving health outcomes.

Several strategies can be implemented to control the costs of health care. For example, payers may increase restrictions on access to costly drugs by using preferred drug lists and prior authorization.[2] Another strategy may involve increasing patients' cost sharing, resulting in greater financial burden to plan beneficiaries.[3,4] Healthcare providers are also affected by payers' cost-control strategies. For example, healthcare providers are pressured to engage in generic substitution and therapeutic interchange of less costly drugs.[5] In addition, pharmacy benefits managers have been aggressive in establishing the deepest discounts in reimbursement formulas for drugs.[6] Because of the discounts, profit margins for pharmaceuticals are decreased.[7] Hence, pharmacies may have to increase their volume in order to maintain the same level of profits and obtain different venues to earn their revenues.

In addition to controlling healthcare costs, payers have begun to focus on improving patient outcomes.[8-11] Health promotion and disease prevention activities have been implemented by many health plans. For instance, medication therapy management (MTM) services are examples of patient care services that provide pharmacists with ample opportunities to improve health outcomes while being able to receive reimbursement for the services.

In short, as a result of rising healthcare costs, payers have implemented various strategies to control costs and improve health outcomes. These strategies have left pharmacists with both threats and opportunities. The threats relate to decreasing profit margins for pharmaceuticals, and the opportunities relate to the provision of patient care services. These opportunities call for change from a traditional product focus to a patient focus.

Mechanisms to Change Pharmacy Practice

Optimizing patient outcomes is a goal of pharmacy practice.[12] To achieve this goal, the practice of pharmacy needs to shift its focus from traditional dispensing activities to patient care activities. One approach is to change the attitudes, skills, and behaviors of individual pharmacists so as to deliver innovative patient care services. Using the individual approach, numerous studies have shown that during the intervention period, patient outcomes and pharmacist satisfaction improved.[13-16] However, these innovative services were not sustained beyond the intervention period.[17,18] Some have suggested that the reason may be that the individual approach does not consider the complexity of organizations.[17,19,20]

An alternative approach to facilitate pharmacy practice change is to target the change at the organizational level. This organization-level approach recognizes that (1) individuals have limited capabilities to make independent decisions regarding adoption and implementation of patient care services, and (2) individuals' values and behaviors are influenced by the organization and the environment.[20] A better understanding of change at the organizational level may help organizational leaders and pharmacists effectively initiate, manage, and sustain change in their organizations from a product focus to a patient focus.

ORGANIZATIONAL CHANGE IN PHARMACY PRACTICE

Change at the organization level can be unplanned or planned. Unplanned change generally happens over a period of time. An unplanned change typically is not instigated by leaders in the organization, but rather is influenced by the external environment. Examples of unplanned change include a growth in part-time pharmacists, an increase in the number of female pharmacists in the workforce, and new federal and state laws and regulations. Even though this type of change is not planned by leaders in the organization, it shapes the way work is scheduled, organized, and managed. In contrast, a planned change occurs as leaders recognize the need for the organization to change and carefully design a plan to accomplish the change. This planned change can be used to improve organizational performance or solve problems within the organization. Typically, in planned-change situations, members of the organization are conscious and aware of the change. In this chapter, organizational change is referred to as a planned change within an organization, such as a plan to implement an MTM service.

LEWIN'S CHANGE MODEL

Most organizational change theories originated from Lewin's change model.[21] This model suggests that organizational behavior is the results of two sets of forces: driving forces and restraining forces (Fig. 8-1). *Driving forces* include forces or factors that initiate and push for change. Conversely, *restraining forces* can be thought of as barriers to change. These forces resist a change and seek to maintain the status quo (i.e., the current state of affairs). At the status quo, both sets of forces are about equal.

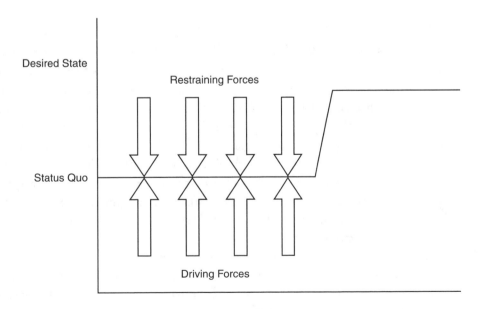

FIGURE 8-1   Balance of Driving Forces and Restraining Forces

Therefore, at the status quo, the state of organizational behavior is maintained and stable. To shift from the status quo to the desired state, the driving forces must exceed the restraining forces.

To ensure that driving forces exceed the restraining forces, the following options can be implemented: increasing the strength of the existing driving forces, adding new driving forces, reducing the strength of the existing restraining forces, or a combination of these options. For instance, the number of prescriptions dispensed in a pharmacy is stable because group norms maintaining the status quo are equivalent to the manager's pressure for change to a higher dispensing rate. This level can be increased to the manager's desired level by increasing the manager's pressure to dispense prescriptions at a higher rate, by modifying the group norms to support higher levels of efficiency, or by using a combination of both strategies.[22] It is important to note that addressing driving forces without modifying restraining forces may increase the strength of the restraining forces. Therefore, it is recommended that restraining forces be modified during the change process. Organizations can choose to modify restraining forces alone or in conjunction with driving forces.

Lewin developed a three-stage model of planned change that explained how to initiate, manage, and stabilize the change process. The three stages are unfreezing, changing, and refreezing.[21]

Unfreezing

Unfreezing is the stage at which change is initiated. As previously stated, the current level of organizational behavior is stabilized because of the balance between restraining forces and driving forces. Hence, in order to make any organizational change, the balance of these forces needs to be modified. At this stage, various strategies can be implemented to ensure that the driving forces exceed the restraining forces. Leaders can begin the unfreezing process by introducing information that shows discrepancies between behaviors desired by leaders and employees' current behaviors. For example, to get pharmacy technicians interested in improving the accuracy of the dispensing process, organizational leaders and pharmacists could compare the pharmacy's current dispensing error rate with the error rates among the competitors. By doing so, the discrepancies will disconfirm the usefulness or appropriateness of technicians' present behaviors or attitudes and hence create the motivation to change. The leaders and pharmacists may also introduce rewards to strengthen the driving forces at this stage. Rewards are used to motivate pharmacy technicians to move toward change. Rewards can be in monetary or nonmonetary form.

Changing

The changing stage happens when the existing behavior shifts to the desired level. During this stage, employees learn new concepts and new ways of doing things. They develop new behaviors, values, and attitudes. To be successful in shifting to the desired level, it is important that employees be provided with information, assistance, and encouragement during the change process. It is highly recommended that organizational leaders communicate clearly and openly with employees on the benefits of changing their behaviors and on how the change will affect them and the organization as a whole. Furthermore, leaders must pay attention to problems that arise during the change process. Once problems are discovered, leaders must deal with them immediately.

Refreezing

Organizational leaders stabilize change during the refreezing stage by helping employees integrate the changed behavior or attitude into their normal way of doing things. This is accomplished by using positive reinforcement, such as rewards, to encourage the desired behavior. Further, organizational leaders can establish feedback systems as a way to reinforce desired behaviors and prevent employees from relapsing to the previous behavior. Additional coaching and modeling are also used at this point to reinforce the stability of the change.

Lewin's model provides a framework to explain the change processes within an organization. Because the model is rather broad in nature, it may not identify specific actions for any particular plans. To determine specific actions to accomplish a desired goal, a force field analysis can be used.

FORCE FIELD ANALYSIS

A force field analysis is a method for listing, discussing, and evaluating the various forces for and against a proposed change. Force field analysis derives from Lewin's three-step model of change in that it recognizes two types of factors affecting organizational change: restraining forces and driving forces. Force field analysis helps leaders look at the big picture by analyzing all of the forces affecting the change and weighing the strength of restraining forces and driving forces. Once the strength of the forces is identified, strategies to reduce the impact of the opposing forces and strengthen the supporting forces can be developed.

To conduct a force field analysis, start with describing the current situation and determining a goal or change to be implemented. Second, list all the restraining forces that hinder the change and the driving forces that promote the change in two different columns. Examples of driving forces are pressure from leaders, monetary and nonmonetary rewards, and new mandates. Examples of restraining forces include the investment cost of new automated technology, limited space and resources, and fear of automated processes. The list of restraining forces and driving forces can be compiled through various methods such as questionnaires, interviews, observations, and records.[22] Once all driving forces and restraining forces are identified, the next step is to assign a score to each force affecting change in terms of its strength, from 1 (weak) to 5 (strong). The strength of each force is based on personal belief and input from organizational members.[22] After rating each force, calculate a total score for each of the two columns. The total score for restraining forces reflects the strength of forces that act against change. Likewise, the total score for driving forces reflects the strength of forces that promote change. After the total scores for driving forces and restraining forces are calculated, leaders must decide whether the goal or change is still feasible. If so, the next step is to develop a manageable course of action to strengthen the existing driving forces, create new driving forces, weaken existing restraining forces, or a combination of these actions.

Figures 8-2 and 8-3 illustrate how a force field analysis can be used to determine a course of action related to the adoption of a new automated dispensing machine in a community pharmacy. Figure 8-2 shows the list of restraining forces and driving forces and their strengths, from which the total scores for driving forces and

DRIVING FORCES (STRENGTH)	Goal: Adoption of a new automated dispensing machine	RESTRAINING FORCES (STRENGTH)
Free up pharmacists' time to develop and implement patient care services (4)		Staff frightened of new technology (4)
Reduce dispensing errors (3)		Cost of new technology (3)
Improve efficiency of dispensing service (2)		Staff resistance to change to automated processes
Increase number of prescriptions dispensed (2)		Loss of staff overtime (2)
		Disruption of workflow during change (2)
Total score = 11		Total Score = 14

Strength of each force is on a scale of 1 (weak) to 5 (strong).

FIGURE 8-2 Force Field Analysis for the adoption of an automated dispensing machine: Assessing the possibility of change

restraining forces are calculated. The current situation shows that the total score for the driving forces is lower than the total score for the restraining forces. Thus, in the current situation, the goal may not be accomplished. Figure 8-3 shows how an action plan is determined using the results of the force field analysis. As previously stated, to make an effective change, the total score for the driving forces must be greater than the restraining forces. This can be accomplished by taking appropriate actions. For example, the community pharmacy could implement a communication plan to address concerns about resistance to change and a training session on the new automated dispensing machine to allow employees to familiarize themselves with it and reduce their fear. After possible actions are developed, the next step is to determine the new scores, assuming that these actions successfully take place. Please note that in this example only the restraining forces are modified. It is possible to develop other action plans to increase the strength of the driving forces or add new driving forces. Figure 8-3 illustrates that after the action plans are implemented, a change to an automated dispensing process is possible because the total score for the driving forces is higher than the total score for the restraining forces.

In summary, a force field analysis allows organizational leaders and pharmacists to look at a planned change in terms of forces for and against the change and to proactively design actions to effectively manage the change. Organizational leaders of pharmacy and pharmacists are encouraged to use Lewin's change model and force field analysis as guidance when developing a plan to implement patient care services. Once patient care services are implemented, leaders of the organization and pharmacists must ensure that effective patient care services are sustained in the practice.

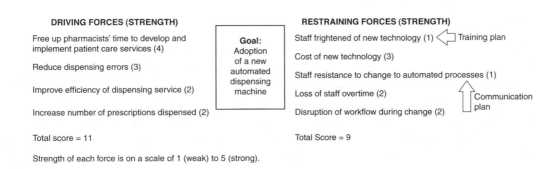

FIGURE 8-3   Force Field Analysis for the adoption of an automated dispensing machine: After the implementation of action plans

SUSTAINABILITY OF PATIENT CARE SERVICES _____

Patient care services, like other innovations, have a life cycle.[23-26] Generally, new services proceed through a series of overlapping stages.[23,24,26] The first stage, initiation, occurs when an organization senses demands on the current system, searches for possible alternatives, and evaluates these alternatives.[26] The second stage, development and adoption, happens when the service is put to the test in a real context.[26] At this stage, to be successful, the service should be reinvented or modified to accommodate the organization's needs and structure.[24] The service then proceeds to the third stage, implementation, during which the program is put into full practice.[26] At this stage, the adopting organization needs to allocate its resources to ensure success.[24,26] The next stage, sustainability, occurs when organizational members no longer think of the service as a new idea and the service becomes part of the organization.[24] Finally, the dissemination stage involves the diffusion of the service to other practice sites.[26]

After a new service is implemented, discontinuation of the program can occur at any stage.[24] Premature termination of effective services can be costly to the organization because substantial time and resources have been invested in the services, to pharmacy staff because discontinuation of services may affect them emotionally or financially, and to customers because they may have counted on the continuation of the services.[27] Hence, organizational leaders and pharmacists should not undermine the sustainability of patient care services. This section provides guidance for building sustainable patient care services. Specifically, the importance and the definition of sustainability are discussed and factors influencing greater sustainability are identified. Leaders and pharmacists should take these factors in consideration during the planning phase.[27,28]

Sustainability

Many pharmacies are conducting patient care services that are new to their organizations. Some of these new services will enjoy long-term survival, and some will be terminated after an initial operating period.[29] In this chapter, *sustainability* is defined as "a service's ability to continue delivering intended services to their targeted audience over the long term and to keep with their goals and objectives for their service."[30] Using this definition, patient care services that cannot achieve the set goals and objectives after proper implementation should not endure for a long time.[31]

After developing and initially implementing a new patient care service, leaders of the pharmacy and pharmacists make a decision regarding whether to continue or reject the service.[24] The decision to continue program delivery increases the sustainability of the service. In contrast, the pharmacy may make a decision to reject the service. There are two types of rejection: replacement and disenchantment.[24] *Replacement* happens when the pharmacy rejects one type of patient care service in order to adopt a better service that supersedes the previous one. *Disenchantment* refers to a pharmacy rejecting the service as a result of dissatisfaction with its performance, without replacing it with any other patient care services.[24] Dissatisfaction can arise from many reasons. For example, the pharmacy may decide, after proper implementation and careful evaluation, that the service did not meet set goals and objectives and therefore should be terminated. In this case, the service was well implemented but did not bring desired benefits to the pharmacy; hence, it is logical to discontinue the service. In other situations, however, dissatisfaction can be the result of poor planning or an improper implementation. In these cases, rejection as a result of dissatisfaction could have been prevented had the service been better planned and implemented.

Research shows that failure to sustain services is often caused by not incorporating a focus on sustainability during the planning phase.[32-34] Goodman and Steckler observed that sustainability is often a latent concern in many health promotion programs.[27] That is, organizations hope to see the services continue; however, in the absence of early and active planning, the conditions that would enhance the degree of sustainability are not created, and as a result, sustainability does not occur.[27] Hence, in order to heighten program sustainability, organizational leaders must move from a passive approach to sustainability to an active use of programmatic approaches that maximize long-term sustainability. Organizational leaders and pharmacists thus need to have a clear understanding of the factors influencing greater sustainability.[28] The following subsection describes five factors that are consistently supported as important factors influencing the extent of sustainability.[26]

Factors Facilitating Program Sustainability

Champions

Program champions are influential individuals within the implementing organization who act as program advocates.[28] Champions make decisive contributions by actively and enthusiastically promoting the service.[29,35] Effective champions must overcome indifference or resistance that the new idea may provoke in an organization.[24] Service sustainability is greatly facilitated when the champion has three specific attributes: (1) a mid- to upper-level administrative position within the organization, (2) an acute sense of the types of tradeoffs that are necessary to influence others to support the service, and (3) negotiating skills that facilitate the formation of coalitions among those individuals who are favorably disposed toward the service.[29]

Literature has shown strong evidence of the effect of champions on increasing the success of innovations[24,35,36] and service sustainability.[23,26,29] That is, the presence of a champion who strongly advocates the continuation of the service increases the service's sustainability. In fact, sustainability is almost guaranteed if there is a champion.[23] For example, results of a study of discontinuation of the fluoride mouth rinse program in public school districts showed that an internal champion played a key role in initial adoption of the service and in preventing it from discontinuation.[25] Accordingly, to ensure the success of patient care services, leaders of the organization should consider developing a champion to advocate for the sustainability of the services.

An example of the role of a champion in pharmacy follows.[29] John Howard is a medication therapy management service coordinator for a large chain pharmacy. Pharmacist Howard successfully facilitates the sustainability of MTM services among participating pharmacies. Before the implementation of MTM services, he first has to understand how managers and staff pharmacists at the participating pharmacies perceive the MTM services. By appreciating the perceptions that members of the pharmacies hold in relation to the service, Howard is in a position to negotiate with each member to foster a favorable impression of the service. Once favorable perceptions begin to emerge, he establishes links among individuals who jointly advocate for the service. Because each member may have different interests in supporting a particular service, a coalition is formed among different individuals. By forming a coalition to support the implementation of MTM services, individual interests become mutual interests. During the implementation phase, Howard frequently visits the participating pharmacies to ensure that they have the necessary resources to carry out the MTM services. Furthermore, he continues to influence upper-level management to support the continuation of MTM services.

Modifiability of Patient Care Services

As previously discussed, sustainability is the ability of patient care services to continuously deliver intended services to clients over time. This suggests important notions of continuation without being limited to any particular form.[28] That is, a service must adjust or adapt to new needs and circumstances if it is to continue.[26] Research studies consistently show that services that are modifiable are more likely to be sustained.[23,28,31,37] O'Loughlin and colleagues found that programs that underwent modification during implementation were almost three times more likely to be sustained than those that remained in their original format.[32]

In pharmacy practice, in order to have patient care services with a high level of sustainability, patient care services should be modifiable to fit with organizational operations. This is especially true if the services have been developed elsewhere (e.g., by professional organizations, academia, or other practice sites). Because these services may not fit well within the new context, leaders of the organization and pharmacists must engage in thoughtful modifications of components of the service to fit the new organizational context. On the other hand, if the service is developed internally, it is suggested that the service be designed in such a way that it can be subdivided, can be delivered in a variety of sequences or formats, or has alternative content and educational materials.[32]

Fit Within the Host Organization

To increase sustainability of the service, fit between service and organization is necessary.[23,29,32,38] *Organizational fit* refers to a service's compatibility with the organization's mission, values, norms, and core operations.[29] Results from various research studies consistently suggest that services that fit well within an organization were more likely to remain viable than those that required adjustment within the organization to accommodate the intervention.[23,29,32,38] This could be because services that could be sold as contributing to the organization's goals were more likely to receive internal support and resources that allowed them to be sustained.[26] Furthermore, activities that could readily fit into existing tasks and procedures were more likely to have the support of operating staff members.[26]

To illustrate the importance of a service–organization fit, consider the case of a health promotion program in a community mental health center.[29] The mental health center's mission was oriented to clinical services in mental health and substance abuse. The health promotion program was a newer concept and ancillary to this mission. Because of the poor fit between the organization's mission and the promotion program, the program became isolated from the center's core functions. Because the program was not a principal concern of the organization, the health promotion program was underfunded, had high staff turnover, lacked consistent implementation, and was eventually rejected.

Similar scenarios could happen in a pharmacy if leaders fail to determine the fit between their organization and patient care services. For example, if a pharmacy is oriented to dispensing, a patient care service that requires intensive scheduled sessions with patients may not be sustainable and eventually may be terminated. To prevent this type of scenario from occurring, leaders and pharmacists should examine how closely the service aligns with the organizational mission, values, and core operations.

Integration with Existing Operations

The fourth factor is related to integration between patient care services and core operations. Research has consistently shown that stand-alone services are less likely to be sustained than services that are well integrated with existing operations.[31,37,39]

This may be because stand-alone services tend to create jealousy and are less likely to attract funding from the central pool.[39] Therefore, leaders and pharmacists should plan to incorporate a new service as an integral part of core functions rather than as a stand-alone activity.[37]

Integrated and nonintegrated patient care services in pharmacy practice can be illustrated by two types of pharmacy-based vaccination services. Generally, a pharmacist or a pharmacy can be involved in vaccination services through two different mechanisms: (1) contracting with outside providers, generally nurses, to administer vaccines in community pharmacies, and (2) using staff pharmacists to administer vaccines at their practice site.[40,41] The first mechanism is referred to as an *outsourced vaccination service*, and the second as an *in-house vaccination service*. Generally, in-house vaccination service providers offer walk-in services or service by appointment,[40] which requires a greater degree of integration with existing workflow and scheduling. Because an outsourced vaccination service is normally offered as a stand-alone service and offered for fewer than four days a year,[40] it is easier to terminate than an in-house vaccination service, which requires a greater degree of integration with existing organizational operations. Therefore, to foster greater sustainability among vaccination services, organizational leaders and pharmacists should incorporate vaccination services into an existing workflow by offering in-house vaccination services rather than outsourced services.

Program Assessments and Evaluations

To ensure that the service meets the set objectives and is correctly implemented, the organization needs to conduct continuous assessments and evaluations.[28,31,32,42] The use of assessment and evaluation allows organizations to continuously monitor and revise both objectives and processes to improve the delivery of the service. Information obtained from the assessments and evaluations can be used to inform decision makers whether any improvements need to be made to the service. The importance of evaluation was supported by Evashwick and Ory, who interviewed 20 organizations that implemented successful sustainable innovative health services.[37] Their study suggested that outcomes and process evaluations were vital to the services' success.[37]

In pharmacy practice, after a patient care service is implemented, it is strongly recommended for the leaders and pharmacists to conduct routine assessments of the process and outcomes of the service. For example, in assessing a pharmacy-based diabetes management service, success in patient recruitment should be assessed by reviewing the number of new patients who successfully enrolled in the service and by reviewing the number of patients with diabetes who could have been recruited. Furthermore, patient outcomes such as blood glucose levels and adherence should also be assessed. Data obtained from the routine assessments can be used to inform the decision makers, champions, and pharmacists who are involved in the diabetes management service whether modifications are necessary and to convince the decision makers to continue their support for the diabetes management service.

Organizational leaders and pharmacists play critical roles in making decisions related to initiating, managing, and sustaining patient care services. In some instances, decision makers are not able to make the most rational decision because they are susceptible to cognitive biases or use mental shortcuts to simplify or oversimplify decisions.[43] The following section discusses the cognitive biases and mental shortcuts that can prevent decision makers from making effective decisions.

HIDDEN TRAPS IN DECISION MAKING

Making decisions is the most important job of organizational leaders.[44] Every day, decisions are being made. Decisions in pharmacy practice can range from small, such as when to place an order for a cold medication, to big, such as whether to implement an MTM service. A number of factors can affect how organizational leaders make decisions. Because of the complexity inherent in decision making, decisions cannot be made completely objectively and rationally.[45] Rather, decision makers usually bring cognitive biases from their beliefs and experiences into the situation or use mental shortcuts to help make decisions.[46,47] Mental shortcuts are typically used when decision makers face complex problems or incomplete information. These shortcuts are simple and usually effective, but sometimes they can mislead decision makers or cause them to choose a different outcome than they might otherwise.[48] Hence, decision makers must be cautious regarding the traps affecting how they make decisions. This section describes three common decision traps and how to overcome them.

Status Quo Trap

In a decision-making context, the *status quo* refers to the existing state of affairs.[49] In business settings, it refers to existing goals or objectives and the existing plans, strategies, and tactics for attaining those goals.[49] Research has consistently shown that decision makers prefer to continue with existing goals and plans instead of other, better alternatives.[49-53] As a result, organizations avoid making changes or breaking with the status quo despite the opportunity to put those resources to more effective use.[44,49]

March and Simon provided an explanation for why organizations prefer maintaining their status quo over choosing other alternatives.[45] They suggested that the retention of the status quo is likely when a current stage is satisfactory.[45] That is, as long as the status quo stage produces positive outcomes, it is unlikely that decision makers will search for superior alternatives. Additionally, even if decision makers are presented with information about superior alternatives, they may, in fact, refuse to invest further time on exploring the better alternatives.[49] Furthermore, research shows that, in some cases, despite negative outcomes produced by the status quo, decision makers discount the negative information, change organizational goals to fit the situation, or retain hope in the eventual success of the status quo.[49]

As in other organizations, decision making in pharmacy may be affected by the status quo trap. Hence, decision makers need to recognize and overcome the status quo tendency. For example, decision makers should be vigilant in examining alternatives by regularly reviewing how organizational goals are achieved by the status quo when compared with other alternatives.[47,49] It is important that decision makers objectively and rationally explore and evaluate all alternatives, including the status quo alternative.[54] To reduce potential status quo tendency, it may be helpful to have an outside, independent, or separate review of the status quo.[49] Selection of one best alternative should only come after complete evaluations of all possible alternatives.

Sunk-Cost Trap

Sunk costs are defined as costs that have already been incurred and cannot be recovered to any significant degree.[55] Decision makers have a tendency to continue an endeavor once an investment in time, money, or effort has been made, even though the endeavor may no longer be producing satisfactory outcomes.[44,56] In other words, decision makers affected by the sunk-cost trap feel as if they have too much invested to quit.[57] They thus have a tendency to continue to invest more money and personnel in a poor performance plan with the hope of seeing an improvement in the outcomes.

Sunk costs are taken into consideration in the decision-making process because decision makers perceive sunk costs as losses; this often results in risky behaviors such as continuing the same endeavor to avoid these losses.[55] Therefore, it is crucial that organizational leaders be aware of the influence of past decisions and past investments and do not allow the effects of sunk costs to cloud their judgment. The following two scenarios, adapted from Arkes and Blumer,[55] illustrate the sunk-cost effect in pharmacy practice.

- *Scenario 1:* As the owner of an independent pharmacy, you have invested $40,000 of the pharmacy's money into remodeling a patient consultation room, purchasing computer software and hardware, and training staff pharmacists in order to provide state-of-the-art MTM services. Your pharmacy's goal is to secure a contract with a large self-insured employer to provide MTM services for its employees. When the project is 80% completed, another pharmacy begins to market its MTM services to the self-insured employer that your pharmacy is targeting. It is apparent that the competitor's services are much better and more attractive to the target employer than the services that your pharmacy is developing. Because this employer is the only possible target group, the question is, should you invest the last $10,000 to finish your plan for the MTM services?

- *Scenario 2:* As the owner of an independent pharmacy, you have received a suggestion from one of your staff pharmacists. The suggestion is to use $10,000 of the pharmacy's money to invest in remodeling a patient consultation room, purchasing necessary computer software and hardware, and training staff pharmacists in order to provide state-of-the-art MTM services. These actions will help the pharmacy to secure a contract with a large self-insured employer to provide MTM services for its employees. However, another pharmacy begins to develop its MTM services for the self-insured employer that your pharmacy is targeting. It is apparent that the competitor's services are much better and more attractive to the target employer than the services that your pharmacy could develop. Because this employer is the only possible target group, the question is, should you invest $10,000 to develop the MTM services?

What was your answer to each of the scenarios? A higher proportion of people would choose to continue to invest in the MTM services in the first scenario and would opt out in the second scenario. As previously stated, this phenomenon is referred to as the sunk-cost effect. Decision makers have a greater tendency to continue an endeavor once an investment in time, money, or effort has been made. In the first scenario, $40,000 has already been invested in developing MTM services; therefore, decision makers are likely to continue to invest resources in this endeavor.

Sunk-cost traps can be avoided if decision makers seek out and listen to people who were not involved in the previous decision making or past investments. Such people are in a more neutral position to make decisions when sunk costs are present. Furthermore, in order to prevent employees from perpetuating mistakes and justifying their past actions, decision makers must develop a nonpunitive culture.[47] In this way, organizations do not tie negative consequences to the outcome of decisions, especially when the individual has little control over the outcomes.[49]

Confirming-Evidence Trap

The confirming-evidence trap is a bias that leads decision makers to seek out information to support their existing beliefs and points of view, while avoiding any contradictory information.[44,58,59] Research has shown that once a single idea is chosen, decision makers typically spend little time exploring other alternatives.[60] This trap not only affects how decision makers seek information but also how they interpret evidence.[44] When decision makers are affected by the confirming-evidence trap, they put too much weight on supporting information and too little on information that is conflicting,[44] or unintentionally select or distort facts to suit their preferences.[43] The confirming-evidence trap happens because people are drawn to information that supports their subconscious beliefs, thoughts, and opinions.

To avoid this trap, a key is to avoid a limited search for alternative solutions.[54] Generally, when decision makers promote a single idea, the search is focused on the single idea rather than expanded to consider other alternatives.[54,61] Hence, decision makers should seek advice from others who are objective in their decision making and are not emotionally attached to a particular idea. In this way, others can help uncover options that would otherwise be undiscovered.[54] It is crucial for decision makers to gather all evidence from multiple perspectives, examine it with equal rigor, and avoid the tendency to accept confirming evidence without questioning it thoroughly.[58] Furthermore, decision makers may find it helpful to build counter-arguments themselves by asking the reasons for choosing different options or asking someone to argue against the option that decision makers are contemplating.[44]

The status quo trap, sunk-cost trap, and confirming-evidence trap are common psychological traps that can mislead people when they make decisions. Decision makers should keep in mind that these traps work in concert with each other. Typically, the effect of traps is more prominent when a decision is made quickly, uncertain, or based on gut instincts. Hence, organizational leaders and pharmacists should avoid these traps in order to make effective decisions.

SUMMARY

Optimizing patient outcomes is a goal of pharmacy practice. To achieve this goal, the practice of pharmacy needs to shift its focus from traditional dispensing activities to patient care activities. Organizational leaders and pharmacists are encouraged to use an organization-level approach to initiate, manage, and sustain change in their organizations. Lewin's change model and force field analysis can be used as guidance to develop a course of action to accomplish changes within the organization.

It is important that organizational leaders incorporate five factors contributing to the sustainability of patient care services into the plan at an early stage of the planning process. Organizational leaders must ensure that a patient care service that is implemented (1) has a champion, (2) fits well within the organization, (3) can be modified, (4) can be integrated with existing operations, and (5) is regularly assessed and evaluated. Further, organizational leaders and pharmacists must be cautious about decision-making traps. Common traps discussed in this chapter were the status quo trap, sunk-cost trap, and confirming-evidence trap. Strategies to overcome these traps were also discussed in this chapter.

REFERENCES

1. Poisal J, Truffer C, Smith S, Sisko A, Cowan C. Health spending projections through 2016: modest changes obscure Part D's impact. Health Aff (Millwood) 2007;26(2):w242-53.

2. Soumeral S. Benefits and risks of increasing restrictions on access to costly drugs in Medicaid. Health Aff (Millwood) 2004;23(1):135-46.

3. Wright BJ, Carlson MI, Edlund T, et al. The impact of increased cost sharing on Medicaid enrollees. Health Aff (Millwood) 2005;24(4):1106-16.

4. Artiga S, Rousseau D, Lyons B, et al. Can states stretch the Medicaid dollar without passing the buck? Lessons from Utah. Health Aff (Millwood) 2006;25(2):532-40.

5. Wallack SS, Weinberg DB, Thomas CP. Health plans' strategies to control prescription drug spending. Health Aff (Millwood) 2004;23(6):141-8.

6. Lipton H, Kreling DH, Collins T, Hertz K. Pharmacy benefit management companies. Annu Rev Public Health 1999;20:361-401.

7. Garis RI, Clark BE. The spread: pilot study of an undocumented source of pharmacy benefit manager revenue. J Am Pharm Assoc 2004;44(1):15-21.

8. Fireman B, Bartlett J, Selby J. Can disease management reduce health care costs by improving quality? Health Aff (Millwood) 2004;23(6):63-75.

9. Galvin R. Pay-for-performance: too much of a good thing? A conversation with Martin Roland. Health Aff (Millwood). 2006;25:w412-9.

10. Health care quality. Health Aff (Millwood) 2005;24(5):1367-9.

11. Buffington DE. Future of medication therapy management services in delivering patient-centered care. Am J Health Syst Pharm 2007;64(15):S10-12.

12. Hepler C, Strand L. Opportunities and responsibilities in pharmaceutical care. Am J Hosp Pharm 1990;43:533-43.

13. Huyghebaert T, Farris KB, Volume CI. Implementing pharmaceutical care: insights from Alberta community pharmacists. Can Pharm J 1999;132:41-5.

14. Herborg H, Soendergaard B, Frokjaer B, et al. Pharmaceutical care value proved. Int Pharm J 1996;10:167-8.

15. Shibley MC, Pugh CB. Implementation of pharmaceutical care services for patients with hyperlipidemias by independent community pharmacy practitioners. Ann Pharmacother 1997;31(6):713-9.

16. Barner JC, Brown CM, Shepherd MD, et al. Provision of pharmacy services in community health centers and migrant health centers. J Am Pharm Assoc 2002;42(5):713-22.

17. Farris KB, Schopflocher DP. Between intention and behavior: an application of community pharmacists' assessment of pharmaceutical care. Soc Sci Med 1999;49:55-66.

18. Odedina FL, Segal R, Hepler CD, et al. Changing pharmacists' practice pattern: pharmacists' implementation of pharmaceutical care factors. J Soc Adm Pharm 1996;13(2):74-88.

19. Baldridge JV, Burnham RA. Organization innovation: individual, organizational, and environmental impacts. Adm Sci Q 1975;20(2):165-76.

20. Scott WR. Organizations: rational, natural, and open system. 5th ed. Upper Saddle River, NJ: Prentice Hall, 2003.

21. Lewin K. Field theory in social science. New York: Harper and Row, 1951.

22. Cummings TG, Worley CG. Organization development and change. 5th ed. St. Paul, MN: West Publishing Company, 1993.

23. Goodman RM, Steckler AB. A model for the institutionalization of health promotion programs. Fam Community Health 1989;11(4):63-78.

24. Rogers EM. Diffusion of innovation. 5th ed. New York: Free Press, 2003.

25. Scheirer MA. The life cycle of an innovation: adoption versus discontinuation of the fluoride mouth rinse program in schools. J Health Soc Behav 1990;31(2):203-15.

26. Scheirer MA. Is sustainability possible? A review and commentary on empirical studies of program sustainability. Am J Eval 2005;26(3):320-47.

27. Goodman RM, Steckler AB. The life and death of a health promotion program: an institutionalization case study. Int Q Community Health Educ 1987-1988;8(1):5-21.

28. Shediac-Rizkallah MC, Bone LR. Planning for the sustainability of community-based health programs: conceptual frameworks and future directions for research, practice and policy. Health Educ Res 1998;13(1):87-108.

29. Steckler AB, Goodman RM. How to institutionalize health promotion programs. Am J Health Promot 1989;3(4):34-44.

30. Bamberger M, Cheema S. Case studies of project sustainability: implications for policy and operations from Asian experience. Washington, DC: The World Bank, 1990.

31. Glaser EM. Durability of innovations in human service organizations: a case study analysis. Knowledge 1981;3:167-85.

32. O'Loughlin J, Renaud L, Richard L, et al. Correlates of the sustainability of community-based heart health promotion interventions. Prev Med 1998;27:702-12.

33. Yin RK. Changing urban bureaucracies: how new practices become routinized. Lexington, MA: Lexington Books, 1979.

34. Shediac MC, Bone LR. Planning for the sustainability of community-based health programs: conceptual frameworks and future directions for research, practice and policy. Health Educ Res 1998;13(1):87-108.

35. Achilladelis B, Jervis P, Robertson A. A study of success and failure in industrial innovation. Sussex, England: University of Sussex Press, 1971.

36. Howell JM, Higgins CA. Champions of technological innovation. Adm Sci Q 1990;35:317-41.

37. Evashwick C, Ory M. Organizational characteristics of successful innovative health care programs sustained over time. Fam Community Health 2003;26(3):177-93.

38. Gladwin J, Dixon RA, Wilson TD. Rejection of an innovation: health information management training materials in east Africa. Health Policy Plan 2002;17(4):354-61.

39. Bossert TJ. Can they get along without us? Sustainability of donor-supported health projects in Central America and Africa. Soc Sci Med 1990;30:1015-23.

40. Chamnanmoh S. Adoption of immunization services in pharmacies [Dissertation]. Social and Administrative Sciences in Pharmacy, University of Wisconsin-Madison, 2004.

41. Savino LB. Your pharmacy and immunizations. America's Pharmacist 1998;120(7):49-53.
42. Stange KC, Goodwin MA, Zyzanzki SJ, Dietrich AK. Sustainability of a practice-individualized preventive service delivery intervention. Am J Prev Med 2003;25:296-300.
43. Teach E. Avoiding decision traps. CFO 2004;20:97-9.
44. Hammond JS, Keeney RL, Raiffa H. The hidden traps in decision making. Harvard Business Rev 2006;84:118-26.
45. March JG, Simon HA. Organizations. New York: Free Press, 1957.
46. Kahneman D, Tversky A. Prospect theory: an analysis of decision under risk. Econometrica 1979;47(2):263-92.
47. Anderson K. Making all of the right decisions. Food Manuf 1999;74:2-4.
48. Tversky A, Kahneman D. Judgment under uncertainty: heuristics and biases. Science 1974;185(4157):1124-31.
49. Silver WS, Mitchell TR. The status quo tendency in decision making. Organ Dyn 1990;18(4): 34-46.
50. Hambrick DC, Geletkanycz MA, Fredrickson JW. Top executive commitment to the status quo: some tests of its determinants. Strategic Manage J 1993;14(6):401-18.
51. Geletkanycz MA. The salience of culture's consequences: the effects of cultural values on top executive commitment to the status quo. Strategic Manage J 1995;18(8):615-34.
52. Samuelson W, Zeckhauser R. Status quo bias in decision making. J Risk Uncertainty 1998;1:7-59.
53. Schweitzer M. Multiple reference points, framing, and the status quo bias in health care financing decisions. Organ Behav Hum Decis Process 1995;63(1):69-72.
54. Nutt PC. Expanding the search for alternatives during strategic decision-making. Acad Manage Exec 2004;18(4):13-28.
55. Arkes H, Blumer C. The psychology of sunk cost. Organ Behav Hum Decis Process 1985;35: 124-140.
56. Zeelenberg M, Van Dijk E. A reverse sunk cost effect in risky decision making: sometimes we have too much invested to gamble. J Econ Psychol 1997;18:677-91.
57. Teger AL. Too much invested to quit. New York: Pergamon Press, 1980.
58. Anderson K. Decision-making traps. Broadcast Engineering 1999;41:106.
59. Anderson K. Decisions. Food Manuf 1999;74:2-4.
60. Nutt PC. Why decisions fail. San Francisco: Berrett-Koehler, 2002.
61. Nutt PC. Averting decision debacles. Technol Forecast Soc Change 2004;71:239-65.

CHAPTER 9

Prescribing Behavior

Kent E. M. Groves, PhD, CChem, Neil J. MacKinnon, PhD, FCSHP, and Ingrid Sketris, PharmD, MPA (HSA)

The factors influencing physicians'* prescribing behavior and the context or system in which they work, including medical, nonmedical, physician, and nonphysician variables, have been extensively studied by various disciplines.[1-18] Although there remain gaps in the literature, specifically in the areas relating to the interdependency between marketing activities and physician-specific characteristics, the goal in this chapter is to bring the insights from the existing body of literature together into one place. This chapter identifies the primary models that provide insight into our understanding of the variables that influence prescribing behavior. Additionally, it presents models used by the pharmaceutical industry in their development of marketing strategy to increase sales of prescription pharmaceuticals.

The traditional marketing approach, followed by the pharmaceutical industry globally, was to target efforts toward physicians (Fig. 9-1).[19] This model still exists, especially in markets in which direct-to-consumer (DTC) advertising is not permitted. Even in markets in which DTC marketing is not permitted, DTC advertising produced within the United States has a spillover or halo effect in many Western cultures through print, broadcast, and electronic media.

DTC advertising in the United States over the last 10 to 15 years has resulted in a two-pronged marketing approach. This new strategy consists of a continued focus on the physician while targeting a complementary (and concurrent) message toward

---

*Although there are many prescribers in the health professions, physicians account for the majority of prescriptions written.

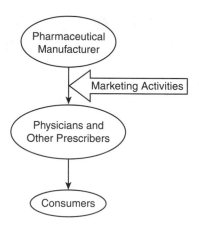

FIGURE 9-1   Traditional Pharmaceutical Industry Marketing Strategy

the consumer† (Fig. 9-2), with the objective of educating and informing the end user and, peripherally, influencing (reinforcing) the physician's interpretation of the message.[20] In markets such as the United States, the two channels are acknowledged and pursued. In other Western markets, DTC advertising is more restricted,‡ with the exception of New Zealand.[21,22]

In the European Union, brands cannot be promoted through advertising that tries to stimulate consumer–physician interaction, although providing education is permitted. A push to weaken this ban was defeated in 2004. At the time of writing this chapter, a new proposal to reform DTC advertising was in progress.[23] In the absence of a DTC-friendly regulatory environment, traditional marketing efforts may be complemented through the efforts of voluntary health agencies who may lobby to have particular drugs added to a jurisdictional formulary.

In addition to the targeted promotion shown in Figures 9-1 and 9-2, there is another level of consideration, as outlined in Figure 9-3. In this scenario, primary influences typically include physician-specific factors, and secondary influences include nonphysician characteristics, such as those individuals or groups that may influence the physician's decision.

---

†This chapter uses the term *consumer* exclusively because consumers are the end target of a marketing message. Thus, consumers may be health professionals as well as patients.

‡In Canada, drugs may be advertised to consumers, but either the name of the drug appears with no medical condition mentioned, or the medical condition appears with no drug named.[155]

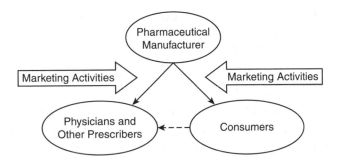

FIGURE 9-2 Pharmaceutical Industry Marketing Strategy in 2009

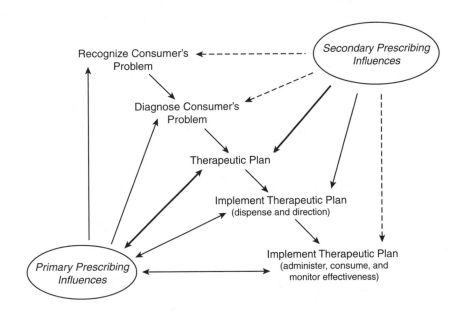

FIGURE 9-3 Flow of Influence Within the Medication Use System Model (Prescribers Decision Process)
Source: Adapted from: Hepler CD, Grainger Rousseau TJ. Pharmaceutical care versus traditional drug treatment. Is there a difference? Drugs 1995;49(1):1–10.

Understanding the extent to which primary and secondary factors influence prescribing activity is critical, because these factors, to a greater or lesser extent, predicate the defined market size for a specific product. That is, the professional identification and diagnosis of a condition, the association of that condition with a specific intervention, the development of a list of possible therapeutic options, and the subsequent selection of one intervention over another will be direct artifacts of the activities and nature of the physician population. More important, these will be a direct artifact of the success of the pharmaceutical company in reaching and influencing that group of prescribers. Ultimately, the complexity of prescribing behavior is a function of the relationship between physician variables, consumer variables, and the environment.

Although there are numerous factors that may influence a physician's prescribing behavior, the factors that influence a consumer's decision process (Fig. 9-4) regarding his or her request for use of a pharmaceutical intervention for an identified condition must also be recognized and considered. Within the context of healthcare consumers, we can see that the decision process involves recognition of a problem, which may

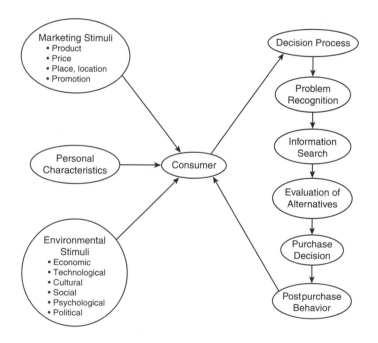

FIGURE 9-4   Consumer Decision-Making Process
Source: Adapted from: Kotler P, Armstrong G and Cunningham PH. *Principles of Marketing*, 6th Canadian Edition. Toronto: Pearson, 2005.

lead to evaluation of alternatives prior to visiting a physician, followed by a conscious decision to accept the physician's recommendation. This decision process is subsequently influenced by external stimuli as well as consumers' own characteristics.[24,25]

The consumer's role in influencing the physician is recognized, and one approach is to consider employing the traditional business-to-consumer marketing approach. Although the model in Figure 9-4 is a construct based on the consumer decision-making literature,[26-30] this direction of strategic evaluation involves another entire body of literature, one that is not directly related to the focus of this chapter—that is, developing an appropriate marketing mix within the context of the existing external stimuli to ultimately influence the consumer's decision process.

THE PHYSICIAN AS A CONSUMER

We typically think of consumers as one of two types: those who buy for their own consumption or those who buy for someone else. Marketers tend to position their messages to target one of these two types of consumers. Physicians, however, are unique in their "consumer/consumption" role in that they are neither the consumer nor the purchaser. Although they may recommend (prescribe) a product, they are not necessarily concerned or influenced by the price of the product. Their reward for the "purchase" may be vicariously provided through seeing improvements in the health of a patient (in this case, the ultimate consumer) or, in some situations, through incentives from the manufacturer or purchaser. Of course, many other factors influence this as well—for example, other reward systems such as pay for performance in some U.S. healthcare settings or budget incentives in the United Kingdom.[31]

Given the unique nature of the physician as a consumer, the marketing strategies employed in the pharmaceutical industry are in sharp contrast to those used in other markets. The primary reason for this is that in the prescription drug market, the physician is the decision maker who identifies the product category and selects a specific product from the alternatives within that category on the consumer's behalf. The most appropriate description of the physician as a consumer is that of an agency relationship, in which, in this case, the physician is the agent,[19,32-34] or advocate, for the consumer.[35] Although it is the physician who makes the decision in collaboration with the consumer, it is still the consumer who uses the product and ultimately takes responsibility for payment for the product.

Because of their role as intermediaries and key decision makers in the prescribing process, it is to be expected that physicians would become the target of marketing activities associated with prescription drugs. For years, a variety of means available to the pharmaceutical industry to communicate their message to physicians has been employed.[36,37] The metric against which the industry measures the success of its marketing effort is the volume of drugs sold, or more specifically, the number of prescriptions written by the physician. The actual writing of a prescription is thus indicative of a physician's recognition that a product is the best alternative to address the consumer's condition, and it is also the primary metric that measures prescribing behavior.

Although it is not within the scope of this chapter to discuss government or specific jurisdictional policy relative to prescribing, it needs to be recognized as an influencing variable on prescribing behavior. The primary issues of policy relate to the eligibility of patients for benefits, the comprehensiveness of prescription drug coverage (formulary listings, cost-sharing mechanisms, etc.), and the pricing of prescription drugs.

INFLUENCES ON PRESCRIBING BEHAVIOR

Given that the most intuitive measure of prescribing behavior is prescribing, we need to consider this action at its basic level, namely, the adoption of an innovation by the physician. The concepts of innovation diffusion and adoption provide insight into the nature of the prescribing metric. Three areas of consideration relative to prescribing behavior are pharmaceutical marketing activity (direct to consumer and direct to professional), the practice characteristics or the clinical profile, and the physician profile or related demographics.

Innovation Diffusion and Adoption

Given that, in the end, the question is really "to prescribe or not to prescribe," it is important to gain insight into current thought on diffusion and adoption and their role in issues related to influencing prescribing behavior. This portion of the chapter thus focuses on the adoption of new technologies in general, not specifically innovations associated with health care. Although an extensive literature review on the topic of spreading and sustaining service innovations in health service delivery organizations was authored by Greenhalgh and associates,[38] this chapter provides information more specific to the adoption of prescription drugs. A review of the adoption of technology provides insight into key variables that may be directly involved in physician adoption, or more specifically, the variables likely to influence prescribing behavior.

The first step in any discussion on diffusion and adoption is to ensure an understanding of the stages and definitions associated with this process. *Diffusion* is defined as the process by which an innovation is communicated through certain channels over time among the members of a social system.[39]

- The *innovation* is an idea, practice, or object that is perceived as new by an individual or other unit of adoption.
- *Communication* is the process by which participants create and share information with one another in order to reach a mutual understanding.
- A communication *channel* is the means by which messages get from one participant to another.
- *Time* is an important element in diffusion, because it is involved in the process by which an individual passes from first knowledge to adoption or rejection, as well as in the speed with which an innovation is adopted relative to other members of the social system.
- The *social system* is considered to be a set of interrelated units that are engaged in joint problem solving to accomplish a common goal.

Initially, adoption was studied by various research traditions. By the late 1970s, they had effectively merged. Several disciplines became integral to studying prescribing behavior, namely, marketing, public health, and medical sociology. A study commissioned by the Charles Pfizer Company established our fundamental understanding of the diffusion and adoption of new drugs by physicians.[40] Although some elements of this diffusion model have been questioned,[41] much of the initial research conducted by Coleman and colleagues remains relevant. The success of marketing managers in launching a new product is often measured by rate of adoption and retention among a target audience.

Physicians are not passive recipients of innovations. They seek them out, they experiment with them and evaluate them, they worry about them, they collaborate with peers and seek reinforcement, they modify them and attempt to adapt them to their specific circumstances, they challenge them, and they may even become emotionally attached to them. Physicians may do this in isolation or with other members of their social system. Within the context of prescribing behavior, we need to recognize that the adopter is an actor who interacts purposefully and creatively with a complex innovation[38] and plays a critical role in the diffusion of innovations, both within health service organizations and the medical community at large.

Probably two of the more important considerations for adoption, as proposed by Peay and Peay, are preparedness to prescribe the new drug and presentation of particular circumstances that are appropriate for its use.[42] An individual's preparedness to prescribe a "new" drug is an independent variable that may be predicted, depending on the physician, consumer, and environmental information available.

To appreciate the variables that may influence physician adoption, one must revisit the innovation-decision process.[39] Prior conditions required to create an environment that will lead to the physician innovation-decision process taking place include previous practice, felt needs or problems, innovativeness, the norms of the social system, and the presence of circumstances appropriate for trial. If these conditions are met, it is more likely that an individual or group will seek out knowledge, be open to persuasion, decide to initiate trial, and implement and evaluate the innovation, as described in Table 9-1.

When considering the traditional approach to adoption, one might determine that the characteristics of the adopter and the adoption environment are stable over time. Waarts and coworkers, however, suggest that the driving factors in adopting innovations will change as the diffusion of the innovation within the market progresses.[43] That is, although it is well known that different groups of adopters have different characteristics concerning the rate of adoption of innovations,[39] the factors explaining the adoption of innovations will not be stable over the diffusion process

---

TABLE 9-1   Steps in the Innovation-Decision Process

1. Knowledge (characteristics of the decision-making unit)*
   a. Socioeconomic characteristics
   b. Personality variables
   c. Communication behavior
2. Persuasion (perceived characteristics of the innovation)
   a. Relative advantage
   b. Compatibility
   c. Complexity
   d. Trialability
   e. Observability
3. Decision
   a. Adoption
   b. Rejection
4. Implementation
5. Confirmation
   a. Adoption—continued
   b. Adoption—discontinuance
   c. Rejection—continued
   d. Rejection—later adoption

*In this case, the decision-making unit is typically the physician, but may also be considered the combination of the physician and the consumer.

but will change as larger numbers of individuals adopt the innovation. Waarts and colleagues suggest that in the first stages of adoption of innovation by organizations, the most important stimulating factors are a combination of internal drivers (personal characteristics), whereas subsequent adopters are more influenced by a mix of stimulating factors focusing on practical issues.[43] This insight is supported by the marketing mix used by industry, in which combinations of direct-to-consumer, journal, and physician advertising change with the nature and "perceived innovativeness" of the drug.[44]

Another consideration in the adoption process relates to individual versus team decisions. Contrary to the traditional five steps associated with individual trial and adoption proposed by Rogers,[39] Wozniak suggests that adoption and technical acquisition decisions are made jointly by team members, and that the influences of the determinants of that decision differ with the timing of adoption and the channels of information dissemination.[45] The traditional steps may not occur successively, but different stages may need to occur concurrently to achieve maximum response. His work also concurs with earlier research with respect to differences between individuals at various stages of adoption. He indicates that early adopters find information more useful in the early stages of adoption decision process rather than in the later stages.

Olshavsky and Spreng question the individual approach to innovation evaluation.[46] The traditional marketing assumption has been that individuals faced with a new stimulus engage in some type of attribute-by-attribute evaluation, in which the interpretation of the innovation is a function of the elements or attributes of the stimulus. Olshavsky and Spreng suggest that people may be more inclined to establish evaluative criteria by placing the new stimulus into an existing category, thus simply giving the innovation the same evaluation that they give other category members. This suggests that not all innovations are adopted using an attribute approach as suggested in Rogers' step 2, "persuasion (perceived characteristics of the innovation)" (Table 9-1). Olshavsky and Spreng suggest that there are four other processes influencing evaluation: forming evaluative criteria, forming expectation about the innovation concept, assessing satisfaction with an old product, and comparing the new and the old products.

An intuitive consideration in adoption is that early adopters are more likely to adopt, and consequently, that early prescribers are more likely to prescribe. Health research in this area has been limited.[47] Shih and Venkatesh found that adopters with higher use-diffusion levels (i.e., those who use a newly adopted product more often and in a greater variety of ways) are not only more satisfied with the current innovation but also are more interested in adopting future innovations.[48] Marinova determined that innovation effort takes shape over time under two opposing forces: market knowledge diffusion ("How will I use this product in the future?"), which propels innovation, and satisfaction with past performance ("I am content and am not interested in new applications or innovations"), which hinders innovation.[49] This, in turn, may affect adoption of "perceived similar" products within a product category.

If intention to engage in a behavior predicts the behavior, preparedness to prescribe a new drug, as proposed by Peay and Peay, thus becomes a critical step in the process leading to actually prescribing.[42] A number of behavioral variables may influence the likelihood of prescribing. These may include, among others, individual prescribing habits, the size of the practice, the location of the practice, and the nature of an individual's social groups. The role of collective behavior on individual adoption[50] and the role of social networks on diffusion and adoption[51] are recognized.

Often it is the multiple interactions that arise in various settings that determine the success or failure of an innovation and its subsequent dissemination. Different product markets may exhibit different adoption characteristics, thus affecting the extrapolation of insights regarding the relationships between products and markets.

Pharmaceutical Marketing Activity

Manufacturers must determine how to strategically present new drugs to target audiences. New product success is dependent on many variables, some that they can control (promotion, price, channels of distribution, etc.) and some that they cannot control (regulation, scientific evaluation leading to publication, independent third-party reviews, etc.). Additionally, success of the new drug depends on the nature of the prescribing physicians (primary influences) and whether they will perceive the new product as a radically differentiated offering (discontinuous innovation) or as a minor variation of existing functionalities (dynamically continuous innovation).[46,52,53] These primary influences are identified within the context of the environment in which the physician practices or may relate to the characteristics of the physicians themselves.

The relationship between a physician and a patient has some differences (e.g., professional codes of conduct) but also some similarities to the relationship that exists between a variety of suppliers and customers in any given market. Marketing has shifted much of its dominant logic away from the exchange of tangible goods and toward the exchange of intangibles (specialized skills and knowledge) and processes.[54] This, in effect, moves marketing toward a more inclusive dominant logic, one that integrates goods with services and provides a broader foundation for the development of marketing theory. Scharitzer and Kollarits suggest that the level of satisfaction expressed between physicians and pharmaceutical sales representatives (personal and professional compatibility) influences the subsequent prescribing behavior of the former.[55]

Direct-to-Physician Marketing

It seems intuitive to suggest that the probability of prescribing a drug is a function of the marketing effort expended on that particular product. This marketing effort may be more specifically defined as corporate or academic detailing (a core of individuals who visit physicians' offices) and the associated drug "trial samples," as well as other commercial sources of information to promote a particular drug. The use of free drug samples is a long-standing industry practice[56] and has been demonstrated to be an excellent way to introduce new products or dislodge a market leader.[57] The two categories of detailing and product sampling are complementary and together typically account for over 80% of total drug promotional expenditures.[44,58]

Although there is some disagreement on the impact that drug promotion has on adoption (some physicians go so far as to suggest that they are not influenced by pharmaceutical marketing, but they believe that their colleagues are influenced[59]), if a particular promotional tactic does not work, the pharmaceutical industry would most likely discontinue its use. Hawkins and Hoch suggest that low-involvement processing leads to poorer memory, but greater belief.[60] That is, the less time individuals spend thinking about a given point or observation, the more likely they are to consider it true; however, they may be less likely to remember it. This work is supported in part by Prosser and associates, who defined general practitioners as largely reactive recipients, rather than active searchers of new drug information, who in many instances relied heavily on the pharmaceutical industry as their major information source.[61]

Given the pharmaceutical industry's approach to its market (brief, frequent visits), we now start to gain insight into why physicians believe that they are not influenced by the marketing activities of industry, even though research would tell us otherwise.[62,63] Watkins and coworkers assert that general practitioners who receive information and visits from the pharmaceutical industry are responsible for higher prescribing costs and prescribe in a less rational manner than their peers who function without direct pharmaceutical industry influence.[64] Additionally, Muijrers and associates found a negative relationship between prescribing according to evidence-based general practical guidelines and the frequency of visits by pharmaceutical sales representatives.[65]

An extension of the physician's perceived resilience or imperviousness to advertising is the consensus among both high- and low-prescribing populations of physicians that they like to prescribe drugs with which they are familiar, which means that there may be some reluctance to prescribe new medications.[66] When considering the definition and application of the word *familiar*, we know that brand names have greater impact on choice in situations where minimal quality information is available on product alternatives.[67] That is, when choosing between two similar products, the familiar brand name is often considered when less qualitative information is available for the comparator. This, in turn, can have a significant impact on usage (prescription) when that brand name is associated with a pioneer or first-to-market-in-category product.[68] Leffler suggested that brand loyalty may result from the high costs of acquiring new information or of learning by experience and subsequently may generate persistence in prescribing patterns, thus influencing physician responsiveness to promotional efforts.[69]

There is support for the relationship between physicians' satisfaction with their pharmaceutical sales representatives and their prescribing behavior,[55] and for the influence of drug company representatives through product information dissemination.[70] Work by Watkins and colleagues suggested that frequent contact with a drug representative was significantly associated with a greater willingness to prescribe new drugs and to agree to consumers' requests for drugs that may not be clinically indicated.[71] Additionally, promotional impact should not be limited to the perception that a manufacturer is simply communicating its message. Although publication of new evidence may be associated with modest changes in individual practice, industry-led promotional activity appears to have a greater influence on the adoption of this new evidence.[72]

Changes in prescribing behavior are not simply a function of the marketing or advertising dollars spent, but more a function of the message and the target audience. Kerr and associates noted that the increase in prescribing cyclooxygenase-2 (COX-2) inhibitors in Australia coincided with a period of energetic marketing to the medical profession, which promoted the message that the new drugs were "safer" than traditional nonsteroidal anti-inflammatory drugs (NSAIDs).[73] Additionally, retrospective work by Van den Bulte[41] on the original study done by Coleman[40] with respect to the medical community's understanding of tetracycline suggests that it was through aggressive marketing efforts targeted at the physician population, and not social contagion, that this product gained in popularity and application.

With the exception of work by Mizik and associates, limited academic literature documents the efficiency of marketing directly to physicians through detailing. Mizik and coworkers quantified the impact of detailing, and determined that detailing and free drug samples have a modest influence on the number of new prescriptions issued by a physician.[74] Interestingly, this impact is only significant when one considers the lagged effect (future response resulting from a current action). That is, immediate impact is less significant than future impact. Mizik and colleagues demonstrated the residual impact of marketing activity 6 months after the fact, but other studies have demonstrated a persistent effect on product sales for more than 12 months.[75]

Gonul and coworkers, interpreting feedback from a panel of physicians, found that a certain level of detailing positively influences prescribing, but that excessive detailing becomes counterproductive.[76] Their work is supported by the work of Manchanda and Chintagunta, who demonstrated that there are optimal levels of marketing, after which incremental increases are negatively elastic.[77] That is, the percentage increase in prescribing declines relative to a similar percentage increase in marketing expenditure.

When pursued by governments, hospitals, and health management organizations, detailing is referred to as academic detailing. Although this form of detailing has been shown to be a very effective technique to encourage adoption of clinical practice guidelines,[78-82] its widespread use is less likely because it is expensive[83] and, as noted by Mizik and others,[74,84,85] physicians are not always receptive to this approach.

Although a positive impact of product detailing, free drug samples, and journal advertising on the prescribing of drugs has been found, it is often difficult to quantify, because their activity is not mutually exclusive. Jones and associates found no clear relationship between the extent of drug advertising and the amount of prescribing by general practitioners[86] and suggested that although advertising in journals is one of many factors that influence general practitioners to prescribe, it is probably not a major influence. Interestingly, there is very little work discussing the impact of drug samples independent of the pharmaceutical representative. Schumock and colleagues made an attempt to quantify this, and their results suggested that free samples influenced prescribing decisions, but that the information disseminated by pharmaceutical sales representatives had no significant impact. It would seem that it is difficult to separate one from the other,[87] and the covariance, or relationship, between the two cannot be discounted.

Although it may be difficult to separate journal advertising from the marketing mix and relate it to response, it is an element of the pharmaceutical industry's approach to the market and probably needs to be evaluated concurrently with total marketing spending versus sales (prescriptions). Majumdar and coworkers suggested that new evidence published in peer-reviewed journals is associated with modest changes in clinical practice but that more active promotional strategies are required to accelerate the adoption of new evidence in routine clinical practice.[72] The use of active promotional strategies was supported in earlier work by Hurwitz and Caves, who demonstrated that promotional outlays by market entrants contribute to expanding their market share, but that price discounts have only a weak short-run effect on entrants' market share.[88] Additionally, the predictable decline in promotional expenditure that is linked to an impending loss of patent status has been associated with a decline in prescriptions.[89] In general, all pharmaceutical marketing activities have been documented to have some effect on prescribing behavior, but detailing has been found to be particularly effective.

Direct-to-Consumer Marketing

Although DTC advertising may be perceived as being a U.S. phenomenon, the reality is that there is extensive overlap of the media and images of U.S.-targeted DTC advertising on Western consumers, and subsequently on their physicians' prescribing decision. One of the few studies that determined the impact of U.S. DTC advertising outside of the United States found that in Vancouver, Canada, 87.4% of consumers in the study had actually seen U.S. prescription drug advertisements.[90]

Physicians often state that they are not influenced by any form of targeted marketing,[62,91] be it pharmaceutical representatives, journal advertisements, or consumers themselves. Despite this, there has been much written about the marketing efficiency of DTC advertising and its subsequent impact on prescribing behavior through the medium of the consumer who makes a direct brand or product category request to his or her physician.[92] Even prior to the advent of DTC advertising, physicians indicated that one of the most common reasons for the use of many medications was consumer demand.[93]

In 1997, the Food and Drug Administration (FDA) in the United States loosened the regulations associated with DTC advertising. Annual spending on DTC advertising for prescription drugs tripled between 1996 and 2000, when it reached nearly $2.5 billion.[58] By 2004, this figure had exceeded $4 billion.[94] Despite the increase from less than $500 million in 1995, DTC advertising still accounts for less than 15% of the total pharmaceutical marketing spending; the majority of pharmaceutical spending in this category continues to be targeted at the physician, indicating that the industry still recognizes that physician-targeted activity has more impact.

Initially, it was unclear what impact advertising targeted directly at the consumer would have. In 1998, shortly after the advertising regulations changed, Peyrot and associates performed a random telephone survey of 440 central Maryland residents in an effort to determine prescription drug knowledge and drug-requesting behavior.[95] Their study suggested that although DTC advertising had an effect on drug requesting, it was unclear whether requesting led to changes in prescribing behavior. This work was supported in part by that of Mehta and Purvis, who determined that a broad range of individuals value DTC advertising, but also determined that there was some variance among demographics (age, education, gender) with respect to comprehension, agreement with the message, and the expected impact of the message on the individual's anticipated exchange with his or her physician.[96]

Zachry and colleagues took the approach of using a time series design to analyze specific products advertised from January 1992 to December 1997.[97] Their results suggested that the DTC advertising expenditure was associated with physician diagnosing and physician prescribing only for certain drugs and drug classes. However, even when a statistically significant association was found, DTC advertising was deemed to account for only a modest amount of the variance associated with diagnosing and prescribing. They note that the relationship between DTC advertising and physician prescribing and diagnosing is a complex one that is not well understood.

Vogel and coworkers assessed the effects of DTC advertising on the pharmaceutical industry's approach to marketing in the United States using economic models.[98] Although their models suggest that DTC advertising affects the price and quantity demanded of pharmaceutical products indirectly via its effect on changes in consumer demand, they gained little insight into the impact the pharmaceutical industry's approach to marketing has on prescribing trends.

Rosenthal and associates measured the impact of DTC advertising on market share within a therapeutic class, as well as on an entire therapeutic class, which is effectively a multistage budgeting structure.[20] They examined monthly data from August 1996 to December 1999 for five therapeutic classes, including all the drugs in each class. Their results suggest an average advertising elasticity of 0.1, in which one would realize a 1% increase in sales following a 10% increase in DTC spending, with variation between drug classes.

Mintzes and colleagues linked DTC advertising to increased prescribing.[90] They surveyed a split population of physicians and their consumers, with one study taking place in Vancouver, Canada, and the other in Sacramento, California. Although consumers in both markets reported seeing DTC advertising, Sacramento consumers reported more advertising exposure and requested more advertised drugs than consumers in Vancouver; in both settings, however, consumers with higher exposure to advertising requested more advertised drugs. Consumers with higher self-reported exposure to advertising had conditions that were potentially treatable by advertised drugs and/or had greater reliance on advertising and subsequently requested more advertised medicines. The results of this study suggest that more advertising leads to more requests for advertised medicines, and ultimately to more prescriptions. This study corroborates work by Donohue and associates, whose research on the effects of DTC advertising suggested that not only was DTC advertising of antidepressants associated with an increase in the number of people diagnosed with depression, but also was associated with an increase in the number who initiated medication therapy.[99]

In summary, the weight of evidence in the United States suggests that DTC advertising has a primary impact on the consumer, followed by a secondary influence on the physician and his or her prescribing behavior.

Practice Characteristics: Clinical Profile

This section considers those elements of a physician's practice that relate to consumer demographics, the physical location of the practice, and the nature of the practice (sole practitioner or multiple-practitioner clinic) and their subsequent influence on prescribing behavior.

Consumer Profile and Demographics

Stevenson and colleagues indicated that in interviews with 21 general practitioners (GPs) in the Birmingham Health Authority, 100% of the respondents believed they had experienced pressure for a prescription from consumers, and all indicated that they had prescribed when they would not have otherwise done so.[100]

Britten and associates considered the variables that influence consumers with respect to their attitudes toward medicines and their expectations for a prescription.[101] The study took place in south London, England, and surveyed 544 consumers waiting in GPs' offices. Because they were in England, the influence of DTC advertising was likely limited. The primary factors influencing consumers' expectations for a prescription were determined to be as follows:

1. Demographic variables, which included gender, age, marital status, period of time at the same address, age leaving school, ethnic group, employment status, and prescription status (extent of coverage)
2. Organizational variables, which included day of the week and appointment status
3. Illness variables, including symptoms, reason for the visit, and self-medication
4. Attitudes toward medicine, as measured by individuals' level of agreement with a variety of statements about medicines and their role in health and wellness

Unlike Britten and colleagues, Mamdani and coworkers suggested that demographics, particularly age and household income, did not play a role in consumer expectations, but did appear to influence physician prescribing.[102] This study determined that physicians in the province of Ontario, Canada, practicing in low-income neighborhoods were more likely to prescribe lower-priced generic drugs for their elderly consumers, regardless of the consumers' drug coverage. This work is consistent with research by Soumerai and associates on the impact of copayments among lower-income populations[103] and by Tamblyn and associates on the impact of cost sharing among elderly persons and welfare recipients.[104] In both studies, cost sharing contributed to a decrease in the use of essential drugs.

Stewart and colleagues in the Netherlands assessed the effects of general practitioner and consumer characteristics on prescribing behavior.[105] They measured adherence to the global World Health Organization (WHO) pharmacotherapeutic guide-lines[106] in combination with Barber's good prescribing guidelines.[25] The study of 251 general practitioners from 190 practices suggested that adherence to prescribing guidelines (effectively, factors influencing prescribing behavior) were influenced by two sets of variables: practice characteristics and consumer characteristics. Consumer characteristics were either directly related to the consumer or were aggregated to a categorized consumer level. Directly related variables of age and gender were shown to influence adherence to prescribing guidelines, whereas the aggregated variables of mean costs, mean volume, and different WHO anatomic, therapeutic, and chemical classifications of drugs (effectively, variance in drug selection for given conditions) were shown to influence prescribing.

Bradley suggested that consumer factors such as age, ethnicity, social class, and education influence prescribing; however, factors that are equally important are the physician's prior knowledge of the consumer, the physician's feelings toward the con-sumer, communication problems, and the doctor's desire to try to preserve the doctor–consumer relationship.[107] Additional work by Bradley[15] and by McKinlay and associates,[108] while recognizing the many considerations (including medical, social, and logistic) that influence the decision to prescribe in general practice, notes that prescribing depends on the complex interaction of many disparate influences.

Bennett and coworkers focused on the variables that might influence the likeli-hood of switching a consumer from one drug to another.[109] Their work focused on switching consumers from nonselective to newer selective NSAIDs. A surprisingly low percentage (17%) of incumbent nonselective NSAID users were switched to selective NSAIDS or COX-2 inhibitors. Older female consumers were more likely to be switched from nonselective NSAIDs to COX-2 inhibitors, but one of the reasons may be that physicians believe women are more prone to gastrointestinal toxicity.

Tamblyn and colleagues suggested that a high proportion of elderly patients in a practice was associated with a greater likelihood of prescribing any new drug, but at the same time, there was a lower rate of new drug utilization among members of this cohort with multiple prescriptions.[110] Again, although it may seem intuitive that the consumer's age might influence prescribing, this influence may simply be a function of the consumer's current drug regimen, and subsequently it is just as likely to influ-ence more prescribing as it is to influence less prescribing.

Another demographic variable, education, may have some influence on pre-scribing, but this has not been tested. Mehta and Purvis did, however, determine that individuals with advanced education are more open to new approaches to health care, and most likely have insight and interest in new drugs,[96] but it is unknown whether this converts into a change in prescribing.

In summary, although there is a large amount of research that supports the impact of consumer demographics on physician prescribing, the results are inconsistent and seem to reinforce the requirement that geographic variables be taken into consideration. That is, extrapolations between similar populations in different geographic areas may be less representative than previously thought, and the inconsistency in influence simply reinforces the need for geographic-specific (and geodemographic-specific) analysis.

Location of Practice

Following consumer demographics, the second practice consideration has to do with how the population influences the practice. One example of population influence that has been studied is whether practices are in a rural or urban setting. This location in turn may have an impact on a variety of factors, including the characteristics of the physicians and the consumers, relative access to new information and continuing medical education, and possibly the extent of contact with industry representatives. Another issue with respect to rural practitioners is their individual profiles and those of their practices. Rural physicians tend to be older and more likely to be male than their urban counterparts.[18,111,112] Additionally, the consumer profile of the rural practice tends to be more elderly than that of the urban practice. These variances may in turn have an effect on prescribing given the influence of consumer age and physician gender on prescribing.

Tamblyn and associates' research indicated that new drug utilization was lower among generalists and specialists practicing in rural Quebec, and suggested that this may be a function of the characteristics of physicians who elect to practice in rural areas, their isolation from the influence of peers and colleagues, or possibly the reduced frequency of visits from pharmaceutical marketing representatives.[110] One deficiency with this observation, however, relates to what is defined as rural and urban. Tamblyn and coworkers indicated that Quebec uses "tarification" territories, which are classified as remote, rural and urban, to establish levels of physician remuneration. Unfortunately, these territories are not further defined by population density.

Stewart and colleagues defined rural practices as physicians operating in an area with a population density of fewer than 1,500 addresses per square kilometer, and urban as those with more than 1,500 addresses per square kilometer.[105] Although this work suggested that the location of the practice was significant with respect to adherence with prescribing best practices, the investigators did not indicate the extent to which physicians in rural or urban practices were likely to prescribe.

Rural practitioners in Australia (obtained from a defined database of the rural workforce agency) felt that their remoteness and the remoteness of their consumers had an influence on their prescribing activities.[111] The work of Cutts and Tett further suggested that for the 142 responding doctors practicing in rural Queensland (55% survey response rate), the propensity to prescribe a new drug was inversely proportional to the amount of monitoring required of the consumer following prescription. In general, rural physicians in this study had prescribed fewer new medicines than their urban counterparts, but again we have a similar problem with the definition of *rural*. In another paper, Cutts and Tett suggested that prescribing of recently marketed drugs was more likely by doctors practicing in less remote rural areas.[113]

Nature of Practice

There are many considerations related to the nature of the practice. These include organizational factors (whether the practice is solo or group), access to other health professionals (e.g., nurse practitioners), types of information technology available, and types of patients in the practice (e.g., number and types of diseases, socioeconomic status). The organizational factor relates to the opportunity the physician has to interact with other practitioners, and also addresses the influence of knowledge opinion leaders on prescribing behavior. This is not to say that sole practitioners do not interact with their peers, but merely suggests that there is a greater opportunity for informal interaction among individuals working in the same clinic.

Practice Size: Number of Consumers

Although it may seem intuitive, the frequency of opportunities available to prescribe a new drug influences whether it can be adopted into practice and used. As Peay and Peay suggest, in order for a drug to be prescribed, the doctor must be prepared to use it, and the treatment situation must be appropriate for its use.[42] Effectively, the presence of more consumers likely to benefit from a specific drug in a physician's practice increases the likelihood of drug trial.

The increase in the number of situations available in which to prescribe a given drug influences the likelihood of trial. However, as the number of drugs introduced into a given consumer's regimen increases, the likelihood of prescribing a new drug into that consumer's mix decreases. Tamblyn and coworkers suggest that one explanation may be a function of the physician's lack of confidence and understanding of comorbidity and contraindications between multiple interventions.[110] Interestingly, Redelmeier and colleagues suggested that there is an inverse correlation between the presence of a chronic disease and the likelihood of treatment of an unrelated disorder.[114] Howlett and associates suggested that although effective medical treatment is not likely withheld, depending on physician specialty there may be varying degrees of adoption of new interventions for specific conditions (in this case, congestive heart failure).[115]

The presence in a physician's consumer population of health conditions for which a given drug is recommended is likely to have an influence on trial of that drug. The experience from this initial trial will have a significant effect on continued use (adoption) or, conversely, discontinued use (relinquishment) of a drug. This was supported by work by Buban and colleagues, who suggested that, in the case of new agents to treat cancer, one of the most significant influences on the adoption of paclitaxel was physician experience with paclitaxel to treat late-stage breast cancer.[116] Buban and coworkers also suggested that perceptions of the relative advantages of a new drug are formed through individual experience with the drug and through interactions with other practitioners.

Practice Size: Number of Physicians

Although drug trial resulting from interaction was supported through early research by Coleman and colleagues,[117] as mentioned previously, the implications of this study were subsequently questioned by Van den Bulte and associates, who suggested that the social influence was overstated and that it was more than likely simply aggressive marketing that let to the rapid adoption of tetracycline.[41] Despite this work by Van den Bulte and colleagues, the fact that people act in accordance with a frame of reference produced by the groups to which they belong is a long-accepted premise and is supported throughout the literature.[118] Peers and individuals from the physician's normative social group have influence, as supported by Ajzen's work on planned behavior.[119] Although improving prescribing requires physician education, the types of educational interventions and continuing professional development that are most effective is still being determined.[120,121]

Steffensen and coworkers determined that although physicians in single-person practices and those in partnerships both adopted new drugs, the median time for adoption (as defined by their first prescription) in partnership practices was 10 days (mean = 41), whereas in single-person practices it was 52 days (mean = 119).[122] With partnership practices adopting new drugs faster, Steffensen and his team concluded that continuous professional stimulation and other social factors are responsible for the accelerated adoption. These findings were supported by Dybdahl and colleagues, who reduced the number of independent variables and also found that larger practice size had a positive influence on adoption time, with partnership practices demonstrating the most rapid rate of new product adoption.[47]

The rate of relinquishment of trial if initial observations are less than favorable may also be influenced by practice size. Cranney and colleagues surveyed 76 physicians in an attempt to determine why GPs do not implement evidence-based guidelines.[123] Although their work suggested that solo GPs were enthusiastic about peer-based continuing medical education because it provided them with the peer interaction they lacked, this study was qualitative, lacked an adequate sample size, and was not really representative. Interestingly, Peay and Peay suggested earlier that the inclination to innovate is not related to the number of other doctors with whom the doctor practices, but is more likely to be influenced by commercial advertising.[42] Prosser and associates supported both the work of Peay and Cranney and demonstrated that prescribing of new drugs is related to the mode of exposure to pharmacologic information, the social influences on decision making, risk perception, frequency of pharmaceutical representative visits, and individual experience with the drug.[61,124]

In Finland, a government-sponsored program aimed at changing clinical practice to enhance rational prescribing has proven to be effective when using GPs as facilitators of their continuing medical education programs, and results at the local level have suggested that critical thinking and willingness to consider change of practice have been achieved.[125] This approach has been subsequently supported through research by Maue and colleagues suggesting that implementation strategies that utilize well-respected physician champions (key opinion leaders, educational influencers) in the practice sites may improve guideline compliance,[126] and by Cutts and Tett, who identified factors such as access to continuing medical education and specialists as having an influence on prescribing.[113]

There is a greater possibility of seeing or hearing about new products if there is more than one individual in an office or peer group or if the physician regularly interacts with peers and opinion leaders through other associations. This interaction is also an opportunity for professional development, as suggested by Pearson and colleagues in their study of interns,[127] by which every prescription charted is an opportunity for learning and subsequently influences their development as effective practitioners. This notion of practical application and trial to establish prescribing and therapeutic insight is supported by the steps in adoption and by the work of Jones and colleagues, who found that the progression from first use to regular use is an important step in the drug innovation process.[70]

Previous experience with a drug that has resulted in a positive or favorable outcome may lead to a less than thorough investigation of the consumer's condition and evaluation of other options available to treat a consumer prior to prescribing. Denig and coworkers' in-depth interviews with 61 general practitioners determined that fully 40% made recommendations out of habit, without undertaking any specific contemplation of the consumer's condition.[128] Schwartz and associates also noted that prescribers asserted that their own clinical experience indicated that these drugs were actually the therapies of choice in the conditions presented, despite contrary research evidence.[93] Physicians may remain with their previous prescribing patterns as defined by habit and experience in spite of new literature suggesting other alternatives.

Allery and associates considered physician characteristics from the perspective of changing their practice. In a study of 50 general practitioners, they found that organizational factors, education, and contact with professionals were influential in changing their clinical practices.[129] The weakness of this study is that the aforementioned variables account for less than 50% of the changes in clinical behavior. Additionally, the small sample size and the large number of independent variables make it difficult to confidently measure the influence of professional contact.

Landon and colleagues suggested that physicians in solo and two-person practices appear to have a more aggressive treatment style than those physicians in group practices.[130] Although the definition of *aggressive* is associated with the propensity to request clinical tests, there is no indication that this activity is causal to prescribing. Additionally, this study is limited by the use of physician-reported behavior based on vignettes rather than measures of actual clinical decisions. A similar observation was made by O'Neill and Kuder, who noted that being in a solo practice had a greater association with the ordering of services (tests);[131] however, as with Landon and colleagues, it was not indicated whether this was associated with actual prescribing.

Ashworth and colleagues considered physician motivation to change within the context of GPs who had joined a general practice covering a geographic locality in south London.[132] Within the context of the United Kingdom's Primary Care Commissioning Group structure, it appears that one of the lead motivators for change was related to a collectivist (team) perspective among GPs who are prepared to consider the prescribing implications for their fellow GPs. Contrary to Ashworth, however, Simon and associates demonstrated that both group and individual academic detailing improved antihypertensive prescribing over and above usual care,[81] and Watkins and colleagues suggested that the effects of interventions in larger practices appear to be less significant given the logistics of getting all the physicians together at one time.[84]

Although it seems logical that general practitioners who have access to an informal peer network may be more likely to prescribe new interventions, the opposite may also be true. That is, informal feedback from peers may result in a tendency to decrease their levels of prescribing. Research by Watkins and coworkers has suggested that there may be a greater tendency to prescribe innovations among sole practitioners practicing in markets of individuals with low income, with minimal academic detailing.[64] This insight was supported in part by Peay and Peay, who determined that the number of other doctors with whom a doctor practices was not a significant predictor of innovativeness.[42] Carthy and associates suggested that some physicians did not consult with their colleagues because they were either confident in their own decisions or did not want to subject themselves to potential criticism.[133]

Outside of the influence of colleagues in a practice environment is the issue of the influence of individuals in peer groups—colleagues operating in different clinics, markets, or environments—as well as opinion leaders whose experience and insight is respected and deemed relevant. Soumerai and colleagues suggest that working with opinion leaders and providing performance feedback can accelerate the adoption of some alternative acute myocardial infarction (AMI) therapies.[134] This suggests that local physicians have the potential to be influenced by local peers and opinion leaders. The weakness of this study, however, was the inability to control for a variety of other factors that might have led to the adoption of the alternative AMI therapies. Soumerai and colleagues' proposal on the influence of local opinion leaders was supported by Sbarbaro.[4] While Sbarbaro suggested that the endorsement of national professional guidelines by local opinion leaders may have a positive influence on the impact of professional guidelines, it may also be effective to provide performance feedback comparing the physician's results to peers.

Hepler reinforced the value of the opinion leader among health professionals by suggesting that physicians tend to value autonomy and being socially powerful.[8] To this end, institutional pharmacists are well advised to seek out opinion leaders who have power and know how to use it. Having the support of such an individual can increase the ability to influence appropriate drug use (prescribing behavior) within a physician population.[8]

Physician Profile

The final area within the context of practice characteristics relates to a number of physician-dependent factors. This area has always been recognized as playing a role in the likelihood of a physician prescribing a particular product, given a specific condition. An extensive review of physician influences by Hemminki categorized influencing variables as education, advertising, colleagues, regulations and control measures, societal and consumer demands, and doctor characteristics.[135] Although there are a number of areas of influence, this chapter considers only the areas of gender, age, training and background, and experience.

Gender

Although there is very little in the literature that considers the influence of gender on prescribing, there are also relatively few studies that have been conducted in the area of consumer behavior on gender differences.[136] Most research in this area tends to focus on the female (or collective) consumer because of such consumers' significant purchasing power, and in the case of some of the benchmark studies on consumer styles and decision making, the influence of gender on the consumer decision-making process is not even weighted.[137,138] Thus, the research in this area is inconclusive and often contradictory. Although the challenge is to determine the influence of gender on prescribing, when considering the physician as a consumer we must recognize that men and women want different products and are likely to have different ways of thinking about obtaining them.

A review of the consumer behavior literature[139-141] identifies men as more independent, confident, competitive, externally motivated, and willing to take risks. A study of 358 male and female shoppers between the ages of 18 and 44 further suggests that men use more information and communication technology products than women and show a greater interest in these products.[136] Even though the age profile in this study is not truly reflective of the physician population, this observation suggests that we might anticipate a greater propensity among male physicians to have an interest in new technology (new medications) and, subsequently, the prescribing of new drugs.

Tamblyn and associates found that male general practitioners had higher rates of new drug use than women, but this trend was not significant after adjusting for other physician and practice characteristics such as year of graduation and the profile of the consumers in their practice.[110] This pattern, although not significant, relates to work by Mitchell and Walsh that suggests that male physicians are more confident than female physicians in initiating new medical treatments[136] and to work by Groves indicating a greater propensity among men to prescribe COX-2s relative to their female counterparts.[18]

Work by Steffensen and colleagues concurs with Tamblyn and coworkers' research and suggests that there is an association between late adoption and the independent variables of female gender, smaller practice, low diagnostic activity per consumer, and a general restrictive attitude toward pharmacotherapy.[122] Although this study was qualitative, and as such did not have the ability to test for these variables independently, it does suggest that the characteristics of the "light" prescriber (i.e., a physician who issues fewer prescriptions per patient visit than the general physician population) tend to fit into the conservative physician typology.

Inman and Pearce divided a sample of physicians involved in the United Kingdom's prescription event monitoring scheme into six segments, defined by the relative values of prescriptions of new drugs issued per consumer over a 7-year period, commencing in 1984.[142] From an initial sample of over 28,000 physicians, they selected representative subsets from each segment. Their results suggest that female gender was strongly associated with the likelihood of not prescribing, or of prescribing less than their male colleagues. Although this is significant, given the low relative prescribing ratios, the logic here suggests that women may have more part-time practices and spend more time with their patients. Subsequently, they have less propensity to test new drugs and have less time to do so. The propensity to not prescribe was also supported through research by Duetz and associates, who found that female physicians were more inclined to discontinue antihypertensive drug therapy than their male counterparts.[143]

Thus, although we seem to have a trend, none of the studies has conclusively developed a relationship between gender and prescribing. Additionally, the research in this area does not appear to identify gender as a primary focus but as an artifact that was identified following testing against previously defined primary hypotheses.

Age

In consideration of the influence of age, sociologists, psychologists, and marketers have done much to document the resistance to change common among the elderly.[144] The combined observations from the literature are best summarized with the recognition that the older the consumer, the more negative the view toward technology, and the lower the use of various technologies (including new prescription drugs).

Although Peay and Peay's work demonstrates a level of agreement with the consumer literature and suggests that age was significant in predicting innovativeness in high-risk therapy, it also suggests that the results are not stable when controlling for specialty or a specific drug.[42] Despite this, they did suggest that older doctors are less innovative than younger ones. Hemminki summarized the influence of age with the suggestion that more appropriate prescribers were younger, more cosmopolitan, and modern,[135] albeit the definition of *appropriate* is subjective and is not necessarily reflective of the degree of adoption. This observation is supported by the work of Lacy and colleagues, who determined that older physicians prescribed proton pump inhibitors more often than younger physicians for mild or intermittent gastroesophageal reflux disease, without really giving consideration to nonprescription solutions.[145]

The work of Steffensen and colleagues supported the commonly held belief that rate of adoption is a function of physician characteristics, but suggested that the rate of adoption may be influenced by the drug's characteristics as well.[122] Within this context, they identified several physician variables that may influence prescribing (gender was mentioned earlier), including age. In this case, physicians older than 50 years were more likely to be categorized as late prescribers (although the validity of these results may be questionable due to the small sample size). Freiman's work supported this proposal by demonstrating that the likelihood of prescribing a new drug decreases as the physician ages.[146]

Although Tamblyn and coworkers did not specifically measure for age, they did consider year of graduation from medical school, which may be considered as a relative age variable.[110] Given this, their results suggested that year of graduation had no influence on rates of adoption among general practitioners. Using a similar approach to Tamblyn and associates, the work of Helin-Salmivaara and colleagues on the adoption of COX-2s demonstrated that the clinical experience of the physician, measured as the number of years since graduation, had no significant effect on adoption.[147] Although age may play a role in prescribing behavior, research has been unable to consistently establish the extent of its influence. Thus, age is probably best considered a factor influencing prescribing on a situation-by-situation basis.

Training, Background, and Experience

Hemminki's review of the literature on the influence of education on drug prescribing led her to conclude that education positively influences the quality of prescribing.[135] Quality of prescribing, however, is subjective with respect to the level of prescribing, and as a result means little in our attempt to measure educational influence on prescribing. Work by Landon and associates suggested that there is no evidence of a consistent practice style across general practitioners when presented with representative clinical scenarios.[130] This was supported through research by Tamayo-Sarver and colleagues with emergency physicians and the study of their prescribing practices for opioids, which noted that although some physicians tended to interpret information provided in similar ways across conditions, they could not find any physician or practice characteristics that were significantly associated with physician responses.[148]

In effect, Hemminki's review of the literature (pre-1975) simply suggested that there was no significant difference in prescribing among doctors graduating from different medical schools. This observation is supported in part by Tamblyn and colleagues, whose physician sample was representative of four medical schools in Quebec.[110] Her results demonstrated no variance between the traditional schools. However, the school that uses a problem-oriented medical curriculum has demonstrated higher relative prescribing rates of new drugs versus those using the traditional curriculum format.

Although Tamblyn and colleagues have suggested that the type of educational format offered by the medical school may influence prescribing, they also demonstrated that specialists had higher relative rates of drug utilization than general practitioners. Helin-Salmivaara and colleagues suggested that this early adoption and more frequent utilization of drugs may be related to the concept that prescribing a new drug may enhance reputation better than prescribing an older drug.[147]

The dynamics of a physician's practice may be correlated to physician age and experience, and as such may be interchangeable. As their practice becomes more stable or predictable and physicians become more familiar with their patients and their specific conditions, the physicians may become more risk averse and less inclined to try new drugs or interventions with which they do not have much experience. Contrary to this logic, however, is the acknowledgment that familiarity may lead to the desire to try alternative products among that portion of a physician's patient population that has not responded to traditional treatments. Work by Armstrong and associates suggested that behavior change follows a dramatic or conflictual clinical event (e.g., a product doesn't work),[149] whereas Bennett and colleagues suggested that physicians with a patient's history (experience and knowledge of the patient's health and drug regimen over time) are more likely to switch patients to new drugs, particularly if they have personal experience or insight into the results associated with previously prescribed interventions.[109]

This latter body of research ties in with the notion that when physicians know what works for them, they are less likely to actively consider all possible alternatives and are likely to go with the familiar, given that the effect on patients' health outcomes is likely to be similar.[133,150,151] Conversely, when an intervention isn't working in their own trials, they are more likely to seek out new alternatives.

SUMMARY

As stated in the introduction to this chapter, physician prescribing behavior is complex. It is a function of the relationship between physician factors, consumer factors, and the environment. The body of literature in this field has grown substantially in recent years, from the early work of Hemminki in the 1970s to Segal and Hepler in the 1980s to a critical mass of researchers such as Denig, Tamblyn, and others over the past 20 years. With this growth has come greater understanding of the role of these various factors and their influence on prescribing behavior. Although more knowledge about physician decision making is beneficial in its own right, there are at least three critical caveats about prescribing behavior.

First, one of the challenges associated with the isolation of physician and consumer (patient) characteristics is the fact that these variables do not function in isolation of each other, and tend to exhibit varying degrees of covariance. Additionally, influence may further be a function of nonmeasured variables such as practice geography, jurisdiction, beliefs and values, or even sampling bias. Thus, it is obvious from the literature that there are physician characteristics that influence prescribing, but the challenge is determining which have the greatest influence and their weight of influence relative to the presence of other variables and given sets of circumstances or prescribing situations. For example, Jones and associates made the observation that practice variables explain only a small proportion of the variance in prescribing, and that prescribing decisions are complex and idiosyncratic and will not be fully explained by easily identifiable general practitioner characteristics.[152] McKinlay and colleagues suggested that variability in decision making is not entirely accounted for by strictly rational Bayesian inference.[108]

Second, patient involvement in the decision-making process regarding prescribing has increased as there has been movement away from the paternalistic medical model; however, there is still much work to be done to determine the optimal role for the patient in this process. As per the discussion in this chapter, there are times when patients can influence prescribing for the worse, for example, when asking the physician for a medication they saw on television or that a friend is taking that may not be appropriate for them. Still, patients who are knowledgeable about their disease and medications and who demonstrate optimal adherence can greatly increase the probability of an optimal outcome from a prescription. A study by Gardner and colleagues highlighted the difference between physician and patient preferences in the choice of drugs.[153] Patients and family physicians were surveyed about the perceived importance of 12 differentiating factors when selecting an antidepressant. Overall, there was moderate disagreement between the patients and physicians, including considerable disagreement on the importance of uncommon serious side effects, cost, and dosing schedule.

Third, although influencing prescribing can result in improved patient outcomes, prescribing is only one part of the medication-use system. Other essential elements of this system include timely recognition of drug indications and other signs and symptoms relevant to drug use; safe, accessible, and cost-effective medicines; distribution, dispensing, and administration of drug products with appropriate patient advice; optimal adherence; monitoring; documentation and communication; and performance measurement.[154] Even a prescription that is entirely appropriate and evidence-based does not guarantee an optimal outcome. As Segal and Wang note, "the medical literature supports the assertions that prescribing 'the drug of choice' does not guarantee a good patient outcome and that poor outcomes probably have more to do with what happens after a drug is prescribed."[2] Finally, perhaps we can take some assurance in the fact that these problems and issues are not unique to modern medicine. For centuries, patients have struggled with suboptimal healthcare interventions.

ACKNOWLEDGMENTS

Special thanks to Jocelyn LeClerc and Tiffany Nguyen for their work on this chapter. We would also like to recognize the contributions of Tony Schellinck, Jim McNiven, and Carolyn Watters to Kent Groves' PhD thesis which helped to form the basis of this chapter.

REFERENCES

1. Groves K, Flanagan P, MacKinnon N. Why physicians start or stop prescribing a drug: literature review and formulary implications. Formulary 2002;37:186-94.
2. Segal R, Wang F. Influencing physician prescribing. Pharm Pract Manage Q 1999;19(3):30-50.
3. Gill PS, Makela M, Vermeulen KM, et al. Changing doctor prescribing behaviour. Pharm World Sci 1999;21(4):158-67.
4. Sbarbaro JA. Can we influence prescribing patterns? Clin Infect Dis 2001;33(suppl 3):S240-4.
5. Parrino TA. Controlled trials to improve antibiotic utilization: a systematic review of experience, 1984–2004. Pharmacotherapy 2005;25(2):289-98.
6. Pippalla RS, Riley DA, Chinburapa V. Influencing the prescribing behaviour of physicians: a metaevaluation. J Clin Pharm Ther 1995;20(4):189-98.
7. Wilson AL. Influencing prescribers. Top Hosp Pharm Manage 1994;14(3):40-6.
8. Hepler CD, Segal R, Freeman RA. How physicians choose the drugs they prescribe. Top Hosp Pharm Manage 1981;1(3):23-44.
9. Raisch DW. A model of methods for influencing prescribing: part II. A review of educational methods, theories of human inference, and delineation of the model. DICP 1990;24(5):537-42.
10. Raisch DW. A model of methods for influencing prescribing: part I. A review of prescribing models, persuasion theories, and administrative and educational methods. DICP 1990;24(4):417-21.
11. Grol R, Grimshaw J. From best evidence to best practice: effective implementation of change in patients' care. Lancet 2003;362:1225-30.
12. Anderson GM, Lexchin J. Strategies for improving prescribing practice. CMAJ 1996;154(7): 1013-7.
13. Carter AO, Strachan D, Appiah Y. Physician prescribing practices: what do we know? Where do we go? How do we get there? CMAJ 1996;154(11):1649-53.
14. Vuckovic N, Nichter M. Changing patterns of pharmaceutical practice in the United States. Soc Sci Med 1997;44(9):1285-302.
15. Bradley CP. Uncomfortable prescribing decisions: a critical incident study. BMJ 1992; 304(6822):294-6.
16. Weiss MC, Fitzpatrick R, Scott DK, Goldacre MJ. Pressures on the general practitioner and decisions to prescribe. Fam Pract 1996;13(5):432-8.
17. Einarson TR. The authority/pharmacotherapy care model: an explanatory model of the drug use process in primary care. Res Soc Adm Pharm 2005;1:101-17.
18. Groves KEM. The influence of pharmaceutical marketing activity, practice characteristics and physician profile on physician prescribing behaviour [PhD dissertation]. Dalhousie University, Canada, 2006.

19. Gonul FF, Carter F, Petrova E, Srinivasan K. Promotion of prescription drugs and its impact on physicians' choice behavior. J Marketing 2001;65:79-90.

20. Rosenthal MB, Berndt ER, Donohue JM, Epstein AM, Frank RG. Demand effects of recent changes in prescription drug promotion. Menlo Park, CA: Henry J. Kaiser Family Foundation, 2003.

21. Semin S, Aras S, Guldal D. Direct-to-consumer advertising of pharmaceuticals: developed countries experiences and Turkey. Health Expect 2007;10(1):4-15.

22. Mintzes B. What are the public health implications? Direct to consumer advertising of prescription drugs in Canada. Ottawa: Health Council of Canada, 2006.

23. Health Action International. Direct to consumer advertising revisited by European commission, "Deja-vu all Over Again?" October 4, 2006. (Accessed at http://www.haiweb.org/05102006/PressReleaseDTCARevisited.pdf.)

24. Jenkings KN, Barber N. What constitutes evidence in hospital new drug decision making? Soc Sci Med 2004;58(9):1757-66.

25. Barber N. What constitutes good prescribing? BMJ 1995;310(6984):923-5.

26. Horton LR. Some relationships between personality and consumer decision making. J Marketing Res 1979;16(2):233.

27. Turley WL, LeBlanc PR. Evoked sets: a dynamic process model. J Marketing Theory Pract 1995;3(2):28.

28. Kotler P, Armstrong G, Cunningham PH. Principles of marketing. 6th Canadian ed. Toronto: Pearson, 2005.

29. Solomon M, Zaichkowsky J, Polegato R. Consumer behaviour. Toronto: Prentice-Hall, 2004.

30. Olshavsky RW, Granbois DH. Consumer decision making—fact or fiction? J Consumer Res 1979;6(2):93.

31. Landon BE. Is pay-for-performance moving north? P4P prospects in the Canadian healthcare system. Healthc Pap 2006;6(4):28,33; discussion 72-4.

32. Rochaix L. The physician as perfect agent: a comment. Soc Sci Med 1998;47(3):355-6.

33. Mooney G, Ryan M. Agency in health care: getting beyond first principles. J Health Econ 1993;12(2):125-35.

34. Mott DA, Schommer JC, Doucette WR, Kreling DH. Agency theory, drug formularies, and drug product selection: implications for public policy. J Public Policy Marketing 1998;17(2):287-95.

35. MacLeod SM. Improving physician prescribing practices: bridge over troubled waters. CMAJ 1996;154(5):675-7.

36. McTavish JR. What did Bayer do before aspirin? Pharm Hist 1999;41(1):3-15.

37. Angus DE, Karpetz HM. Pharmaceutical policies in Canada. Issues and challenges. Pharmacoeconomics 1998;14(suppl 1):81-96.

38. Greenhalgh T, Robert G, MacFarlane F, Bate P, Kyriakidou O. Diffusion of innovations in service organizations: systematic review and recommendations. Millbank Q 2004;82(4):581-629.

39. Rogers EM. Diffusion of innovations. New York: Free Press, 1983.

40. Coleman J, Katz E, Menzel H. Medical innovation: a diffusion study. Indianapolis: Bobbs-Merrill, 1966.

41. Van den Bulte C, Lilien GL. Medical innovation revisited: social contagion versus marketing effort. Am J Sociol 2001;106(5):1409-35.

42. Peay MY, Peay ER. Innovation in high risk drug therapy. Soc Sci Med 1994;39(1):39-52.

43. Waarts E, van Everdingen YM, van Hillegersberg J. The dynamics of factors affecting the adoption of innovations. J Product Innov Manage 2002;19(6):412.

44. Ma J, Stafford RS, Cockburn IM, Finkelstein SN. A statistical analysis of the magnitude and composition of drug promotion in the United States in 1998. Clin Ther 2003;25(5):1503-17.

45. Wozniak DG. Joint information acquisition and new technology adoption: late versus early adoption. Rev Econ Statistics 1993;75(3):438.

46. Olshavsky WR, Spreng AR. An exploratory study of the innovation evaluation process. J Product Innov Manage 1996;13(6):512.

47. Dybdahl T, Andersen M, Sondergaard J, Kragstrup J, Kristiansen IS. Does the early adopter of drugs exist? A population-based study of general practitioners' prescribing of new drugs. Eur J Clin Pharmacol 2004;60(9):667-72.

48. Shih C, Venkatesh A. Beyond adoption: development and application of a use-diffusion model. J Marketing 2004;68(1):59.

49. Marinova D. Actualizing innovation effort: the impact of market knowledge diffusion in a dynamic system of competition. J Marketing 2004;68(3):1.

50. Granovetter M. Threshold models of collective behavior. Am J Sociol 1978;83:1420-43.

51. Valente TW. Social network thresholds in the diffusion of innovations. Soc Networks 1996;18(1):69-89.

52. Carpenter GS, Nakamoto K. Consumer preference formation and pioneering advantage. J Market Res 1989;26(3):285.

53. Boulding W, Christen M. Sustainable pioneering advantage? Profit implications of market entry order. Marketing Sci 2003;22(3):371.

54. Vargo SL, Lusch RF. Evolving to a new dominant logic for marketing. J Marketing 2004; 68(1):1.

55. Scharitzer D, Kollarits HC. Satisfied customers: profitable customer relationships: pharmaceutical marketing. How pharmaceutical sales representatives can achieve economic success through relationship management with settled general practitioners—an empirical study. Total Quality Manage 2000;11(7):S955.

56. Groves KE, Sketris I, Tett SE. Prescription drug samples—does this marketing strategy counteract policies for quality use of medicines? J Clin Pharm Ther 2003;28(4):259-71.

57. Marks JL, Kamins AM. The use of product sampling and advertising: effects of sequence of exposure and degree of advertising claim exaggeration on consumers' belief strength, belief confidence and attitudes. J Marketing Res 1988;25(3):266.

58. Rosenthal MB, Berndt ER, Donohue JM, Frank RG, Epstein AM. Promotion of prescription drugs to consumers. N Engl J Med 2002;346(7):498-505.

59. Kondro W. Academic drug detailing: an evidence-based alternative. CMAJ 2007;176(4):429-31.

60. Hawkins SA, Hoch SJ. Low-involvement learning: memory without evaluation. J Consumer Res 1992;19(2):212-25.

61. Prosser H, Almond S, Walley T. Influences on GPs' decision to prescribe new drugs—the importance of who says what. Fam Pract 2003;20(1):61-8.

62. Avorn J, Chen M, Hartley R. Scientific versus commercial sources of influence on the prescribing behavior of physicians. Am J Med 1982;73(1):4-8.

63. Guldal D, Semin S. The influences of drug companies' advertising programs on physicians. Int J Health Serv 2000;30(3):585-95.

64. Watkins C, Harvey I, Carthy P, Moore L, Robinson E, Brawn R. Attitudes and behaviour of general practitioners and their prescribing costs: a national cross sectional survey. Qual Safety Health Care 2003;12(1):29-34.

65. Muijrers PE, Grol RP, Sijbrandij J, Janknegt R, Knottnerus JA. Differences in prescribing between GPs. Impact of the cooperation with pharmacists and impact of visits from pharmaceutical industry representatives. Fam Pract 2005;22(6):624-30.

66. Jacoby A, Smith M, Eccles M. A qualitative study to explore influences on general practitioners' decisions to prescribe new drugs. Br J Gen Pract 2003;53(487):120-5.

67. Jiang P. The role of brand name in customization decisions: a search vs experience perspective. J Product Brand Manage 2004;13(2):73-83.

68. Gorecki KP. The importance of being first: the case of prescription drugs in Canada. Int J Industrial Organ 1986;4:371-95.

69. Leffler KB. Persuasion or information? The economics of prescription drug advertising. J Law Econ 1981;24:45-74.

70. Jones MI, Greenfield SM, Bradley CP. Prescribing new drugs: qualitative study of influences on consultants and general practitioners. BMJ 2001;323(7309):378-81.

71. Watkins C, Moore L, Harvey I, Carthy P, Robinson E, Brawn R. Characteristics of general practitioners who frequently see drug industry representatives: national cross sectional study. BMJ 2003;326:1178-9.

72. Majumdar SR, McAlister FA, Soumerai SB. Synergy between publication and promotion: comparing adoption of new evidence in Canada and the United States. Am J Med 2003;115:467-72.

73. Kerr SJ, Mant A, Horn FE, McGeechan K, Sayer GP. Lessons from early large-scale adoption of celecoxib and rofecoxib by Australian general practitioners. Med J Aust 2003;179(8):403-7.

74. Mizik N, Jacobson R. Are physicians "easy marks"? Quantifying the effects of detailing and sampling on new prescriptions. Manage Sci 2004;50(12):1704.

75. Hanssens MG, Dekimpe DM. The persistence of marketing effects on sales. Marketing Sci 1995;14(1):1.

76. Gonul FF, Carter F, Wind J. What kind of patients and physicians value direct-to-consumer advertising of prescription drugs. Health Care Manage Sci 2000;3(3):215-26.

77. Manchanda P, Chintagunta PK. Responsiveness of physician prescription behavior to salesforce effort: an individual level analysis. Marketing Letters 2004;15(2-3):129-45.

78. Coenen S, Van Royen P, Michiels B, Denekens J. Optimizing antibiotic prescribing for acute cough in general practice: a cluster-randomized controlled trial. J Antimicrob Chemother 2004;54(3):661-72.

79. Solomon DH, Van Houten L, Glynn RJ, et al. Academic detailing to improve use of broad-spectrum antibiotics at an academic medical center. Arch Intern Med 2001;161(15):1897-902.

80. Zwar N, Wolk J, Gordon J, Sanson-Fisher R, Kehoe L. Influencing antibiotic prescribing in general practice: a trial of prescriber feedback and management guidelines. Fam Pract 1999;16(5):495-500.

81. Simon SR, Majumdar SR, Prosser LA, et al. Group versus individual academic detailing to improve the use of antihypertensive medications in primary care: a cluster-randomized controlled trial. Am J Med 2005;118(5):521-8.

82. Schuster RJ, Terwoord NA, Tasosa J. Changing physician practice behavior to measure and improve clinical outcomes. Am J Med Qual 2006;21(6):394-400.

83. Fretheim A, Oxman AD, Havelsrud K, Treweek S, Kristoffersen DT, Bjorndal A. Rational prescribing in primary care (RaPP): a cluster randomized trial of a tailored intervention. PLoS Med 2006;3(6):e134.

84. Watkins C, Timm A, Gooberman-Hill R, Harvey I, Haines A, Donovan J. Factors affecting feasibility and acceptability of a practice-based educational intervention to support evidence-based prescribing: a qualitative study. Fam Pract 2004;21(6):661-9.

85. Polinski JM, Brookhart MA, Katz JN, et al. Educational outreach (academic detailing) regarding osteoporosis in primary care. Pharmacoepidemiol Drug Safety 2005;14(12):843-50.

86. Jones M, Greenfield S, Bradley C. A survey of the advertising of nine new drugs in the general practice literature. J Clin Pharm Ther 1999;24(6):451-60.

87. Schumock GT, Walton SM, Park HY, et al. Factors that influence prescribing decisions. Ann Pharmacother 2004;38(4):557-62.

88. Hurwitz AM, Caves ER. Persuasion or information? Promotion and the shares of brand name and generic pharmaceuticals. J Law Econ 1988;31(2):299.

89. Stafford RS, Furberg CD, Finkelstein SN, Cockburn IM, Alchegn T, Ma J. Impact of clinical trial results on national trends in alpha-blocker prescribing, 1996–2002. JAMA 2004;291(1): 54-62.

90. Mintzes B, Barer ML, Kravitz RL, et al. How does direct-to-consumer advertising (DTCA) affect prescribing? A survey in primary care environments with and without legal DTCA. CMAJ 2003;169(5):405-12.

91. Scott IA. On the need for probity when physicians interact with industry. Intern Med J 2006;36(4):265-9.

92. Roth MS. Media and message effects on DTC prescription drug print advertising awareness. J Adv Res 2003;43(2):180-93.

93. Schwartz RK, Soumerai SB, Avorn J. Physician motivations for nonscientific drug prescribing. Soc Sci Med 1989;28(6):577-82.

94. Donohue JM. Direct-to-consumer advertising of prescription drugs: does it add to the overuse and inappropriate use of prescription drugs or alleviate underuse? Int J Pharm Med 2006; 20(1):17-24.

95. Peyrot M, Alperstein NM, Van Doren D, Poli LG. Direct-to-consumer ads can influence behavior. Advertising increases consumer knowledge and prescription drug requests. Market Health Serv 1998;18(2):26-32.

96. Mehta A, Purvis SC. Consumer response to print prescription drug advertising. J Adv Res 2003;43(2):194-206.

97. Zachry WM, Shepherd MD, Hinich MJ, Wilson JP, Brown CM, Lawson KA. Relationship between direct-to-consumer advertising and physician diagnosing and prescribing. Am J Health Syst Pharm 2002;59(1):42-9.

98. Vogel RJ, Ramachandran S, Zachry WM. A 3-stage model for assessing the probable economic effects of direct-to-consumer advertising of pharmaceuticals. Clin Ther 2003;25(1):309-29.

99. Donohue JM, Berndt ER, Rosenthal M, Epstein AM, Frank RG. Effects of pharmaceutical promotion on adherence to the treatment guidelines for depression. Med Care 2004;42(12): 1176-85.

100. Stevenson FA, Greenfield SM, Jones M, Nayak A, Bradley CP. GP's perceptions of patient influence on prescribing. Fam Pract 1999;16(3):255-61.

101. Britten N, Ukoumunne OC, Boulton MG. Patients' attitudes to medicines and expectations for prescriptions. Health Expect 2002;5(3):256-69.

102. Mamdani MM, Tu K, Austin PC, Alter DA. Influence of socioeconomic status on drug selection for the elderly in Canada. Ann Pharmacother 2002;36(5):804-8.

103. Soumerai SB, Avorn J, Ross-Degnan D, Gortmaker S. Payment restrictions for prescription drugs under Medicaid. Effects on therapy, cost, and equity. N Engl J Med 1987;317(9):550-6.

104. Tamblyn R, Laprise R, Hanley JA, et al. Adverse events associated with prescription drug cost-sharing among poor and elderly persons. JAMA 2001;285(4):421-9.

105. Stewart RE, Vroegop S, Kamps GB, van der Werf GT, Meyboom-de Jong B. Factors influencing adherence to guidelines in general practice. Int J Technol Assess Health Care 2003; 19(3):546-54.

106. World Health Organization. World Health Organization of experts on the rational use of drugs. Geneva: World Health Organization, 1987.

107. Bradley CP. Factors which influence the decision whether or not to prescribe: the dilemma facing general practitioners. Br J Gen Pract 1992;42(364):454-8.

108. McKinlay JB, Potter DA, Feldman HA. Non-medical influences on medical decision-making. Soc Sci Med 1996;42(5):769-76.

109. Bennett K, Teeling M, Feely J. "Selective" switching from non-selective to selective non-steroidal anti-inflammatory drugs. Eur J Clin Pharmacol 2003;59(8-9):645-9.

110. Tamblyn R, McLeod P, Hanley JA, Girard N, Hurley J. Physician and practice characteristics associated with the early utilization of new prescription drugs. Med Care 2003;41(8):895-908.

111. Cutts C, Tett SE. Doctors' perceptions of the influences on their prescribing: a comparison of general practitioners based in rural and urban Australia. Eur J Clin Pharmacol 2003;58(11):761-6.

112. Baldwin LM, Rosenblatt RA, Schneeweiss R, Lishner DM, Hart LG. Rural and urban physicians: does the content of their Medicare practices differ? J Rural Health 1999;15(2):240-51.

113. Cutts C, Tett SE. Influences on doctors' prescribing: is geographical remoteness a factor? Aust J Rural Health 2003;11(3):124-30.

114. Redelmeier DA, Tan SH, Booth GL. The treatment of unrelated disorders in patients with chronic medical diseases. N Engl J Med 1998;338(21):1516-20.

115. Howlett JG, Cox JL, Haddad H, Stanley J, McDonald M, Johnstone DE. Physician specialty and quality of care for CHF: different patients or different patterns of practice? Can J Cardiol 2003;19(4):371-7.

116. Buban GM, Link BK, Doucette WR. Influences on oncologists' adoption of new agents in adjuvant chemotherapy of breast cancer. J Clin Oncol 2001;19(4):954-9.

117. Coleman J, Menzel H, Katz E. Social processes in physicians' adoption of a new drug. J Chronic Dis 1959;9(1):1-19.

118. Bearden WO, Etzel MJ. Reference group influence on product and brand purchase decisions. J Consumer Res 1982;9(2):183.

119. Ajzen I. The theory of planned behavior. Organizational Behav Hum Decision Proc 1991; 50(2):179.

120. Rosenstein AH, Shulkin D. Changing physician behavior is tool to reduce health care costs. Health Care Strateg Manage 1991;9(9):14-6.

121. Grimshaw J, Eccles M, Tetroe J. Implementing clinical guidelines: current evidence and future implications. J Contin Educ Health Prof 2004;24(suppl 1):S31-7.

122. Steffensen FH, Sorensen HT, Olesen F. Diffusion of new drugs in Danish general practice. Fam Pract 1999;16(4):407-13.

123. Cranney M, Warren E, Barton S, Gardner K, Walley T. Why do GPs not implement evidence-based guidelines? A descriptive study. Fam Pract 2001;18(4):359-63.

124. Prosser H, Walley T. New drug uptake: qualitative comparison of high and low prescribing GPs' attitudes and approach. Fam Pract 2003;20(5):583-91.

125. Helin-Salmivaara A, Huupponen R, Klaukka T, Hoppu K, Steering Group of the ROHTO programme. Focusing on changing clinical practice to enhance rational prescribing—collaboration and networking enable comprehensive approaches. Health Policy 2003;66(1):1-10.

126. Maue SK, Segal R, Kimberlin CL, Lipowski EE. Predicting physician guideline compliance: an assessment of motivators and perceived barriers. Am J Manag Care 2004;10(6):383-91.

127. Pearson SA, Rolfe I, Smith T. Factors influencing prescribing: an intern's perspective. Med Educ 2002;36(8):781-7.

128. Denig P, Haaijer-Ruskamp FM, Wesseling H, Versluis A. Impact of clinical trials on the adoption of new drugs within a university hospital. Eur J Clin Pharmacol 1991;41(4):325-8.

129. Allery LA, Owen PA, Robling MR. Why general practitioners and consultants change their clinical practice: a critical incident study. BMJ 1997;314(7084):870-4.

130. Landon BE, Reschovsky J, Reed M, Blumenthal D. Personal, organizational, and market level influences on physicians' practice patterns: results of a national survey of primary care physicians. Med Care 2001;39(8):889-905.

131. O'Neill L, Kuder J. Explaining variation in physician practice patterns and their propensities to recommend services. Med Care Res Rev 2005;62(3):339-57.

132. Ashworth M, Armstrong D, Colwill S, Cohen A, Balazs J. Motivating general practitioners to change their prescribing: the incentive of working together. J Clin Pharm Ther 2000;25(2):119-24.

133. Carthy P, Harvey I, Brawn R, Watkins C. A study of factors associated with cost and variation in prescribing among GPs. Fam Pract 2000;17(1):36-41.

134. Soumerai SB, McLaughlin TJ, Gurwitz JH, et al. Effect of local medical opinion leaders on quality of care for acute myocardial infarction: a randomized controlled trial. JAMA 1998;279(17):1358-63.

135. Hemminki E. Review of literature on the factors affecting drug prescribing. Soc Sci Med 1975;9(2):111-6.

136. Mitchell V, Walsh G. Gender differences in German consumer decision-making styles. J Consumer Behav 2004;3(4):331-46.

137. Sproles GB, Kendall EL. A methodology for profiling consumers' decision-making styles. J Consumer Aff 1986;20(2):267.

138. Sproles KE, Sproles BG. Consumer decision-making styles as a function of individual learning styles. J Consumer Aff 1990;24(1):134.

139. Chang J, Samuel N. Internet shopper demographics and buying behaviour in Australia. J Am Acad Business 2004;5(1/2):171.

140. Dholakia RR. Going shopping: key determinants of shopping behaviors and motivations. Int J Retail Distrib Manage 1999;27(4):154.

141. Fischer E, Arnold SJ. Sex, gender identity, gender role attitudes, and consumer behavior. Psychol Marketing 1994;11(2):163.

142. Inman W, Pearce G. Prescriber profile and post-marketing surveillance. Lancet 1993; 342(8872):658-61.

143. Duetz MS, Schneeweiss S, Maclure M, Abel T, Glynn RJ, Soumerai SB. Physician gender and changes in drug prescribing after the implementation of reference pricing in British Columbia. Clin Ther 2003;25(1):273-84.

144. Gilly MC, Zeithaml VA. The elderly consumer and adoption of technologies. J Consumer Res 1985;12(3):353-7.

145. Lacy BE, Crowell MD, Riesett RP, Mitchell A. Age, specialty, and practice setting predict gastro-esophageal reflux disease prescribing behavior. J Clin Gastroenterol 2005;39(6):489-94.

146. Freiman MP. The rate of adoption of new procedures among physicians. The impact of specialty and practice characteristics. Med Care 1985;23(8):939-45.

147. Helin-Salmivaara A, Huupponen R, Virtanen A, Klaukka T. Adoption of celecoxib and rofecoxib: a nationwide database study. J Clin Pharm Ther 2005;30(2):145-52.

148. Tamayo-Sarver JH, Dawson NV, Cydulka RK, Wigton RS, Baker DW. Variability in emergency physician decision making about prescribing opioid analgesics. Ann Emerg Med 2004; 43(4):483-93.

149. Armstrong D, Reyburn H, Jones R. A study of general practitioners' reasons for changing their prescribing behaviour. BMJ 1996;312(7036):949-52.

150. Denig P, Witteman CL, Schouten HW. Scope and nature of prescribing decisions made by general practitioners. Qual Safety Health Care 2002;11(2):137-43.

151. Nazareth I, Freemantle N, Duggan C, Mason J, Haines A. Evaluation of a complex intervention for changing professional behaviour: the Evidence Based Out Reach (EBOR) trial. J Health Serv Res Policy 2002;7(4):230-8.

152. Jones MI, Greenfield SM, Jowett S, Bradley CP, Seal R. Proton pump inhibitors: a study of GPs' prescribing. Fam Pract 2001;18(3):333-8.

153. Gardner DM, MacKinnon N, Langille DB, Andreou P. A comparison of factors used by physicians and patients in the selection of antidepressant agents. Psychiatr Serv 2007;58(1):34-40.

154. MacKinnon NJ. The eight essential elements of an optimal medication-use system. Ottawa: Canadian Pharmacists Association, 2007.

155. Health Canada. Legislative renewal—issue paper; direct to consumer advertising (DTCA) of prescription drugs. Ottawa: Government of Canada, 2003.

CHAPTER 10

Patient Decision Making: Responses to Illness and Treatment

Nathaniel M. Rickles, PharmD, PhD, BCPP, Nicky Britten, PhD,
Janine Morgall Traulsen, PhD, and Paul Bissell, PhD

Earlier chapters in this book have presented theories that show us that certain health beliefs lead to different preventive and treatment behaviors; however, these theories tend to provide little insight into how patients interpret their symptoms and illness experiences and how such interpretations affect their decision making regarding treatment and their involvement with pharmacists. Therefore, this chapter explores patients' interpretation of their symptoms and their treatment responses to symptoms, how individuals make sense of their illness and treatment experience within a social context, and how the pharmacist–patient relationship can affect patients' decision-making process. By the end of the chapter, the reader will gain perspective on what might be going through a patient's mind with regard to his or her illness and how the relationship with the patient can alter perspectives on symptoms and treatments.

INTERPRETATION OF SYMPTOMS

Based on past cognitive psychology research, we have learned how individuals subconsciously process and selectively attend to certain information. For example, in the late 1950s Broadbent proposed the concept that people use both their sensory and perceptual systems to attend to various stimuli.[1] In the sensory system, the senses receive information from several sources simultaneously (visual, auditory, gustatory, olfactory, and tactile) and briefly retain it. In the perceptual system, the individual's subconscious selectively attends to one or more of these sensory stimuli. This latter process of selective attention allows individuals to attend to only those sensory stimuli that have physiologic and psychosocial importance to their environmental needs.

Such cognitive psychology research can be applied to how individuals might perceive health-related stimuli such as symptoms. The journey from person to patient, in the words of Zola,[2] usually begins when the person notices symptoms, some kind of bodily discomfort, or the inability to carry out his or her normal activities. Patients will use both their sensory and perceptual systems to take in what they are sensing at the moment and then subconsciously attend to those symptoms that are most serious or problematic. It is therefore no surprise to clinicians when patients report certain symptoms and omit others they may have felt or are feeling currently.

Patients use the symptoms they selectively attend to in order to form mental pictures and cognitive representations or schematas of their illness and treatment options. Health psychologists have theorized that these cognitive representations are based on people's possession of an implicit, organized knowledge base about various illnesses and treatments.[3] These researchers further suggest that patients construct "illness prototypes" or templates as standards to which they match and evaluate existing symptoms.[4] Such templates are likely more common among individuals with greater awareness of the health literature, personal health experiences, and other self-learning efforts (such as the increasing use of the Internet for health information). These patient-constructed illness templates can also lead to confusion or added worry because symptoms may overlap with other templates they possess. For example, a patient may selectively attend to symptoms such as a running nose, aches and pains, cough, fatigue, and fever and suggest these symptoms match his or her "flu template." The patient may also think such symptoms are related to his or her "sinus allergy template."

Bishop suggests that an illness template has five dimensions: identity, cause, time line, consequences, and cure.[3] *Identity* is the label the patient places on the disease and the symptoms associated with it. For example, the patient labels a set of symptoms as part of a flu or sinus allergy. *Cause* refers to the individual's perception of how the disease state is obtained. A patient identifying symptoms as related to the flu may think the cause is bacteria spread from a family member. The *time line* of an illness template is associated with the patient's sense of how long the disease will last. The fourth dimension of an illness template, *consequences*, reflects the patient's expectations of the manifestations and outcome of disease. The common flu template would indicate a period of multiple symptoms followed by several days of improvement, ultimately resulting in full recovery. The final dimension of an illness template involves the patient's perceptions of how an illness can be therapeutically resolved. Patients may believe that the flu can be resolved with medications, fluids, and bed rest. Based on the patient's perception of how the illness can be cured, he or she will decide how to respond to the illness symptoms. These different responses to symptoms are explored in more detail in the next section.

TREATMENT RESPONSES TO SYMPTOMS

Having perceived a symptom or symptoms, a person can respond in a number of ways. This includes doing nothing, engaging in some kind of self-care such as resting or self-medicating, or consulting a healthcare provider.[5] In some cases these responses may be appropriate from a clinical point of view. Relatively little is known about how people make these kinds of treatment choices, although significant others are often influential.

Use of Self-Care

Studies carried out in the 1970s and 1980s established that people living in community settings experienced many symptoms that they did not report to clinicians; this phenomenon was referred to as the "clinical iceberg." For example, Banks and associates carried out a diary-based study of 516 women in the United Kingdom and found that respondents recorded 37 symptom episodes for every patient-initiated consultation with her general practitioner.[6] The likelihood of consultation varied with the type of symptom, with only 1 in 184 headaches leading to a consultation, compared with 1 in 14 symptoms of chest pain. Laypeople experiencing symptoms make their own judgments about when to consult healthcare practitioners. This requires them to have sufficient discrimination to make appropriate consulting decisions, but once in a healthcare practitioner's office, they are not usually regarded as having appropriate expertise. Bloor and Horobin described this as the "double bind."[7]

More recently, Heritage and Robinson have described how patients need to present their problems as "doctorable," that is, worthy of medical attention.[8] Because laypeople often make judgments that differ from those of practitioners, some seemingly serious symptoms are not brought to the attention of practitioners, whereas other, seemingly trivial, symptoms are. Help-seeking behavior may be influenced by a person's psychological makeup, family and social circumstances, and the healthcare system as well as the nature of his or her health condition. In between doing nothing and deciding to consult a practitioner, laypeople may carry out self-care activities or may self-medicate. Community pharmacists have a potential role to play in contributing to people's self-management strategies, provided they are consulted or initiate consultations with patients. Patients with already diagnosed chronic illnesses may also carry out self-care activities or self-medicate at the same time as taking prescribed medications. Decisions regarding self-care include choosing to use over-the-counter (OTC) treatments, seeking complementary and alternative therapies, and self-adjusting prescribed therapies.

Use of Over-the-Counter Treatments

One of the main approaches to self-care involves the use of OTC products for various remedies. OTC products often involve doses and drugs that have been deemed safe and effective for consumer self-medication. These medications are often similar to prescription medications but at lower doses, are the same as medications that have been previously available only as prescriptions but were found to have few side effects or drug interactions, or are long-term remedies that have been found to be safe for the general public. An interview-based study of the general population in Finland found that, in the two days preceding the interview, the most commonly used OTC medicines were vitamin and mineral supplements, nonsteroidal anti-inflammatory drugs (NSAIDs), and analgesics.[9]

The role of pharmacists in relation to OTC products partly depends on the patient. Some people have made up their own minds about what product they want to buy and have no expectations that the pharmacist will do anything more than sell it to them. Others may want some advice about the product itself or choice of product, whereas still others may ask for advice about how best to respond to their symptoms. For minor ailments, pharmacists may be seen as a more appropriate healthcare practitioner to consult, either because of their expertise or because the physician's time is perceived as too valuable to waste (if free) or else unaffordable (if not). If patients do not ask pharmacists for advice, there may be problems because people often do not realize that by taking several different preparations with the same or similar ingredients, they are effectively increasing the dose. People may also be unaware of potential interactions between OTCs and prescribed drugs. Herxheimer and Britten argued for a formulary for self-care that could promote collaboration between general practitioners and community pharmacists and ensure consistent advice for patients from whomever they ask.[10] It is important to note that although patients have an important role in deciding to access a pharmacist's OTC advice, pharmacists also need to make themselves more accessible to patients and talk to them about OTC products. In many situations the pharmacist appears "too busy," and patients may perceive this as the pharmacist not being open to communicating with them.

Use of Prescription Medicines

Once a person has decided to consult a healthcare practitioner about his or her problem, there is a good chance that the individual will be prescribed a medication. For example, Himmel and colleagues found that 68% of patients consulting German general practitioners on randomly selected days of the week received prescriptions.[11]

Britten and coworkers found that prescriptions were written in two thirds of study consultations in a U.K. study.[12] Patients play a role in physicians' treatment decisions, because their expectations have been shown to influence prescribing. In a study of general practice in Australia, Cockburn and Pit found that patients who expected medication were nearly three times as likely to receive it; when general practitioners thought that the patient expected medication, they were 10 times more likely to write a prescription.[13] Some of these expectations are based on previous experience, and there is some evidence that patients' expectations are higher in high-prescribing practices.[14] Patients' expectations may themselves be influenced by direct-to-consumer (DTC) advertising in countries where this is permitted. In a survey of primary care physicians in the United States and Canada, Mintzes and associates found that patients with higher self-reported exposure to advertising, conditions potentially treatable by advertised drugs, and/or those who used advertising as an information source were more likely to request advertised medications.[15] Even in those countries where DTC advertising is not officially permitted, patients' expectations for medications may be influenced by advertising on the Internet.

Although some consumers may not perceive pharmacists to have a professional role in relation to OTC products, this is less likely to be the case in relation to prescription medications. Even so, it has been shown that some people either have low expectations of the roles of pharmacists or actively resent pharmacists' questioning or advice about prescription medications. In a survey of 19 community pharmacies and 355 pharmacy consumers, Chewning and Schommer found that barriers to question asking by patients included embarrassment and ignorance about the appropriateness of doing so.[16] Patients may prefer physicians to give them information about prescription medications, but it is often the case that physicians do not consistently provide such information. In the survey by Chewning and Schommer, clients were asked what questions they wanted the answers to when obtaining a new prescription.[16] The majority wanted information about possible side effects and directions for taking the medication. If prescribers are not providing this information, pharmacists need to do so.

Once a medication has been prescribed and dispensed, the patient has to decide, often on a daily basis, whether to take it or not. Conrad used the term *self-regulation* to describe the ways in which people with epilepsy developed their own medication practices.[17] His criteria for self-regulation, based on the ways in which people managed their medications, were reducing or raising the daily dose of prescribed medicines for several weeks or more; skipping or taking extra doses regularly under specific circumstances, such as when drinking alcohol or staying up late; or stopping taking medications for three consecutive days or longer. Using these criteria, he found that nearly half his sample self-regulated their medication for epilepsy. From a professional point of view, patients' decisions to self-regulate their use of medications may be seen as a form of nonadherence. Donovan, however, has cogently argued that patient decision making is the missing ingredient in compliance research, and that patients make decisions about treatment that fit with their own beliefs and personal circumstances.[18] Donovan further argues that the traditional concept of adherence is outmoded in modern healthcare systems, where chronic illness and questioning patients predominate.[18]

A review of qualitative research regarding lay perspectives on medications characterized various ways in which laypeople test their medications.[19] These included weighing costs and benefits; dealing with adverse effects; judging the acceptability of the regimen in terms of their daily lives; stopping the medication and seeing what happened; observing others; and using objective or subjective indicators. Not all patients' concerns can be addressed by this kind of consumer testing of medications. For example, it is difficult for consumers to test such concerns as dependence, the potential for harm over the longer term, or the possibility that taking medications might mask symptoms of disease.

The synthesis carried out by Pound and colleagues produced a comprehensive model of medication taking.[19] It showed that once a medication is prescribed and dispensed, people use the medication in a number of ways. Those described as *passive accepters* may take the medication without question, possibly because they trust the prescriber and are willing to do as he or she suggests. These people follow the prescription and constitute the group normally referred to as adherent. In Vrijens and Urquhart's terms, these are the people who both accept their medication and persist with it.[20] Other people carry out their own process of evaluating medications as described previously to address their specific worries and concerns. If their concerns can be dealt with in this process—for example, if fears about side effects are not warranted—they may subsequently accept their medication. These people then become *active accepters*. The medication-taking behavior of passive and active accepters may appear similar, but they have taken a different route to the same destination.

Still others may actively modify their regimen following a period of testing, for example, by reducing the dose to minimize side effects or by taking regular drug holidays. These people do take their medications, but not as prescribed, typically reducing the dose. In the model of Pound and coworkers, these latter individuals are referred to as *active modifiers*.[19] Modification of medication taking has several rationales: to minimize intake, to decrease adverse effects and addiction, to make the regimen more acceptable, to reduce cost, to manage symptoms, for strategic reasons such as avoiding interactions with alcohol, and to replace or supplement medications with nonpharmacologic treatments. People who do not accept the medication in the first place, or who subsequently stop taking the medication altogether, are known as *rejecters*.

The model of Pound and associates is not intended to suggest that these categories are stable over time, or that they label groups of people in a static way. Rather, they represent the range of ways in which people may use their medications at different times and in different circumstances. Not enough longitudinal research has been carried out to know the extent to which people's medication decisions change over time and in different circumstances.

NARRATIVES AND THE MEANING OF THE ILLNESS AND TREATMENT EXPERIENCE

The first part of this chapter focused on how the individual cognitively perceives illness and approaches treatment but provided little context relating to how individuals make sense of, understand, and attribute meaning to their illnesses and treatment experiences. However, we know that to achieve a greater understanding of the process individuals use to identify and respond to symptoms, it is necessary to see how such individual decision making relates to our self and/or our identity. After all, when we become ill and have to undergo medical treatment, including taking medicines, this affects how we feel about ourselves and how we experience our bodies; and this shapes our relationships with significant others. We also have to account—both to ourselves and others—for how and why we became ill. In this part of the chapter, we describe how some sociologists have attempted to explore this area of social life. In doing so, we return to a critique of the biomedical model in order to provide some context for this.

Sociological interest in the experience of illness needs to be seen in the context of the dominance of the biomedical model. With its origins in the development and growth of laboratory science in the 18th and 19th centuries, the biomedical model consists of a number of fundamental assumptions about the etiology and management of disease, and it is widely acknowledged that these assumptions have shaped how the patient is conceptualized within medicine.[21] From the 1920s onward in Western societies, biomedicine became the most widely accepted model for treating the afflictions of disease and for explaining health. However, as numerous sociological commentators have made clear, one of the problems with this model is that it obscures or overlooks the perspectives or experiences of the individual diagnosed with illness. As we know, living and coping with illness is often profoundly painful and unpleasant, can involve having to deal with stigmatizing labels, can result in exclusion from work and social activities, can affect our identities and our close relationships, and can have many other significant impacts. Equally important, the ill often seek explanations for their illness beyond the limited explanations provided by biomedical practitioners; they seek to ascertain the meaning behind their illness, asking questions about why illness struck them and why it struck when it did. Whereas biomedicine is effectively silent on these issues, medical sociologists have had much to say about them.

The Experience of Illness and Concern with Self

How illness affects one's sense of self and identity has been an enduring theme in the sociology of health and illness.[22] For example, Charmaz has carried out ground-breaking work into how people with physical disabilities experience social interaction with others and the impact this has on their sense of self.[23] She suggests from her research that people with physical disabilities are concerned about the sense of self they have lost, and the kind of person they find themselves becoming. She identifies four key dilemmas that emerge from this process. First, individuals scrutinize social interactions with others to look for signs of potential "dis-creditation." Second, the illness experience can foster dependence on others to achieve self-definition that can strain personal or familial relationships. Third, as illness increases, sufferers find they may require more intimate contact to preserve what she refers to as their "crumbling" self-image. Charmaz notes: "If they openly reveal their suffering, show self-pity, guilt, anger or other emotions conventionally believed to be negative, they are likely to further estrange those who take an interest in them." A final dilemma is concerned with the conflict with cultural values and norms. Charmaz suggests that Western society is concerned with doing, rather than being, and that those who cannot carry out their conventional tasks tend to lose the means needed to sustain a meaningful social life. Interestingly, Charmaz went on to revise this picture, suggesting that loss of self is not necessarily a pervasive feature for those people who experience physical disabilities.[24] She suggested that some people were able to create "reconstructed" identities by making an active attempt to create their lives and themselves.

What Charmaz is referring to is the set of approaches by which individuals come to terms with living with illness and how illness influences their sense of self. We need to be careful here to highlight the fact that this is clearly far more than a simple set of techniques that help sufferers to cope better with their illness or help them to comply with treatment. Rather, what we are referring to often involves a full-scale reorientation of how a person learns to live in the world.[25,26] It is argued that illness often calls for narrative work to convince others in society that the ill person's place in the world has changed. As Bury points out, "Not only do language and narrative help sustain and create the fabric of everyday life, they figure prominently in the repair and restoring of meanings when they are threatened. Under conditions of adversity, individuals often feel a pressing need to examine and refashion their personal narratives in an attempt to maintain a sense of identity."[21] In other words, when illness strikes, individuals typically need to make sense of their illness in personal and social terms, and they seek to draw links between their own life story and the wider social system they inhabit. This process often involves people having to answer their own questions about why the illness happened to them when it did, what it means to them, and how it can be explained.

As human beings, we are continuously engaged in striving to create meaning from our individual experiences and to find internal answers to the larger questions of existence: What is the meaning of my life? Why is this happening to me? How can I change things? We employ reflexive thought to explore the meaning of our lives in an attempt to exert some form of control over our feelings, thoughts, actions, and bodies. The stories that we tell ourselves are created via language through our interactions with other people and are shaped by the wider social and cultural context of our lives. These stories are also frequently moral stories about our connection to other people, and in turn that connection is inextricably linked to our concept or sense of self, of who we are. As moral stories, they are often embedded within issues of power and control as we attempt to construct our sense of self.

What this reminds us is that illness is never an entirely personal or individual matter, and that explanations and understanding of illness—at least when we are referring to patients—do not reside solely within the orthodox biomedical model. Indeed, Bury refers to a crisis regarding biomedical narratives, in the sense that there is a "progressive separation of the medical model of disease from the lay experience of illness."[21] He cites a number of factors as contributing to this process, such as the rise in the number of people with chronic illness, the increasingly sophisticated nature of high-tech modern medicine, the growth of complementary and alternative medicine (CAM), the rise in self-help groups, contemporary debates about the medicalization of everyday life and about the effectiveness of modern medicine, the rise of holistic and person-centered approaches to medicine, and the enormous expansion of information about health aimed at the general public. Bury points out that "patients' illness narratives, once silenced by a paternalistic if not overtly authoritarian medicine, suddenly find a new voice. . . . [U]nder all of these conditions it is not surprising to see illness narratives gaining greater attention once again."[21]

Arthur Frank has written extensively about the experience of illness, having had a heart attack and testicular cancer himself.[27,28] One of the basic points Frank makes in his work is that given that many people live for some time with disabling chronic conditions, they clearly need to make sense of their illness at an existential and personal level. One of the ways they do this is through their stories or narratives about illness. Frank suggests that stories about illness are not simply descriptions of what it is like to be ill, and the moral linkage with social values and norms. Rather, he suggests that the narratives ill people construct are a key means by which they actually carry out efforts to restore their sense of self. Narratives are one of the mechanisms patients use to articulate their sense of who they are, how they have come to be what they are, and how they might develop a new and different sense of self.

In his book *At the Will of the Body*, Frank narrates his personal account of illness and the ebb and flow of events that surrounded him.[27] The book provides a powerful illustration of how people experience being ill and how they relate to health professionals and the world of medicine. Like many people experiencing chronic illness, Frank had to come to terms not only with a body that had been transformed, but also with a life that had been transformed. Frank describes the loss of physical functioning and the loss of his younger self that accompanied his illnesses. In particular, Frank identifies the shifts in perception of time that accompany illness: Before he was ill, he was able to see his present as directly linked with the past. But when illness struck, he had to recognize that his past was over and that his future was contingent on medical projections of survival. Frank highlights a disorderliness that occurs with an illness threat and the trajectory nature of illness: with cancer, the fear of sudden death was absent, whereas this was reversed with heart disease, at least in its acute phase.

In *The Wounded Storyteller*, Frank argues that key changes have occurred over the last century, in that vast numbers of people now live with the aftereffects or direct effects of chronic illness.[28] In his words, we now live in a "Remission Society," where people live with chronic illness managed through various technological interventions. This situation has produced a novel set of circumstances: individuals and families now "share the worries and daily triumphs of staying well."[28] For Frank, this means that illness should not be seen as a disruption in one's life but as part of life's map or journey.[28] In short, what Frank is arguing is that "patients" are now reclaiming their bodies from modern medicine. Whereas patients' voices were once silenced by an all-encompassing medical narrative, laypeople can now adopt a postmodernist stance through which they can articulate their experiences without necessarily referring to medicine at all. Frank argues that medical sociology, like medicine, needs to adopt a stance of being a witness to suffering by listening to narratives.

Frank identifies different types of narrative accounts: restitution, chaos, and quest. *Restitution narratives* are those that involve the expectation that the sufferer will become healthy again. *Chaos narratives* are those in which the individual imagines she or he will never get better. *Quest narratives* are those that involve self-transformation and the offering of help to themselves and others through illness. Frank indicates that the quest narrative, with its emphasis on self-transformation, is an important aspect of the healing work achieved through the narrative process. He also argues that illness can help individuals to make clear their own moral values and sense of self,[29] or as Charmaz says, "Chronic illness often crystallizes vital lessons about living."[30]

This use of illness narratives to help individuals make moralistic meaning of their lives has come under attack for its overly romantic view of illness and its almost Christian or religious sense of the virtues of suffering.[31] On a different note and in the context of people living with HIV infection and people surviving sexual abuse, Crossley has drawn attention to some of the wider critiques of narrative, particularly regarding the idea of the therapeutic or redemptive narrative.[32] For example, in the case of survivors of sexual abuse, Crossley argues that some stories based on the notion of healing or redemption, although potentially useful from the point of view of the individuals themselves, may actually serve to depoliticize incest and suffering, thus erasing key feminist questions about the nature of male power in a patriarchal society.[32] To put this more simply, focusing exclusively on illness narratives, with their emphasis on growth, development, and change for the individual, may deflect attention from the structural determinants of ill health and obscure the need to transform social, economic, and political structures. As Crossley has shown in her own work on people with HIV, illness narratives can lead people to being concerned solely with themselves, with "me" and "my needs," often to the detriment of others.[32]

Frank also comments extensively about his relationships with health professionals.[27] He suggests that the disruption in life plans caused by illness as well as the everyday disruptions of illness are often very difficult for health professionals to appreciate or even acknowledge. This may be exacerbated by the growth of evidence-based care in most Western societies, which has resulted in guidelines, protocols, and "evidence" of different sorts to assist health professionals. For patients, however, such evidence fails to take into account the particularities and specificities of chronic illness. As Bury points out, "It is the particularities of experience that give meaning to illness for the individual, but these are almost impossible for others to take on board. How each person in the care giving/care receiving relationship handles these tensions can play a large part in determining the experience." [33] According to Frank, the problem is that caregivers do not face a linear set of problems from patients with chronic illness: they face a stew of panic, uncertainty, fear, denial, and disorientation.[27]

In this situation, Frank suggests that patients are vulnerable, often scared, and dependent, a situation essentially at odds with the tenets of Western culture, based as it is on individual autonomy and control. Charmaz reported that the needs of the chronically ill may strain close personal and familial relationships (as well as those with health professionals).[23] However, as Frank points out, "I needed others more than I ever have and I was also most vulnerable to them."[27] Having to appear positive in front of health professionals could be wearing, where acknowledgment and recognition of pain would have been more authentic and reassuring. In terms of his relationships with professionals, Frank reports that although some were able to acknowledge the concerns he had, many did not. This acknowledgment is perhaps key to understanding the experience of health and illness in contemporary society. Acknowledging another's suffering is a key aspect of being in a relationship with another. As Crossley makes clear in her work on narrative, this acknowledgment, or simply "being present" in a relationship, is an essential attribute that is often absent in many healthcare relationships, but it is something that is often extremely important to those suffering chronic illness.[32] Frank notes that for many health professionals "continuing suffering threatens them, so they deny it exists."[27] These findings highlight how the quality of relationships between healthcare providers and patients can be critical in helping patients make sense of their illnesses and treatment. We will now explore the specific factors affecting the development of pharmacist–patient relationships and how such relationships can affect pharmacist involvement in patient decision making.

PHARMACIST–PATIENT RELATIONSHIPS

A discussion on how patients view and make decisions about their illness and treatment experience would not be complete if it did not explore the relationship between the pharmacist and the patient. This relationship is important in helping patients process their illness experience and make important decisions about how to respond to their treatment options. The pharmaceutical care movement from the 1990s to the present suggested that the fundamental pharmacist–patient relationship is a covenant or "a mutually beneficial exchange in which a patient promises to grant authority to the provider, and the provider promises compromise and commitment" to the patient.[34] Although many pharmacy associations and pharmacy academies have accepted this view of the pharmacist–patient relationship, it is less than clear whether this ideal relationship actually occurs in today's pharmacy practice environment. Before discussing the factors affecting the development of a pharmacist–patient relationship and the extent of their collaboration and decision making, it is important to first identify some context regarding what defines a pharmacist–patient relationship and how this definition has changed in the last 50 years.

Historical Context of the Pharmacist–Patient Relationship

When we think of having a professional relationship with a healthcare practitioner, we begin to ask ourselves a series of questions. First, how do we know we have such a relationship with a provider? Do we have a "relationship" with a provider after only seeing him or her once? Does the quality of that interaction affect whether we consider having a professional relationship with another healthcare provider? When we think of a relationship with any health professional, most of us think of it in a reflective manner, looking retrospectively over a series of interactions. We do not usually say after one or two visits that we have a professional relationship with the provider. However, we might say after several interactions with the same provider that we have a relationship with him or her that began several visits ago. The word *relationship* suggests an ongoing involvement between two or more people that has developed over time. Thus, when we think of the specific pharmacist–patient relationship, it is probably best to think of it as that involvement between a pharmacist and patient that has developed over several visits to the pharmacy. It is also important to recognize that a pharmacist–patient relationship is much more than just the act of communication between two individuals. Pharmacist–patient communication is the basis from which a relationship develops. A relationship is evidenced by a growing connection between the pharmacist and patient that spans time and involves cognitive and emotional investment.

The other major component of a professional relationship is the qualitative aspects of the involvement between two individuals. A person may go to the pharmacy several times and possibly see the same pharmacist each time but engage very little with the pharmacist. This patient may have a difficult time thinking of this limited interaction with the pharmacist as a professional relationship with the pharmacist. Conversely, the patient may clearly report having a professional relationship with the pharmacist who he or she sees at most visits and who asks how the patient is doing (establishing rapport) and gives meaningful assistance regarding his or her treatment. A strong pharmacist–patient relationship can result from the same pharmacist seeing patients multiple times and engaging them in some conversation and helping solve treatment issues. Patients perceive such pharmacists as being "involved" in their care in a genuine way and not for business purposes only.

In the United States, consumers who are middle-aged or older will likely remember the days (especially before the mid-1980s) of the pharmacist who practiced at a small neighborhood pharmacy and to whom their families went for many years. In those times, the pharmacist and patient knew each other well. The patient would frequently ask the pharmacist questions and have much trust regarding the pharmacist's knowledge. Since the 1980s, the U.S. pharmacy practice community has experienced a significant expansion in the number of large chain pharmacies that sell a wide range of sundry goods and expect to process a much greater number of prescriptions per store. Today, most U.S. consumers have witnessed both a sharp decline in the number of small pharmacies independently owned and a corresponding sharp rise in the number of large chain pharmacies in their communities.

The shift from small pharmacies to large chain pharmacies is also associated with changes in the nature and extent of the pharmacist–patient relationship. Many chain pharmacies experience significant prescription volumes and limited staffing. The significant prescription volumes partly stem from an expanding older population with significant prescription medication needs. These heavy prescription volumes make it difficult for a chain pharmacist to realistically spend much time with patients and cultivate a relationship. Such excessive workloads can also contribute to staff turnover, making it more likely that a given chain pharmacist will not stay at a particular location for many years, which also inhibits patients' ability to maintain a relationship with a community pharmacist. A great number of pharmacists often work part-time, which disenables the pharmacist and patient from consistently seeing each other and developing a relationship. Finally, many pharmacies are meeting their shortage of staff pharmacists by hiring temporary pharmacists who float from store to store to meet short-term anticipated needs. Floaters, like part-timers, are often unable to establish any significant relationships with patients they see only seldom or inconsistently. These factors have made it difficult for chain pharmacists to establish relationships with patients. Such difficulty is especially felt hardest by middle-aged or older consumers who remember the days of having such a relationship with their pharmacists and are no longer able to do so.

The Pharmacist–Patient Relationship and Patient Decision Making

In addition to the historical and systemic factors affecting the nature and extent of the pharmacist–patient relationship, there is some literature to suggest there are patient factors that influence the development of this relationship and its subsequent impact on patient willingness to collaborate with pharmacists. Patient factors known to be associated with the quality of the pharmacist–patient relationship include the patient's frequency of contact with the pharmacist, the perceived competence or expertise of the pharmacist, the patient's trust in the pharmacist, the caring nature of the pharmacist, and the patient's satisfaction with the pharmacist.[35-37] These factors are interdependent, because frequency of contact between pharmacist and patient may affect the patient's trust in and perceived competence of the pharmacist. Further, the patient's perceived trust in the competence of the pharmacist may affect his or her satisfaction in the pharmacist and subsequently the pharmacist–patient relationship.

Hermansen and Wiederholt showed that a patient's measure of interpersonal relationship quality (including dimensions of caring, respectfulness, and trustworthiness) was an important variable influencing the patient's willingness to collaborate with the pharmacist.[37] These studies suggest that patients who have a good relationship with their pharmacist may be more inclined to ask questions about medication use and to involve the pharmacist in their decision making regarding medication use. Conversely, patients who have weak or nonexistent relationships with their pharmacist are less likely to involve their pharmacists when making decisions regarding their medication therapy.

In addition to patient factors affecting the pharmacist–patient relationship, it is important to note pharmacist and other factors that can affect the pharmacist–patient relationship. There has been relatively little to no research that has explored pharmacist factors that influence the development of a relationship with a patient. If we assume that the factors affecting the initiation of communication are somewhat similar to those to involving the initiation of a relationship, then it is likely that the following pharmacist variables might affect the development of a pharmacist–patient relationship: the pharmacist's time, the importance of the information to be exchanged, the pharmacist's transfer of the prescription to the patient, and the pharmacist's attitude toward counseling.[38,39] It is very possible that a strong desire by pharmacists to have relationships with patients will increase the probability that they will help patients with making decisions regarding their treatment. Other possible variables include the availability of a private counseling area and how comfortable the pharmacist is with talking about the patient's illness. More research is needed to explore whether any of these factors indeed affect pharmacists' willingness to engage in a professional relationship with patients and subsequently help patients make decisions regarding their medication therapy.

SUMMARY

This chapter began by presenting theoretical and empirical research regarding what we know about how patients initially perceive their symptoms and how patients use these symptoms to build mental representations of what illnesses they have and what treatments might be appropriate for them. The chapter then explored three treatment possibilities: self-care, use of over-the-counter medications, and use of prescription medications. In each of these possibilities, patients are perceived as making choices and considering among alternatives to select the best alternative. This part of the chapter ended with the discussion of a model by Pound and colleagues that summarizes different ways patients might respond to medication use: as passive accepters (who accept medication as prescribed without questioning), active accepters (who accept medication as prescribed only after their concerns have been met), and active modifiers (who independently alter their treatment based on their own sense of treatment).[19]

The chapter then considered how patients make social meaning of both their illness and treatment experiences. In particular, this discussion explored the use of illness narratives as an important way for patients to share how their illnesses have shaped their self-concept and relationship with others, including healthcare providers. The final part of the chapter examined how the pharmacist–patient relationship has changed and what patient and pharmacist factors affect the patient's decision-making process.

The reader should now understand psychosocial aspects of how patient interpretations and experiences regarding illness and treatment can influence the decisions they make before and during their interaction with pharmacists. Further, the reader should also now be able to readily identify ways in which a pharmacist can build a relationship with a patient and subsequently help the patient make appropriate and effective treatment decisions.

REFERENCES

1. Broadbent DE. A mechanical model for human attention and memory. Psychol Rev 1957;64: 205-15.
2. Zola IK. Pathways to the doctor—from person to patient. Soc Sci Med 1973;7:677-89.
3. Bishop GD. Understanding the understanding of illness: lay disease representations. In: Skelton JA, Croyle RT, eds. Mental representations in health and illness. New York: Springer-Verlag, 1991:32-59.
4. Bishop GD, Converse SA. Illness representations: a prototype approach. Health Psychol 1986; 5:95-114.
5. Dean K. Conceptual, theoretical and methodological issues in self-care research. Soc Sci Med 1989;29:117-23.
6. Banks MH, Beresford SAA, Morrell DC, Waller JJ, Watkins CJ. Factors influencing demand for primary medical care in women aged 20–44 years: a preliminary report. Int J Epidemiol 1975;4:189-95.
7. Bloor M, Horobin GW. Conflict and conflict resolution in doctor/patient interactions. In: Cox C, Mead A, eds. A sociology of medical practice. London: Collier Macmillan, 1975.
8. Heritage J, Robinson JD. Accounting for the medical visit: giving reasons for seeking medical care. In: Heritage J, Maynard DW, eds. Communication in medical care: interaction between primary care physicians and patients. Cambridge: Cambridge University Press, 2006.

9. Sihvo S. Utilization and appropriateness of self-medication in Finland [PhD thesis]. Department of Public Health, University of Helsinki, 2000.

10. Herxheimer A, Britten N. Formulary for self-care. Br J Gen Pract 1994;44:339-40.

11. Himmel W, Lippert-Urbanke E, Kochen MM. Are patients more satisfied when they receive a prescription? The effect of patient expectations in general practice. Scand J Primary Health Care 1997;15:118-22.

12. Britten N, Jenkins L, Barber N, Bradley C, Stevenson F. Developing a measure for the appropriateness of prescribing in general practice. Qual Safety Health Care 2003;12:246-50.

13. Cockburn J, Pit S. Prescribing behaviour in clinical practice: patients' expectations and doctors' perceptions of patients' expectations—a questionnaire study. BMJ 1997;315:520-3.

14. Britten N, Ukoumunne O. The influence of patients' hopes of receiving a prescription on doctors' perceptions and the decision to prescribe: a questionnaire survey. BMJ 1997;315:1506-10.

15. Mintzes B, Barer ML, Kravitz RL, et al. How does direct-to-consumer advertising (DTCA) affect prescribing? A survey in primary care environments with and without legal DTCA. CMAJ 2003;169:405-12.

16. Chewning B, Schommer JC. Increasing clients' knowledge of community pharmacists' roles. Pharm Res 1996;13:1299 1304.

17. Conrad P. The meaning of medications: another look at compliance. Soc Sci Med 1985;20:29-37.

18. Donovan JL. Patient decision making: the missing ingredient in compliance research. Int J Technol Assess Health Care 1995;11:443-55.

19. Pound P, Britten N, Morgan M, et al. Resisting medicines: a synthesis of qualitative studies of medicine taking. Soc Sci Med 2005;61:133-55.

20. Vrijens B, Urquhart J. Policy questions posed by pervasive short persistence with chronic-use drug dosing regimens. Paper presented at the Conference on Pharmaceutical Policy Analysis, Zeist, The Netherlands, 2007.

21. Bury M. Illness narratives: fact or fiction? Sociol Health Illness 2001;23(3):263-85.

22. Annandale E. The sociology of health and medicine: a critical introduction. Cambridge, MA: Polity Press, 1998.

23. Charmaz K. Loss of self: a fundamental form of suffering in the chronically ill. Sociol Health Illness 1983;5(1):168-95.

24. Charmaz K. Struggling for a self: identity levels of the chronically ill. In: Roth JA, Conrad P, eds. Research in the sociology of health care. Greenwich, CT: JAI Press, 1987.

25. Bury M. Chronic illness as biographical disruption. Sociol Health Illness 1982;4:167-82.

26. Williams G. The genesis of chronic illness: narrative reconstruction. Sociol Health Illness 1984;6:174-200.

27. Frank AW. At the will of the body. Boston: Houghton Mifflin, 1991.

28. Frank AW. The wounded storyteller: body, illness and ethics. Chicago: Chicago University Press, 1995.

29. Frank AW. Stories of illness as care of the self: a Foucauldian dialogue. Health 1998;2(3):329-48.

30. Charmaz K. Good days, bad days: the self in chronic illness and time. New Brunswick, NJ: Rutgers University Press, 1991.

31. Atkinson P. Narrative turn or blind alley? Qualitative Health Res 1997;7(3):325-44.

32. Crossley ML. Introducing narrative psychology: self, trauma and the construction of meaning. Buckingham, England: Open University Press, 2000.

33. Bury M. Health and illness. Cambridge, MA: Polity Press, 2005.

34. Hepler C, Strand L. Opportunities and responsibilities in pharmaceutical care. Am J Pharm Educ 1989;53:7S-15S.

35. Berger BA. Building an effective therapeutic alliance: competence, trustworthiness, and caring. Am J Hosp Pharm 1985;50:2399-403.

36. Worley MM, Schommer JC. Pharmacist-patient relationships: factors influencing quality and commitment. J Soc Adm Pharm 1999;16(3/4):157-73.

37. Hermansen CJ, Wiederholt JB. Pharmacist-patient relationship development in an ambulatory clinic setting. Health Commun 2001;13(3):307-25.

38. Schommer JC, Wiederholt JB. A field investigation of participant and environment effects on pharmacist-patient communication in community pharmacies. Med Care 1995;33(6):567-84.

39. Schommer JC, Wiederholt JB. The association of prescription status, patient age, patient gender, and patient question asking behavior with the content of pharmacist-patient communication. Pharm Res 1997;14(2):145-51.

CHAPTER 11

Interpersonal Communication for Pharmaceutical Care

Lourdes G. Planas, PhD

What are the types and extent of communications that might occur between a pharmacist and patient? Interestingly, there are many possibilities, and the likelihood of their occurrences varies based on numerous factors. The type and extent of communication that can take place between a patient and the pharmacist depends on many individual, interpersonal, and environmental factors. For example, what attitudes about patient counseling does the pharmacist possess? What expectations regarding pharmacist–patient communication does the pharmacist believe the patient has? What beliefs about pharmacist–patient relationships does the patient have? How does the pharmacist's work setting facilitate or hinder the provision of pharmaceutical care?

This chapter describes relevant issues pertaining to interpersonal communication for pharmaceutical care. Specific issues that it examines are as follows:

- What is the nature of interpersonal communication for pharmaceutical care?
- To what extent does interpersonal communication for pharmaceutical care occur in practice?
- What factors influence interpersonal communication for pharmaceutical care?

It is important to be aware of these issues because interpersonal communication is a fundamental social and behavioral aspect of pharmaceutical care practice. Therefore, understanding its nature, extent, and influencing factors is critical for pharmacists to help patients optimize their drug therapy outcomes.

NATURE OF INTERPERSONAL COMMUNICATION FOR PHARMACEUTICAL CARE

Effective interpersonal communication is vital for pharmaceutical care practice. Specifically, it is essential in pharmacist–patient interactions to establish rapport, foster therapeutic relationships, promote dialogue for accurate information exchange, and engage patients in collaborative problem solving to identify, resolve, and prevent drug therapy problems (DTPs). Figure 11-1 depicts the interplay between these behaviors and how they contribute to the relationship between interpersonal communication and pharmaceutical care. Interpersonal communication in pharmaceutical care serves two basic functions: (1) to establish rapport between a pharmacist and patient, and (2) to promote information exchange. Establishing rapport using a patient-centered approach is instrumental to building a therapeutic relationship. Likewise, information exchange for the purpose of problem solving is instrumental to implementing the patient care process. Developing a therapeutic relationship with patients and con-

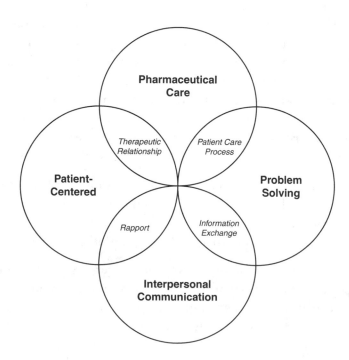

FIGURE 11-1   Nature of Interpersonal Communication for Pharmaceutical Care
Source: Adapted from Cipolle RJ, Strand LM, Morley PC. Pharmaceutical care practice: the clinician's guide. 2nd ed. New York: McGraw-Hill; 2004.

ducting the patient care process are the primary provider roles in pharmaceutical care practice.[1] This section of the chapter examines features of the elements that appear in Figure 11-1. At varying levels, all of these elements contribute to the social and behavioral nature of interpersonal communication for pharmaceutical care.

Interpersonal Communication

Interpersonal communication is the process of interaction that takes place between two people. There are many models of interpersonal communication. Figure 11-2 presents an adaptation of a model that is widely used in pharmacy communication.[2,3] The model includes five elements: sender, receiver, message, feedback, and barriers.

In the interpersonal communication process, a *sender* encodes and transmits a message to a *receiver*, who then decodes and receives the message. The meaning that the receiver assigns to the message might not be the same meaning that the sender intended. However, for effective communication to occur, the receiver must assign the same meaning as the sender intended. The receiver assigns meaning based on his or her experiences, definitions, and knowledge.

The *message* is the element that is transmitted from the sender to the receiver. Messages are transmitted either intentionally or unintentionally. Additionally, messages can be transmitted verbally, nonverbally, in written form, or in some combination of

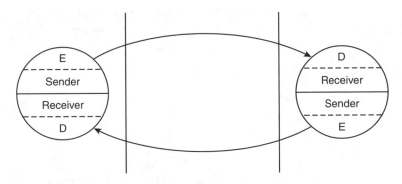

E = Encode; D = Decode; ⇄ = Message/Feedback; | = Barriers

FIGURE 11-2   Interpersonal Communication Model
Source: Adapted from: Shannon CE, Weaver W. The mathematical theory of communication. Urbana, IL: University of Illinois Press; 1949; Schramm W. How communication works. In: Schramm W, editor. The process and effects of mass communication. Urbana, IL: University of Illinois Press; 1954. p. 3–26; Mehrabian A. Silent messages. Belmont, CA: Wadsworth; 1971.

these. Verbal communication consists of actual words that are stated. Nonverbal communication includes eye contact, facial expressions, gestures, posture, proximity (distance between two people), and paralanguage (tone, volume, inflection). The majority of messages that people send are nonverbal in nature, ranging from approximately 55% to 93%.[4,5] Communication also can be provided in written form. Examples of written communication between pharmacists and patients are prescriptions and the medication information leaflets that accompany prescriptions.

Feedback is the process by which the receiver transmits his or her understanding of the message back to the sender. During feedback, the receiver becomes the sender, and the sender becomes the receiver. Feedback can range from a simple head nod to repeating a set of instructions. Feedback is crucial for effective communication and mutual understanding because it permits the sender and receiver to confirm the accuracy of the message.

Barriers in the communication process can distort messages and cause misunderstandings between individuals. There are two major categories of barriers: personal and environmental. Each of these categories consists of many types of barriers (Table 11-1). Some barriers are obvious, whereas others are not. Likewise, some barriers are easier than others to minimize or overcome.

The model presented in Figure 11-2 emphasizes the dynamic and transactional nature of interpersonal communication by acknowledging that messages and feedback

TABLE 11-1	**Common Interpersonal Communication Barriers in Pharmacist–Patient Interactions**	
Category	**Type**	**Example**
Personal	Psychological	Emotional state (e.g., rushed)
	Internal noise	Competing thoughts
	Social	Lack of prior relationship
	Historical	Previous unpleasant encounter
	Cultural	Differences in use of eye contact
	Semantic	Not understanding words (e.g., medical terms)
Environmental	Physical	High prescription counter
	Setting	Lack of private area
	External noise	Phones ringing

Adapted from Mehrabian A. Silent messages. Belmont, CA: Wadsworth, 1971.

can be sent simultaneously between a sender and receiver. In other words, a person may be a sender and a receiver at the same time. The transactional nature of this model is in contrast to a transmission model, in which communication is depicted as a one-way, linear process from sender to receiver. In a transaction model, senders should send messages in their clearest form and ask for feedback to determine whether the message was received as intended. Likewise, receivers should offer feedback to check whether they correctly understood the message. These activities make communication a two-way process intended to establish shared meaning between its participants. It is important to anticipate potential barriers and develop strategies to minimize them so that effective communication can occur.

Rapport for Building Therapeutic Relationships

Figure 11-1 depicts rapport as an interpersonal communication component that, through a patient-centered approach, is instrumental to building a therapeutic relationship. The *American Heritage Dictionary* defines *rapport* as "a relationship, especially one of mutual trust or emotional affinity."[6] Rapport can be synonymous with "understanding."[7] A pharmacist who establishes rapport with a patient, therefore, attempts to develop a relationship that can involve understanding a patient's needs and experiences while developing trust and a positive emotional bond.

Active Listening and Empathic Responding

The major interpersonal communication behaviors for establishing rapport with patients are active listening and empathic responding. Listening is a commonly neglected communication skill, yet it is the communication skill that we use most frequently. Of our time spent communicating, approximately half is spent listening, while the remaining time is divided between talking, reading, and writing.[8,9] Effective listening involves trying to understand another's thoughts and feelings.

Listening can be passive or active. In passive listening, the receiver assumes that he or she has heard and understood correctly. The receiver remains passive and does not verify what has been expressed. In *active listening*, the receiver is genuinely interested in understanding what the other person is thinking and feeling, and in ensuring that his or her perception is accurate before responding with his or her own new message. Active listening involves paraphrasing or summarizing one's understanding of the sender's message and reflecting it back for verification. This verification or feedback process enhances the receiver's ability to decode the sender's message in a way that is congruent with what the sender intended. Also, the reflection to the sender of what he or she conveyed makes the sender feel cared for and understood. Feeling understood by a healthcare provider can lessen patients' negative emotions that accompany illness.

Empathic responding is another interpersonal communication behavior that helps establish rapport. Patients often communicate how they feel, whether directly or indirectly, in the messages they send. Empathy entails experiencing and expressing the feelings, attitudes, and thoughts of another. It involves taking the other person's perspective by imagining one's self in that person's situation.[10] Empathic responses are free from judgment and advice. The main characteristic that distinguishes empathy from active listening is that an empathic response acknowledges feelings (and sometimes content), whereas active listening primarily paraphrases or summarizes content. An example of an empathic response is a pharmacist saying, "Sounds like you're discouraged that your doctor prescribed more medications for you."

Active listening and empathic responding build rapport with patients by helping them feel understood and able to trust a health care provider as someone who genuinely cares about them. Rapport between a patient and a healthcare provider is necessary for patient-centered care. The dimensions of patient-centered care have been defined as understanding a patient's illness experience, perceiving each patient as unique, fostering an egalitarian relationship with a patient, building a therapeutic alliance with a patient, and developing self-awareness of one's personal effects on patients.[11] A central tenet of patient-centered care is involving patients in the decision-making process to meet therapeutic goals that they and their healthcare providers endorse.

THERAPEUTIC RELATIONSHIP

Hepler and Strand described the therapeutic relationship in pharmaceutical care as "a mutually beneficial exchange in which the patient grants authority to the provider and the provider gives competence and commitment (accepts responsibility) to the patient."[12] They characterized this relationship as a covenant, or a solemn and binding agreement between patient and provider.[13] Other notable additions to the description of a therapeutic relationship accentuate greater patient involvement through dialogue and shared decision making. Whereas a covenantal relationship emphasizes the commitment of the provider to the patient, a dialogic relationship recognizes the discourse that must take place between patient and provider for the relationship to be formed and cultivated.[1] During meaningful dialogue, needs are expressed, expectations are shaped, and trust is explored. Additionally, a therapeutic relationship has been described as a participatory relationship in which patients collaborate with providers on treatment decisions.[14] Providers who engage in meaningful dialogue and collaborative decision making with patients deliver care that is truly patient centered.

Information Exchange for the Patient Care Process

Figure 11-1 portrays information exchange as an interpersonal communication component that, when conducted for the purpose of problem solving, is instrumental to the patient care process. Information exchange in this context serves four primary purposes: (1) assessing patients' health, (2) reaching decisions on treatment plans and goals, (3) implementing treatment plans, and (4) evaluating treatment effects. Information *exchange* denotes a back-and-forth pattern of communication between patient and provider. Indeed, the most widely used model for patient counseling is an example of information exchange in action.

Indian Health Service Model of Pharmacist–Patient Consultation

The patient counseling techniques developed by the Indian Health Service (IHS) are widely accepted in pharmacy.[15-17] The IHS patient counseling approach consists of three steps: (1) assess patient knowledge, (2) provide medication information, and (3) verify patient understanding. The ultimate goals are to ensure that patients understand how to use and what to expect from their medications so they can make appropriate decisions regarding their drug therapy.

Pharmacists ask a series of prime questions to ascertain what patients know about their medication (Table 11-2). Based on the answer a patient provides for each prime question and any necessary related follow-up questions, a pharmacist provides appropriate information to fill in the gaps that exist in the patient's knowledge. At the conclusion of the prime question-answer-information sequences, the pharmacist asks the patient to repeat the most pertinent information. This last step in the IHS patient counseling approach is a form of feedback that enables the pharmacist to check that the patient understands what has been discussed.

The three IHS prime questions encompass four drug-related needs that patients may have: indication, adherence, safety, and effectiveness. *Drug-related needs* are any lack of understanding, concerns, or expectations that patients may have regarding a particular medication.[1] Each of these drug-related needs, if not appropriately addressed, can result in a DTP (Table 11-2).[1,18]

For example, informing a patient about what to expect from his medication in terms of effectiveness, instructing him how to monitor his response, and setting goals for his therapy can empower him to know whether the medication is working as intended. Through monitoring symptoms or other parameters (e.g., blood pressure), a patient can detect a lack of medication effectiveness. This deficiency could exist because of a DTP associated with a suboptimal dosage (e.g., low dosage) or because the medication is not the most effective one for this patient (e.g., wrong drug). Unless patients understand how to monitor their response to treatment, they may not be able

TABLE 11-2   Information Exchange in the Patient Counseling and Patient Care Process

IHS Prime Questions	Provide Drug Information	Drug-Related Need	Drug Therapy Problem
What did your doctor tell you the medication is for?	Purpose	Appropriate indication	Need additional drug therapy Unnecessary drug therapy
How did your doctor tell you to take the medication?	Dosage Dosage schedule How to take What to do if a dose is missed Duration of use Precautions for use Proper preparation and storage	Adherence	Nonadherence
What did your doctor tell you to expect?	Common or potentially dangerous side effects What to do to manage side effects	Safety	Adverse drug reaction Dosage too high
	Benefits of medication Techniques and criteria for self-monitoring of response	Effectiveness	Wrong drug Dosage too low

IHS, Indian Health Service.

Adapted from Pfizer I. Pharmacist-patient consultation program. Unit I: an interactive approach to verify patient understanding. New York: National Healthcare Operations, 1991.

to assist with the detection of this type of DTP. In essence, the information exchange that occurs during the IHS patient counseling approach serves as a problem-solving mechanism to identify potential DTPs and prevent or reduce their occurrence.

PATIENT CARE PROCESS

The patient care process has been called the "heart" of pharmaceutical care practice.[1] It is the combination of day-to-day activities that pharmacists perform when inter-acting with patients in a pharmaceutical care practice. The purposes of the patient care process are to attain the most appropriate, effective, safe, and convenient drug therapy for the patient; to identify, resolve, and prevent any DTPs that could inter-fere with this attainment; and to ensure positive patient outcomes. The patient care process comprises three steps: assessment, pharmaceutical care plan, and follow-up evaluation. It is a comprehensive and systematic problem-solving process.[1]

During the assessment step of the patient care process, a pharmacist explores a patient's drug-related needs.[1] This includes asking questions to ascertain what the patient wants, does not want, and knows about his or her drug therapy. A comprehen-sive assessment for the DTPs listed in Table 11-2 is also performed, which can include modifications of the IHS prime questions. To assess drug therapy appropri-ateness, a pharmacist can ask for what purpose each medication is being taken. This questioning helps to identify unnecessary drug therapy such as therapeutic duplica-tions. A modification of the second prime question can be used to assess how the patient is *actually* taking the medication. The third prime question regarding what to expect can be divided into two separate questions addressing safety and effectiveness. Patients can be questioned about the incidence and severity of adverse effects. Additionally, they can be asked about their response to treatment.

The second step of the patient care process is the pharmaceutical care plan.[1] During this step, a patient and pharmacist collaborate to establish a list of possible actions to address all drug-related needs and DTPs. Based on a patient's preferences and guided by a pharmacist's expertise, the most appropriate interventions are selected. Additionally, therapeutic goals are set in conjunction with a patient's needs and values. The planned resolution of DTPs in a pharmaceutical care plan is impor-tant because these problems can interfere with patients achieving their desired thera-peutic goals. Pharmaceutical care plans are also intended to address the prevention of potential DTPs that might minimize the patient's probability of attaining his or her therapeutic goals.

The final step of the patient care process is the follow-up evaluation. This step is conducted to determine the extent of intervention success, whether therapeutic goals were met, and whether any new DTPs have developed.[1] A pharmacist's involvement in the follow-up evaluation is proactive. This step is where the pharmacist assumes responsibility for a patient's drug therapy outcomes. In reassessing for DTPs, the process begins again with the assessment step. Thus, the patient care process is continuous, with the follow-up evaluation acting as a means of feedback.

At its most basic level, information exchange is a dialogue, a series of questions and answers between two individuals. In the context of problem solving, it becomes a means to assess a patient's drug-related needs and ensure he or she understands how to use his or her medication. In a pharmaceutical care practice, the patient care process is a comprehensive and systematic problem-solving process that relies heavily on effective information exchange between a pharmacist and patient.

Feedback is crucial in many aspects of interpersonal communication for pharmaceutical care and is necessary for mutual understanding in the interpersonal communication process. Active listening and empathy are forms of feedback to help patients feel understood and to establish rapport. During patient counseling, verifying that a patient understands aspects of his or her drug therapy is accomplished by eliciting feedback from the patient. Finally, the patient care process becomes a continuous process when follow-up evaluations are conducted to receive feedback on the success of interventions and the achievement of therapeutic goals.

EXTENT OF INTERPERSONAL COMMUNICATION FOR PHARMACEUTICAL CARE

The pharmacy profession has undergone major evolution since the latter part of the 20th century, most notably the clinical pharmacy and pharmaceutical care eras.[12,19] While the social, ethical, and professional roles of pharmacists have changed, so has the extent of interpersonal communication, specifically pharmacist–patient communication. The more that pharmacists have accepted responsibility for patients' drug-related needs and have been held accountable for this commitment,[1] the greater the extent of interpersonal communication that has taken place in pharmacist–patient interactions.

This section of the chapter examines the extent of interpersonal communication in pharmacy practices. To accomplish this, we review different types of studies, including some in which mock patients (secret shoppers) reported what they encountered, pharmacists and patients were surveyed regarding their experiences, and researchers directly observed pharmacist–patient interactions. The extent of written prescription information in community pharmacies also is described. Because the profession's standard has moved to pharmaceutical care, we examine the extent of pharmaceutical care provision in community pharmacies based on pharmacists' self-reports. Additionally, the numbers and types of DTPs identified by pharmacists in pharmaceutical care practices are summarized. The implications of common DTPs and the degree to which pharmacist–patient communication is required to identify them are discussed in the context of pharmaceutical care practice.

Patient Counseling

Extent of Patient Counseling

Few studies of pharmacist–patient communication were conducted until the late 1960s. A 1969 study helped to identify a lack of patient counseling in situations where a potential DTP existed.[20] Posing as patients, these researchers discovered that only 6 of 36 pharmacists (17%) and 1 of 12 pharmacists (8%) refused to dispense prescriptions contraindicated for patients with diabetes and severe depression, respectively.

Following this study, an emerging body of literature attempted to quantify the percentage of patients who receive counseling and information from pharmacists. Studies prior to 1993 reported that approximately 60% to 80% of patients who received a prescription did not receive oral counseling from a pharmacist.[21-26]

Some of these studies used secret shoppers to initiate pharmacist–patient encounters. In a study in which pharmacy students posed as mock patients, 73% of patients received no oral counseling from a pharmacist when they picked up their prescriptions.[21] A Kansas study found that oral counseling did not occur in 69% of encounters.[22] Researchers in Wisconsin found that pharmacists failed to interview 63% of patients.[23]

Other studies have used mail surveys to query consumers. In a mail survey study of North Carolina households, 45% to 70% of consumer respondents reported either "never" or "infrequently" receiving oral counseling on medication directions, side effects, and storage.[24]

Some studies have used direct observation to describe the extent of pharmacist–patient communication in community pharmacy settings. Researchers in Florida observed and rated pharmacist–patient interactions prior to an educational intervention.[25] Of 381 dispensing encounters, 20% included some pharmacist consultation. Similarly, a New Mexico study of different payment methods and practice settings found that only 8% to 13% of patients were counseled, with those in capitation programs receiving significantly less counseling.[26]

These aforementioned studies occurred before the implementation of the Omnibus Budget Reconciliation Act of 1990 (OBRA '90), which required pharmacists to offer to counsel Medicaid patients about their prescriptions and to conduct prospective drug utilization reviews.[27] Since its passage in 1990 and implementation in 1993, 36 states have expanded the scope of the OBRA '90 regulations to all patients, not only Medicaid patients. There has been an upward trend in the extent of patient counseling in community pharmacies since the implementation of OBRA '90. Studies using mock patients or direct observation of interactions have reported counseling occurring in approximately 60% to 70% of pharmacist–patient encounters.[28-32]

Content of Patient Counseling

In addition to the occurrence of patient counseling, some studies have investigated the content of communication between pharmacists and patients. A Florida study reported that the most common types of information relayed pertained to how to take a medication (40%) and side effects (38%).[25] Wisconsin researchers found that the most common types of information provided were directions for medication use (39%), administrative elements such as generic substitutions or price (37%), solicitation of feedback (36%), and purpose of medication (31%).[33]

A study focusing on pharmacist question asking in New Mexico community pharmacies reported that pharmacists asked questions in only 36% of encounters.[30] More than one drug therapy question was asked in only 6% of these encounters. Open-ended questions were asked in only 7% of these encounters. Open-ended questions convey a willingness to listen and increase patient participation, thus using a more patient-centered approach. In contrast, closed-ended questions reduce a patient's degree of openness and increase passivity.[34]

Written Prescription Information

Written prescription information is an important component of communicating with patients. Most pharmacies distribute medication leaflets with patients' prescriptions. Written prescription information should supplement, not replace, verbal patient counseling.

The percentage of patients who receive written prescription information has increased. Fifteen percent and 59% of patients received written prescription information in 1982 and 1994, respectively,[28] and this percentage increased to approximately 89% between 1999 and 2001.[35-37] The most comprehensive study took place in 44 states during 2001.[37] These latest rates of distribution of written prescription information met goals set by the Food and Drug Administration (FDA) in its 1995 Medication Guide Requirements.[38] The FDA proposed a 75% distribution goal for written prescription information by 2000. However, the goal for 2006 was 95%. Therefore, improvements were needed.

In 1996, federal legislation was passed that required the U.S. Department of Health and Human Services to assess not only the distribution, but also the quality, of written prescription information.[39] The legislation authorized the FDA to take action if distribution goals were not met (i.e., 95% in 2006) and written information was not useful. Criteria for evaluating usefulness stated that information must be scientifically accurate, sufficiently specific and comprehensive to inform consumers about medication use, and formatted legibly to be comprehended by and not confusing to users.[39] The comprehensive 44-state study in 2001 found that medication leaflets distributed in pharmacies tended to be scientifically accurate. However, less than 10% met criteria for information specificity, comprehensibility, and legibility.[37]

The extents of patient counseling and medication leaflet distribution have increased in past decades. However, there is still room for improvement. Patient counseling, even when supplemented with written medication information, is usually executed only for new prescriptions and focuses on brief messages pertaining to how to take a medication and potential side effects. These interactions are typically one-way, medication-focused transmissions of information from pharmacists to patients with little opportunity for information exchange and patient involvement.

Patient counseling and provision of written prescription information are intended to ensure that patients understand important aspects of their medications so they can make appropriate decisions to optimize their therapy. Most patient counseling encounters focus on providing information for the immediately prescribed medication. What happens when the patient begins taking the medication? Is the medication effective? Does the patient experience bothersome or severe adverse effects? Does the patient take the medication as prescribed? If not, what factors influence the patient not to adhere to the prescribed regimen? These questions are answered by performing pharmaceutical care activities (i.e., identifying, resolving, and preventing DTPs that interfere with achieving therapeutic goals). Patient counseling and written prescription information are useful communication tools, but they alone do not constitute a pharmaceutical care practice.

PHARMACEUTICAL CARE

This section summarizes the extent of pharmaceutical care provision in practice and in pharmaceutical care intervention studies. First, pharmacists' self-reports of performing specific pharmaceutical care activities are described. Measures of pharmaceutical care activities vary, but generally include screening patient profiles, patient counseling, patient-oriented DTP identification and solving, and documentation.

Second, the numbers of DTPs identified in studies that specifically sought to implement and evaluate pharmaceutical care practices are examined. Because the patient care process in pharmaceutical care practice is a comprehensive problem-solving process, investigating the extent of DTP identification in intervention studies is also a marker of pharmaceutical care provision. But more important, examining the types of DTPs that are commonly identified and comparing this to the types of DTPs that require more direct pharmacist–patient communication offers some insight into the extent of interpersonal communication that occurs in pharmaceutical care practices.

Pharmaceutical Care Provision

Studies attempting to determine the extent of pharmaceutical care provision have generally used self-administered surveys to collect information from community pharmacists. Three such studies are summarized here.

Researchers in Florida surveyed community pharmacists about their implementation of pharmaceutical care services.[40] The Behavioral Pharmaceutical Care Scale was used to quantify the extent of pharmaceutical care provision.[41] Respondents reported moderate levels of patient record screening, patient consultation, and verification of patient understanding. They reported very low levels of patient assessment, implementation of therapeutic objectives and monitoring plans, and documentation.

The extent of pharmaceutical care provision in West Virginia rural community practices was determined by surveying pharmacy owners and managers.[42] Activities that respondents indicated performing most frequently pertained to patient communication, reviewing patients' medication profiles, and obtaining and maintaining patient information. Drug therapy monitoring was the least frequently reported activity. All activities, with the exception of drug therapy monitoring, were typically conducted at the time of dispensing a prescription, especially a new prescription. In contrast, drug therapy monitoring included monitoring a patient's medication adherence, therapeutic effect, and possible adverse effects.

In a North Carolina mail survey, 30% of pharmacists indicated that they provided pharmaceutical care services in their practices.[43] However, only 20% reported providing pharmaceutical care services specified in the Pharmacy Practice Activity Classification (i.e., ensure appropriate pharmacotherapy, ensure patients' understanding of and adherence to their treatment, and monitor and report outcomes).[44]

As these studies demonstrated, pharmaceutical care implementation by community pharmacists is low. Furthermore, activities that are distinct to pharmaceutical care are performed less frequently than those that are more in line with OBRA '90, such as screening patients' medication records and counseling them about their medications.[27]

Amounts and Types of Drug Therapy Problems

In addition to pharmacists' self-reports, the extent of pharmaceutical care provision in studies in which pharmaceutical care services are implemented can be measured by the number of DTPs. In many instances, DTP identification, resolution, and follow-up evaluation rely on pharmacist–patient communication (e.g., medication history, assessing patient's response to treatment).

For example, screening patients' medication records for drug–drug interactions or therapeutic duplications requires very little pharmacist–patient communication. In contrast, interviewing patients about their response to treatment or presence of symptoms (e.g., suboptimal response due to a low dosage, needing an additional medication prescribed for an untreated indication, or nonadherence) requires more information exchange and direct patient contact.

Pharmaceutical care intervention studies that have measured the numbers of identified and resolved DTPs report an average of two to three DTPs per patient per year.[45-48] With regard to types of DTPs, undertreatment appears to be a prevalent problem. Consistently, the most common types of DTPs identified tend to be the following: needing additional drug therapy, low dosage, and nonadherence (Table 11-3). For example, a patient with hypertension whose blood pressure is not at goal may require an additional medication to be added to her regimen (i.e., additional drug therapy) or a dosage increase of a medication she is currently taking (i.e., low dosage). Additionally, a patient may have a suboptimal response as a result of not taking a medication as prescribed (i.e., nonadherence).

The identification of these most common types of DTPs typically requires direct pharmacist–patient communication. These DTPs cannot be identified by merely screening a patient's medication profile, which requires little, if any, pharmacist–patient communication. Furthermore, monitoring of the resolution of these types of DTPs usually requires asking patients about their treatment response and medication adherence. In most community pharmacies, these are best accomplished by moving away from the computer and talking with patients. Medication refill dates in a patient's profile can provide an estimate of adherence, but speaking with a patient can uncover issues such as reasons for nonadherence and preferable solutions.

The last half-century has seen an evolution of pharmacist–patient communication, especially in the contexts of patient counseling and pharmaceutical care. The need for effective interpersonal communication between pharmacists and patients is expected to increase as more pharmacists move toward a patient-centered pharmaceutical care practice. Understanding factors associated with interpersonal communication for pharmaceutical care can help improve its expansion. Such factors are discussed in the following section.

TABLE 11-3	Type and Percentage of Drug Therapy Problems Identified in Pharmaceutical Care Studies			
	Kassam et al.[45] (2001)	McDonough and Doucette[46] (2003)	Doucette et al.[47] (2005)	Isetts[48] (2007)
Indication				
Need additional drug therapy	40	39.8	22.0	20.1
Unnecessary drug therapy	7	3.7	12.9	3.6
Adherence				
Nonadherence	12	31.1	25.9	23.3
Safety				
Adverse drug reaction	11	11.7	11.1	7.8
Dosage too high	7	2.3	5.3	7.5
Effectiveness				
Wrong drug	13	2.2	13.2	8.0
Dosage too low	7	9.2	9.7	29.6
Total number of DTPs per patient per year	**2.7**	**2.2**	**3.0**	**2.3**

DTP, drug therapy problem.

FACTORS ASSOCIATED WITH INTERPERSONAL COMMUNICATION FOR PHARMACEUTICAL CARE

Many factors influence pharmacist–patient communication. These factors can be divided into three types: individual, interpersonal, and environmental.

Individual Factors

Some factors that influence interpersonal communication for pharmaceutical care are specific to an individual pharmacist. These factors include attitudes, self-efficacy beliefs, perceived behavioral control, and perceived responsibility. The word *perceived* appears in some of these categories because the influencing factor is the pharmacist's *perception* rather than an outside perspective.

An attitude is "a learned predisposition to respond in a consistently favorable or unfavorable manner with respect to a given object."[49] Attitudes can be measured as the sum of beliefs about the consequences of performing a behavior, in which each belief is weighed by one's evaluations of these consequences.[49] Using patient counseling as an example, a pharmacist may believe that patient counseling is helpful for patients, is important for pharmacists to do, takes a lot of time, and warrants reimbursement. Each of these beliefs is then weighted by its relative importance to the pharmacist. For example, a pharmacist might believe that helping patients is more important than being reimbursed.

Attitudes are determinants of peoples' intentions to perform behaviors, which are precursors to actual behavior.[49] Because attitudes can be learned, and thus influenced, social and behavioral pharmacy researchers often attempt to measure pharmacists' attitudes about patient care behaviors. Pharmacists' decisions to counsel patients and provide pharmaceutical care are influenced by their attitudes toward the pharmacist's role as a counselor[23,50,51] and attitudes toward pharmaceutical care,[52,53] respectively.

Self-efficacy beliefs are "people's judgments of their capabilities to organize and execute courses of action required to attain designated types of performances."[54] Two important elements of self-efficacy beliefs are (1) an individual's confidence in his or her ability to perform certain tasks and (2) expectations that performing a task will lead to a particular outcome. Studies that have investigated the influence of self-efficacy beliefs on providing pharmaceutical care have asked pharmacists to indicate their level of confidence that they can successfully perform pharmaceutical care behaviors.[40,42,52,55] Self-efficacy beliefs have either directly predicted pharmacists' self-reports of pharmaceutical care provision[55] or influenced them indirectly through past behavior recency.[52] In the case of the latter, the more recently pharmacists had provided pharmaceutical care, the greater their self-efficacy beliefs were (i.e., confidence by doing). Furthermore, pharmacists' confidence in their patient counseling and referral services have shown a large impact on their reports of pharmaceutical care provision.[42]

Perceived behavioral control is another factor that influences pharmacists. This factor relates to the pharmacist's sense of how much control he or she has over the performance of behaviors. Some studies have asked pharmacists to report their perceived ease or difficulty of providing pharmaceutical care.[40,52,55] These pharmacists have reported low perceived behavioral control for providing pharmaceutical care. Other findings related to perceived behavioral control are somewhat inconsistent. For example, one study found that perceived behavioral control directly influenced both intention to provide pharmaceutical care and self-reported pharmaceutical care delivery.[40] However, another study reported that perceived behavioral control did not directly influence pharmaceutical care delivery; instead, it directly influenced pharmacists' self-efficacy beliefs, which in turn directly influenced self-reported pharmaceutical care delivery. For example, pharmacists who lack appropriate models and strategies to implement pharmaceutical care will likely feel a low sense of perceived behavioral control, which may influence their confidence.[55] Therefore, a pharmacist's perceived behavioral control can be an appraisal process that frames how he or she views the work environment and the extent to which he or she sets boundaries for future behavior.

A key component of pharmaceutical care is a pharmacist's acceptance of responsibility for patients' drug therapy outcomes. Pharmacist responsibility has traditionally been described from philosophical and legal perspectives.[1,56-60] However, researchers found that the extent to which pharmacists report they perceive responsibility for patients' drug therapy outcomes is associated with their self-reports of pharmaceutical care provision.[61]

Interpersonal Perceptions

Pharmacists and patients rely on perceptions of one another to define their relationships. Role perceptions also shape expectations of one another, which can influence resulting interactions. Thus, pharmacist–patient communication takes place within the context of interpersonal perceptions.

Pharmacists have reported that patient demand for receiving counseling and pharmaceutical care activities is a major determinant in their decisions to offer these services.[62-64] In fact, pharmacists' perceptions of patient demand are as important as actual patient demand in influencing pharmacists' provision of patient-oriented services.[65] Yet, studies have revealed that pharmacists may not fully understand what patients would like from them.[65-67]

Patients who have not received pharmaceutical care services may not fully understand what pharmacists are capable of providing.[68,69] This shapes patients' perceptions of pharmacists, what they expect from pharmacists, and how they interact with them.

As in effective interpersonal communication, it is vital for both parties to understand one another. To investigate pharmacists' and patients' understanding of each other, some studies have sought to compare responses from both groups. Studies have revealed that patients and pharmacists generally disagree with one another regarding their roles in patient–pharmacist relationships and the benefits of pharmaceutical care services.[70-72] They also misunderstand each others' perceptions.[70,71]

In a Florida study, pharmacists were instructed to respond based on how they thought patients would answer, and patients were instructed to respond based on how they thought pharmacists would answer. "[Both] groups misunderstood each others' perceptions about the benefits of explaining to patients how to use their medications, developing follow-up plans measuring progress toward goals for the medication, and telling patients about other drugs that may cause problems with their medications."[71] The only issue on which both groups understood each other was making sure that patients understand information that is given to them. Generally, pharmacists thought that patients would perceive pharmaceutical care services to be more beneficial than patients actually did, thus overestimating patients' perceptions.[70,71] Additionally, patients underestimated the extent to which pharmacists would perceive these services to be beneficial to patients.[71]

A nationwide study surveyed pharmacists and patients about the following roles in their relationships: information sharing, responsible behavior, patient-centeredness of relationship, communication related to patients taking an active role in health care, and interpersonal communication.[72] Pharmacists and patients agreed on the *pharmacist's* information-sharing role, which included talking with patients about monitoring side effects and about taking medications with over-the-counter products, even if patients do not have any medication questions. However, pharmacists and patients did not agree on the *patient's* information-sharing role. Pharmacists reported stronger agreement than did patients that patients should discuss medication problems that they are having with the pharmacist, keep the pharmacist up to date regarding changes in their health conditions, and tell the pharmacist about any medication side effects.[72] This pattern is consistent with other studies that have found that pharmacists rely on patients to initiate communication by volunteering information or asking questions.[33,42,73] Ideally, pharmacists should be more proactive in initiating communication to identify potential and actual DTPs. This may increase patient expectations and educate them on what pharmacists can do. In turn, patients may be more likely to see the benefits of pharmaceutical care and participate more actively.

Pharmacists' and patients' views were different on a majority of activities that constituted the responsible behavior role. Pharmacists reported stronger agreement than did patients that *pharmacists* should show an interest and desire to assist patients with their healthcare-related and medication-related needs and concerns, as well as medication management needs.[72] Pharmacists also more strongly agreed that *patients* should work with the pharmacist to manage their medications and help them deal with their healthcare needs. These patterns may have emerged because patient respondents were unfamiliar with these services and thus did not know what pharmacists are capable of providing. Patients' knowledge of pharmacists' roles could be increased by exposing them to written materials about pharmacists' activities, such as pharmaceutical care and medication management.[68]

Environmental Factors

The environment in which communication takes places is an important component of the interpersonal communication process. Some environmental factors originate in a specific practice setting, such as workflow issues. Others are more external in nature, such as federal regulations.

External Environment

These types of factors originate at systems levels rather than at a specific pharmacy. Dominant external environmental factors that influence interpersonal communication in pharmaceutical care include federal and state regulations, pharmacy education, and reimbursement.

Over the last two decades, several changes regarding the types of patient-oriented services provided by pharmacists have been mandated in federal and state regulations. As previously described, the passage of OBRA '90 required Medicaid patients to receive an offer of counseling.[27] Since its passage and implementation, a majority of states have extended the counseling requirement to all patients, and counseling rates have increased.[29-32]

The Medicare Modernization Act of 2003 specified that pharmacists or other qualified healthcare practitioners provide medication therapy management (MTM) services for eligible patients enrolled in the Medicare prescription drug benefit.[74] MTM is a strategy that incorporates the philosophy of pharmaceutical care, including the patient care process, into pharmacy practice for a defined patient population.[75] The core elements of an MTM service are designed to, among other things, improve care and enhance communication among patients and pharmacists in community pharmacies.[76,77] Because it is an emerging service, observational research does not yet exist regarding the impact of MTM services on pharmacist–patient communication. Medicare beneficiaries have reported slightly favorable attitudes toward MTM services, compared with more favorable attitudes toward counseling activities.[69]

State regulations vary among states in terms of their intensity, specifically their scope, stringency, and duration.[78] Pharmacies in states with more intense regulations tend to provide patient counseling more often and to a greater extent, including greater numbers of medication information items (e.g., drug name, purpose, directions for use) and asking patients questions to assess their understanding.[32] A state's regulations are considered more intense if they specifically address counseling and cover all patients (scope), require face-to-face counseling by a pharmacist or pharmacy intern/extern for all patients and their agents who present a new prescription (stringency), and were implemented before OBRA '90 (duration).[32]

Regulations also invoke a deterrent effect. Pharmacists' concerns over liability as a result of malpractice suits and disciplinary actions by their state board of pharmacy may influence them to adhere to regulations. A study of Texas pharmacists found their reports of these concerns to be positively related to reports of advising patients about taking contraindicated medications.[62]

Pharmacy education is another external environmental factor that influences interpersonal communication between pharmacists and patients. Pharmacy schools and their accrediting organizations have recognized the importance of developing effective communication skills among student pharmacists in both didactic and experiential learning programs.[79-82] The majority of U.S. schools of pharmacy offer communications courses as part of their required curricula.[80] However, behavioral assessments of pharmacist–patient communication in courses focus more on dispensing a new prescription rather than monitoring ongoing therapy.[83] Expansions of early experiential programs are underway to increase opportunities for student pharmacists to develop their patient communication skills while in pharmacy school.[82]

Lack of reimbursement often has been cited as a barrier to pharmacists providing counseling and pharmaceutical care activities.[84-86] The potential for pharmacists to bill for these types of services is greater now than at any other time in the profession's history.[87] Future tracking of pharmacist billing for MTM core element services (i.e., medication therapy reviews, personal medication records, medication-related action plans, intervention and referral, and documentation and follow-up) is needed to shed light on whether financial incentives influence service provision.[76,77]

Pharmacy Environment

Practice setting characteristics, such as physical layout, workflow, and busyness, influence a pharmacist's activities.[67,85] Workflow, for example, can influence whether or not a pharmacist is the person who hands a prescription and offers counseling to a patient. Prescription transfer by the pharmacist is related to the occurrence of communication.[50] Workflow modifications and adequate numbers of trained staff are usually necessary for a pharmacist to be able to transfer completed prescriptions to patients. Such modifications have increased pharmacists' counseling offers to patients; however, these increases have not resulted in more patients receiving counseling.[88,89] Patient expectations regarding counseling are likely contributors to the lack of increase in counseling despite more offers.

Busyness is another factor that influences the extent of pharmacist–patient communication.[34,50,51,85] To date, the most comprehensive assessment of pharmacy busyness was conducted in a study of 306 community pharmacists in eight states. Pharmacies that were considered more busy had fewer percentages of pharmacists talking with patients, providing any specific medication information, and asking any question to assess the patient's understanding.[32] When busyness has been examined, it has not always been a factor in pharmacist–patient communication, so its influence is unclear.[25] Pharmacists who are very busy may perceive a lack of time to communicate with patients. Indeed, lack of time is commonly cited as a barrier to counseling patients.[50,63,85]

Some environmental factors have less to do with the actual setting and are more related to contextual cues. These situational factors are part of the environment at a particular moment.[63] For example, pharmacists tend to counsel patients more for new prescriptions than for refill prescriptions, especially if the patient is unfamiliar with the medication.[33,90] Additionally, the occurrence of pharmacist–patient communication is influenced by the perceived importance of information relayed during the encounter, particularly if pharmacists perceive potentially serious consequences for the patient.[50,90]

Studies that have evaluated factors that influence pharmacists' provision of pharmaceutical care generally place greater emphasis on individual factors, such as attitude toward trying to provide pharmaceutical care, over environmental factors, such as reimbursement and practice setting characteristics.[40,42,53,86] The primary reason for this preference is because individual factors are within a pharmacist's control, whereas many environmental factors are not.[86] However, the relative importance of practice environment has been argued, largely in part because of its influence on how pharmacists perceive control over their work surroundings. As stated previously, pharmacists typically report low perceived behavioral control to provide pharmaceutical care, which can influence their provision of these services because of low self-efficacy beliefs.[55]

SUMMARY

Effective interpersonal communication is necessary to establish rapport with patients by understanding their needs, concerns, and experiences. Rapport serves as a foundation for fostering a therapeutic relationship with patients and having them participate in decision-making processes to meet their therapeutic goals. Interpersonal communication is also important to promote dialogue between pharmacists and patients so that information can be exchanged. Information exchange is critical for conducting the patient care process to identify, resolve, and prevent DTPs that could interfere with patients' therapeutic goals. In summary, interpersonal communication is a fundamental social and behavioral aspect of pharmaceutical care practice.

The extent of interpersonal communication for pharmaceutical care has increased in past decades. However, improvements in both the quantity and quality of communication are needed. Common DTPs encountered in pharmaceutical care practices require direct pharmacist–patient communication. As more pharmacists become pharmaceutical care providers, they will need effective interpersonal communication skills to help patients optimize their drug therapy outcomes.

A variety of factors influence pharmacist–patient communication. Attempts to increase interpersonal communication in pharmaceutical care practices should incorporate interventions that influence personal, interpersonal, and environmental factors. Both pharmacist and patient perceptions must be included, especially because these two groups often misunderstand one another.

This chapter has sought to describe the nature, extent, and influencing factors of interpersonal communication for pharmaceutical care practice. Understanding these issues is crucial for pharmacists to help patients optimize their drug therapy outcomes.

REFERENCES

1. Cipolle RJ, Strand LM, Morley PC. Pharmaceutical care practice: the clinician's guide. 2nd ed. New York: McGraw-Hill, 2004.
2. Shannon CE, Weaver W. The mathematical theory of communication. Urbana: University of Illinois Press, 1949.
3. Schramm W. How communication works. In: Schramm W, ed. The process and effects of mass communication. Urbana: University of Illinois Press, 1954:3-26.
4. Mehrabian A. Silent messages. Belmont, CA: Wadsworth, 1971.
5. Poytos F. New perspectives in nonverbal communication. New York: Pergamon Press, 1983.
6. Rapport. American Heritage dictionary of the English language, 4th ed. Boston: Houghton Mifflin, 2004. (Accessed February 2, 2008, at http://dictionary.reference.com/browse/rapport.)
7. Rapport. Random House dictionary.com unabridged (v1.1). Random House. (Accessed February 2, 2008, at http://dictionary.reference.com/browse/rapport.)
8. Burley-Allen M. Listening: the forgotten skill. 2nd ed. Hoboken, NJ: John Wiley and Sons, 1995.
9. Adler RB, Rosenfeld LB, Proctor RF. Interplay: the process of interpersonal communication. 10th ed. New York: Oxford University Press, 2006.
10. Rogers CR. A way of being. Boston: Houghton Mifflin, 1980.
11. Mead N, Bower P. Patient-centeredness: a conceptual framework and review of the empirical literature. Soc Sci Med 2000;51(7):1087-110.
12. Hepler CD, Strand LM. Opportunities and responsibilities in pharmaceutical care. Am J Hosp Pharm 1990;47(3):533-43.
13. May WF. Code, covenant, contract, or philanthropy. Hastings Cent Rep 1975;5:29-38.
14. Chewning B, Sleath B. Medication decision-making and management: a client-centered model. Soc Sci Med 1996;42(3):389-98.
15. Pfizer I. Pharmacist-patient consultation program. Unit I: an interactive approach to verify patient understanding. New York: National Healthcare Operations, 1991.

16. Pfizer I. Pharmacist-patient consultation program. Unit II: how to counsel patients in challenging situations. New York: National Healthcare Operations, 1993.

17. Pfizer I. Pharmacist-patient consultation program. Unit III: counseling to enhance compliance. New York: National Healthcare Operations, 1995.

18. Strand LM, Morley PC, Cipolle RJ, Ramsey R, Lamsam GD. Drug-related problems: their structure and function. DICP 1990;24(11):1093-7.

19. Higby GJ. From compounding to caring: an abridged history of American pharmacy. In: Knowlton CH, Penna RP, eds. Pharmaceutical care. New York: Chapman and Hall, 1996:18-45.

20. Knapp DA, Wolf HH, Knapp DE, Rudy TA. An experimental analysis . . . the pharmacist as a drug advisor. J Am Pharm Assoc 1969;9(10):502-5.

21. Rowles B, Keller SM, Gavin PW. Pharmacist as compounder and consultant. Drug Intell Clin Pharm 1974;8(5):242-4.

22. Ross SR, White SJ, Hogan LC, Godwin HN. The effect of a mandatory patient counseling regulation on the counseling practices of pharmacy practitioners. Contemp Pharm Pract 1981; 4(2):64-8.

23. Mason HL, Svarstad BL. Medication counseling behaviors and attitudes of rural community pharmacists. Drug Intell Clin Pharm 1984;18(5):409-14.

24. Carroll NV, Gagnon JP. Consumer demand for patient-oriented pharmacy services. Am J Public Health 1984;74(6):609-11.

25. Berardo DH, Kimberlin CL, Barnett CW. Observational research on patient education activities of community pharmacists. J Soc Adm Pharm 1989;6(1):21-30.

26. Raisch DW. Patient counseling in community pharmacy and its relationship with prescription payment methods and practice settings. Ann Pharmacother 1993;27(10):1173-9.

27. Omnibus Budget Reconciliation Act of 1990. Washington, DC: U.S. Government Printing Office, 1990:152-71.

28. Morris LA, Tabak ER, Gondek K. Counseling patients about prescribed medication: 12-year trends. Med Care 1997;35(10):996-1007.

29. Perri M, Kotzan J, Pritchard L, Ozburn W, Francisco G. OBRA '90: the impact on pharmacists and patients. Am Pharm 1995;NS35(2):24-8, 65.

30. Sleath B. Pharmacist question-asking in New Mexico community pharmacies. Am J Pharm Educ 1995;59(4):374-9.

31. Schatz R, Belloto RJ Jr, White DB, Bachmann K. Provision of drug information to patients by pharmacists: the impact of the Omnibus Budget Reconciliation Act of 1990 a decade later. Am J Ther 2003;10(2):93-103.

32. Svarstad BL, Bultman DC, Mount JK. Patient counseling provided in community pharmacies: effects of state regulation, pharmacist age, and busyness. J Am Pharm Assoc 2004;44(1):22-9.

33. Schommer JC, Wiederholt JB. The association of prescription status, patient age, patient gender, and patient question asking behavior with the content of pharmacist-patient communication. Pharm Res 1997;14(2):145-51.

34. Sleath B. Pharmacist-patient relationships: authoritarian, participatory, or default? Patient Educ Couns 1996;28(3):253-63.

35. Svarstad BL, Bultman DC, Mount JK, Tabak ER. Evaluation of written prescription information provided in community pharmacies: a study in eight states. J Am Pharm Assoc 2003;43(3): 383-93.

36. Stergachis A, Maine LL, Brown L. The 2001 National Pharmacy Consumer Survey. J Am Pharm Assoc 2002;42(4):568-76.

37. Svarstad BL, Mount JK, Tabak ER. Expert and consumer evaluation of patient medication leaflets provided in U.S. pharmacies. J Am Pharm Assoc 2005;45(4):443-51.

38. Federal Register, August 24, 1985 (60 FR 44186).

39. Public Law No. 104-180 (August 6, 1996), Agriculture, Rural Development, Food and Drug Administration, and Related Agencies Appropriations Act of 1997.

40. Odedina FT, Hepler CD, Segal R, Miller D. The pharmacists' implementation of pharmaceutical care (PIPC) model. Pharm Res 1997;14(2):135-44.

41. Odedina FT, Segal R. Behavioral pharmaceutical care scale for measuring pharmacists' activities. Am J Health Syst Pharm 1996;53(8):855-65.

42. Venkataraman K, Madhavan S, Bone P. Barriers and facilitators to pharmaceutical care in rural community practice. J Soc Adm Pharm 1997;14(4):208-19.

43. McDermott JH, Christensen DB. Provision of pharmaceutical care services in North Carolina: a 1999 survey. J Am Pharm Assoc 2002;42(1):26-35.

44. Maine LL. Pharmacy practice activity classification. J Am Pharm Assoc 1998;38(2):139-48.

45. Kassam R, Farris KB, Burback L, Volume CI, Cox CE, Cave A. Pharmaceutical care research and education project: pharmacists' interventions. J Am Pharm Assoc 2001;41(3):401-10.

46. McDonough RP, Doucette WR. Drug therapy management: an empirical report of drug therapy problems, pharmacists' interventions, and results of pharmacists' actions. J Am Pharm Assoc 2003;43(4):511-8.

47. Doucette WR, McDonough RP, Klepser D, McCarthy R. Comprehensive medication therapy management: identifying and resolving drug-related issues in a community pharmacy. Clin Ther 2005;27(7):1104-11.

48. Isetts BJ. Evaluating effectiveness of the Minnesota Medication Therapy Management Care Program: final report. St. Paul, MN: Minnesota Department of Human Services, 2007. (Report no. B00749.)

49. Fishbein M, Ajzen I. Belief, attitude, intention, and behavior: an introduction to theory and research. Reading, MA: Addison-Wesley, 1975.

50. Schommer JC, Wiederholt JB. A field investigation of participant and environment effects on pharmacist patient communication in community pharmacies. Med Care 1995;33(6):567-84.

51. Kirking D. Evaluation of an explanatory model of pharmacists' patient counseling activities. J Soc Adm Pharm 1984;2:50-6.

52. Odedina FT, Segal R, Hepler CD, Lipowski E, Kimberlin C. Changing pharmacists' practice pattern: pharmacists' implementation of pharmaceutical care factors. J Soc Adm Pharm 1996;13(2):74-88.

53. Farris KB, Kirking DM. Predicting community pharmacists' intention to try to prevent and correct drug therapy problems. J Soc Adm Pharm 1995;12:64-79.

54. Bandura A. Social foundations of thought and action: a social cognitive theory. Englewood Cliffs, NJ: Prentice Hall, 1986.

55. Farris KB, Schopflocher DP. Between intention and behavior: an application of community pharmacists' assessment of pharmaceutical care. Soc Sci Med 1999;49(1):55-66.

56. Brushwood DB, Hepler CD. Redefining pharmacist professional responsibility. In: Knowlton CH, Penna RP, eds. Pharmaceutical care. New York: Chapman and Hall, 1996:195-214.

57. Hepler CD. Philosophical issues raised by pharmaceutical care. In: Haddad AM, Buerki RA, eds. Ethical dimensions of pharmaceutical care. Binghamton, NY: Haworth Press, 1996:19-47.
58. Brushwood DB. The duty to counsel: reviewing a decade of litigation. DICP 1991;25(2):195-204.
59. Brushwood DB. The pharmacist's expanding legal responsibility for patient care. J Soc Adm Pharm 1995;12(2):53-62.
60. Lynn NJ, Ellis JM. Pharmacists' liability into the year 2000. J Am Pharm Assoc 1998;38(6):747-52.
61. Planas LG, Kimberlin CL, Segal R, Brushwood DB, Hepler CD, Schlenker BR. A pharmacist model of perceived responsibility for drug therapy outcomes. Soc Sci Med 2005;60(10):2393-403.
62. Sitkin SB, Sutcliffe KM. Dispensing legitimacy: the influence of professional, organizational, and legal controls on pharmacist behavior. Res Sociol Organ 1991;8:269-95.
63. Schommer JC, Wiederholt JB. Pharmacists' perceptions of patients' needs for counseling. Am J Hosp Pharm 1994;51(4):478-85.
64. Latif DA. Situational factors as determinants of community pharmacists' clinical decision making behavior. J Am Pharm Assoc 1998;38(4):446-50.
65. Carroll NV, Gagnon JP. Pharmacists' perceptions of consumer demand for patient-oriented pharmacy services. Drug Intell Clin Pharm 1984;18:640-4.
66. Hirsch JD, Gagnon JP, Camp R. Value of pharmacy services: perceptions of consumers, physicians, and third party prescription plan administrators. Am Pharm 1990;NS30(3):20-5.
67. Herrier R, Boyce R. Why aren't more pharmacists counseling? Am Pharm 1994;NS34(11):22-3.
68. Chewning B, Schommer JC. Increasing clients' knowledge of community pharmacists' roles. Pharm Res 1996;13(9):1299-304.
69. Doucette WR, Witry MJ, Alkhateeb F, Farris KB, Urmie JM. Attitudes of Medicare beneficiaries toward pharmacist-provided medication therapy management activities as part of the Medicare Part D benefit. J Am Pharm Assoc 2007;47(6):758-62.
70. Assa M, Shepherd EF. Interpersonal perception: a theory and method for studying pharmacists' and patients' views of pharmaceutical care. J Am Pharm Assoc 2000;40(1):71-81.
71. Assa-Eley M, Kimberlin CL. Using interpersonal perception to characterize pharmacists' and patients' perceptions of the benefits of pharmaceutical care. Health Commun 2005;17(1):41-56.
72. Worley MM, Schommer JC, Brown LM, et al. Pharmacists' and patients' roles in the pharmacist-patient relationship: are pharmacists and patients reading from the same relationship script? Res Soc Adm Pharm 2007;3(1):47-69.
73. Kirking DM. Pharmacists' perceptions of their patient counseling activities. Contemp Pharm Pract 1982;5(4):230-8.
74. Federal Register, January 28, 2005 (42 CFR Parts 400, 403, 411, 417, and 423).
75. McGivney MS, Meyer SM, Duncan-Hewitt W, Hall DL, Goode JV, Smith RB. Medication therapy management: its relationship to patient counseling, disease management, and pharmaceutical care. J Am Pharm Assoc 2007;47(5):620-8.
76. American Pharmacists Association, National Association of Chain Drug Stores Foundation. Medication therapy management in community pharmacy practice: core elements of an MTM service. J Am Pharm Assoc 2005;45(5):573-9.

77. American Pharmacists Association, National Association of Chain Drug Stores Foundation. Medication therapy management in pharmacy practice: core elements of an MTM service model version 2.0. (Accessed March 19, 2008, at http://www.pharmacist.com/MTM/CoreElements2.)

78. Cook K, Shortell SM, Conrad DA, Morrisey MA. A theory of organizational response to regulation: the case of hospitals. Acad Manage Rev 1983;8(2):193-205.

79. Svarstad BL. Development of behavioral science curricula and faculty in pharmacy: some issues requiring attention. Am J Pharm Educ 1994;58(2):177-83.

80. Beardsley RS. Communication skills development in colleges of pharmacy. Am J Pharm Educ 2001;65(4):307-14.

81. Center for the Advancement of Pharmaceutical Education. Educational outcomes 2004. (Accessed March 12, 2008, at http://www.aacp.org/Docs/MainNavigation/Resources/6075_CAPE2004.pdf.)

82. Accreditation Council for Pharmacy Education. Accreditation standards and guidelines for the professional program in pharmacy leading to the Doctor of Pharmacy degree. (Accessed March 12, 2008, at http://www.acpe-accredit.org/pdf/ACPE_Revised_PharmD_Standards_Adopted_Jan152006.pdf.)

83. Kimberlin CL. Communicating with patients: skills assessment in US colleges of pharmacy. Am J Pharm Educ 2006;70(3):67.

84. Penna RP. Pharmaceutical care: pharmacy's mission for the 1990s. Am J Hosp Pharm 1990; 47(3):543-9.

85. Raisch DW. Barriers to providing cognitive services. Am Pharm 1993;NS33(12):54-8.

86. Campagna KD, Newlin MH. Key factors influencing pharmacists' drug therapy decisions. Am J Health Syst Pharm 1997;54(11):1307-13.

87. Isetts BJ, Buffington DE. CPT code-change proposal: national data on pharmacists' medication therapy management services. Am J Health Syst Pharm 2007;64(15):1642-6.

88. Angelo LB, Ferreri SP. Assessment of workflow redesign in community pharmacy. J Am Pharm Assoc 2005;45(2):145-50.

89. Angelo LB, Christensen DB, Ferreri SP. Impact of community pharmacy automation on workflow, workload, and patient interaction. J Am Pharm Assoc 2005;45(2):138-44.

90. Schommer JC, Wiederholt JB. Pharmacists' views of patient counseling. Am Pharm 1994; NS34(7):46-53.

CHAPTER 12

Pharmaceutical Care: Incorporating the Needs and Perspectives of Caregivers

Felicity Smith, PhD, Sally-Anne Francis, PhD, and Paul L. Ranelli, PhD

The focus of this chapter is on the place of caregivers (also termed carers) in the medication management process and the implications for pharmaceutical care. Pharmacists are unusual among healthcare professionals in that they commonly have face-to-face contact only with the representatives or caregivers of patients rather than the patients themselves. This leads to both opportunities and challenges in the provision of pharmaceutical care. In terms of opportunities, as we hope to show in this chapter, caregivers play a major and often essential role in the management of medications for their care recipients. In performing medication-related activities, caregivers have their own problems and perspectives and require information and support in order to be effective. Thus, the contact that pharmacists may regularly have with a caregiver enables them to identify and respond to medication-related issues that arise in the context of the caregiving relationship. The challenges are apparent. The pharmacist may have to depend on the caregiver for information about the patient and may be unable to make a firsthand assessment of needs.

In developing services in pharmaceutical care, caregivers may need to be a central focus. This chapter first provides a brief overview of the extent of caregiving, highlighting its importance in health and social care. It then describes the roles of caregivers in the management of medications, examining, in particular, caregivers of older people and the young (where most caregiving occurs), the range of medication-related activities that caregivers undertake, and ways in which caregivers and care recipients work together to manage their medications. It concludes with a discussion of the implications of caregiving for pharmaceutical care.

WHO ARE CAREGIVERS?

Caregivers (or carers) have been defined as "people looking after, or providing some regular help for a sick, handicapped or older person living in their own or another private household."[1] Caregivers, who are usually a family member or friend of the person for whom they care (the care recipient), provide a vast proportion of health care. Informal caregiving is believed to be a major component of health care in all parts of the world. In the United States, the value of services provided by caregivers has been estimated at $306 billion per year, which is almost twice as much as that spent on home care and nursing home services combined.[2] In the United Kingdom, the contribution of caregivers to health care alone has been valued at £57.4 million annually.[3] Caregiving is a widespread activity in all communities. In the United States, more than 50 million people are believed to be providing care for a chronically ill, disabled, or older family member during any given year.[4] At the time of the last U.K. census, it was estimated that around 6 million people were providing unpaid care.[5] Figures are similar in other European countries; for example, in Belgium, one in ten of the population is believed to provide informal care.[6]

A high proportion of caregivers care for an older person. The aging of populations, in which rising proportions of the population are older people, is a worldwide phenomenon. The associated increases in morbidity will lead to greater pressure on formal healthcare services. Thus, in the future the value of informal caregiving and the consequent burden on caregivers is likely to rise. Consequently, caregiving is likely to remain an important feature of health care all over the world. At the other end of the age spectrum, caregivers of children and young people, especially those with a chronic condition, also contribute significantly to health care.

Caregivers span all age groups. In the 2001 U.K. census, it was estimated that nearly half of caregivers (45%) were aged between 45 and 64 years. However, 1% of children (aged 5–15 years) and 5% of people aged 85 years or more also provided care.[5] Both men and women are involved in caregiving. Under the age of 65 years a larger proportion of women are caregivers, because in many societies they assume greater responsibility for care in the home. However, many caregivers, especially those in older age groups and those caring for a spouse, are male.

The vast majority of caregivers look after a relative (commonly parents or parents-in-law, or a spouse).[1] Less often, caregivers are friends or neighbors. Although the care provided by these people is likely to be more limited, it may comprise essential assistance from the perspective of the care recipient.

Caregivers of older people are often older themselves and have their own health-care needs, with some consequent functional limitations. An older couple may be supporting each other in different ways. As they get older, disease may progress; the burden on the caregiver may increase at the same time as his or her ability to care diminishes. Family caregivers have been reported to have a chronic condition at more than twice the rate of noncaregivers.[4] Daughters and sons (including in-laws) provide significant help for older people. The assistance they provide has to be accommodated alongside other commitments in their own home and working lives: 59% of caregivers who care for someone older than 18 years either work, or have worked, while providing care. Sixty-two percent have had to make some adjustments to their work life, including switching from full-time to part-time employment and giving up work entirely.[7]

Increasingly, the essential contribution of caregivers to health care is being acknowledged. In 1999, the British government published a "national strategy for caregivers" highlighting the need to provide appropriate support services.[8] However, despite the dependence of formal healthcare systems on the contribution of informal caregivers, and the physical and emotional burden associated with caring, the needs of caregivers receive only limited attention.

The remainder of this chapter focuses on the management of medications in the context of informal caregiving. It draws on research that has been undertaken from the perspectives of caregivers regarding their roles in assisting in medication use. This provides a description of the range of medication-related activities that caregivers undertake together with the problems experienced and their concerns. An important context of caregiving is the partnership that exists between caregivers and care recipients, which has implications for all aspects of caring, including medication use and contact with health services. In providing pharmaceutical care to ensure the best medication use, an appreciation by health professionals of the range of activities undertaken, the associated problems, and the patterns of partnership from the perspective of caregivers (and care recipients) are vital.

ROLES OF CAREGIVERS IN THE MANAGEMENT OF MEDICATIONS _____

The use of medicines is commonly a major component of the management of any medical condition. Older people experience more morbidity for which medications will be required. Children and young people who require long-term medication use are most likely to be principally cared for, and assisted by, their parents. Parents may have additional roles in terms of coordinating medication use outside the home (e.g., in schools, at friends' homes). Whereas young people with a chronic condition may take progressively greater responsibility for the use of their medications as they grow up, an older care recipient may become more dependent. Providing assistance with medication use would be expected to be an important part of the caregiving role. Despite this, research into the medication-related aspects of informal caregiving has been very limited.[9-20]

Studies that have been conducted have shown the broad range of medication-related activities that caregivers undertake. Research has also highlighted the huge variation between caregivers in the level of involvement they have, which will, of course, depend on the needs and wishes of the care recipient. Medication-related activities have been shown to be integral to caregiving; this may explain why there have been so few studies focusing specifically on this aspect. The context of the relationship between the caregiver and care recipient has also been found to be important. The ways in which caregivers and care recipients share responsibilities, and their independent health beliefs and perspectives on medication use, may have an impact on their mutual understanding of medicines, adherence, and decision making.

Only a tiny proportion of medication-related activities undertaken by caregivers are visible to health professionals. In particular, pharmacists are aware that many people collect medication for others, but they are not necessarily aware of the full extent of the medication-related assistance provided. The problem is compounded by the fact that many people providing what they see as limited assistance (picking up prescriptions, opening containers, or reminding someone to take his or her medicines) do not necessarily view themselves as caregivers, even though these activities may be important in enabling the care recipient to take his or her medicines. Family members may view their responsibilities as normal activities of family life. Caregivers have been found to be more proactive in seeking resources and talking to health professionals once they have self-identified as caregivers.[21] In the delivery of effective pharmaceutical care, it is important that pharmacists be aware that they only see the tip of the iceberg of caregivers' involvement unless they take proactive steps to delve further.

All caregiving situations differ depending on the needs of the care recipient, the ability of the caregiver to provide help, and the context of the partnership between caregiver and care recipient governing the dynamics of the caregiving role. While recognizing the varying roles of caregivers in assisting in medication use, in order to address pharmaceutical care issues, we separately discuss patterns of caring for older and young people.

CAREGIVERS OF OLDER CARE RECIPIENTS _____

The vast majority of caregivers providing medication-related assistance for an older person are a close relative. In a U.K. study, these caregivers were most commonly a spouse (45%) or children assisting parents or parents-in-law (40%). Of these caregivers, 61% were female and 39% male. They were from all age groups (up to 81 years).[16]

Medication-Related Assistance Provided by Caregivers of Older People

Table 12-1 gives an overview of the type of medication-related assistance that care-givers provide for older people. The number of different tasks undertaken by care-givers varied. Some caregivers were involved in all the tasks listed in Table 12-1, others in only one or two. For caregivers who assisted with only a small number of tasks,

TABLE 12-1	**Medication-Related Assistance That Caregivers Provide for Older Care Recipients (CR)**
Activity	**Percentage Who Provide This Assistance ($n = 184$)**
Ordering CR's prescriptions from the surgery ($n = 182$)	81
Collecting CR's prescriptions from the surgery ($n = 183$)	81
Taking CR's prescriptions to the pharmacy ($n = 183$)	89
Collecting CR's prescription medication from the pharmacy ($n = 183$)	97
Buying nonprescription medication or other remedies for CR ($n = 167$)	60
Giving or lending medication to CR ($n = 181$)	10
Reminding CR when to take medication ($n = 181$)	55
Opening medication containers for CR ($n = 182$)	51
Assisting CR with taking or using medication ($n = 175$)	34
Deciding how much medication CR should take or how often ($n = 178$)	25
Noticing and managing CR's side effects to medication ($n = 127$)	58
Giving CR any other information or help with medication ($n = 156$)	44

Adapted from Francis S-A, Smith F, Gray N, Graffy J. The roles of informal carers in the management of medication for older care-recipients. Int J Pharm Pract 2002;10:1-9.

these were most likely to be picking up prescriptions, taking them to the pharmacy, and collecting the medications. A high proportion of caregivers were also involved in ordering prescriptions from surgeries (a U.K. term referring to office practices of general practitioners). About half of caregivers were involved in providing some assistance with medicines in the home also. This might be reminding people to take their medications, assisting with opening containers, or other activities related to the administration of medications. Between one third and one half of caregivers provided assistance in decisions regarding medication use. This might be advising on the need for a medication or about side effects. What is clear is that the medication-related activities of caregivers are often considerable. To provide safe and effective assistance, caregivers would be expected to have access to specialist advice. To provide appropriate pharmaceutical assistance and advice, health professionals (commonly pharmacists) need to be aware of the range of responsibilities assumed by individual caregivers.

PROBLEMS EXPERIENCED BY CAREGIVERS IN MEDICATION-RELATED ROLES

Because a high proportion of caregivers of older people are older themselves, it is not surprising that they may also experience some difficulties in medication use, similar to those of their older care recipients. One third of caregivers providing some medication-related assistance rated their own health as either fair or poor, suggesting that they may have their own health needs that affect their ability to care. It was also notable that caregivers whose medication-related responsibilities included providing assistance in the home with the administration of medicines and/or advising on their use were significantly more likely to find their caregiving role stressful.[16]

For the purposes of identifying the problems experienced by caregivers, medication management activities can be categorized into four main groups:[17]

- Activities associated with maintaining supplies of medications, which include monitoring use and quantities in the home and communicating with surgeries and pharmacies in the ordering and collecting of new prescriptions
- Assisting with administration and reminding when doses are due
- Advising on the use of medicines, including interpreting information and making judgments of the need for, and appropriate use of, different products
- Communicating with the care recipient and health professionals

Caregivers have been found to experience problems with all of these activities. Examining the types of problems that arise in relation to each of these categories provides some insight into the pharmaceutical care needs of caregivers, as well as indications of how these might be addressed. The following discussion, and the quotations, are taken from the only U.K. multicenter study that has examined medication-related problems from the perspective of caregivers.[16,17]

Ordering, Collecting, and Maintaining Supplies

Many caregivers experience difficulties in making sure there are always sufficient supplies of medications in the home and that new supplies are ordered so that they arrive in time. This can be more of a problem when the care recipient is taking a number of different products or formulations, each with its own regimen, such that new supplies are needed at different times. For the convenience of the care recipient, medications may also be stored in different parts of the home. This complicates the monitoring of supplies. Caregivers find that careful organization is required to ensure that medications are always available. This is often a time-consuming task.

> She doesn't need all the tablets every time so I have to go through and see how many she's got left because the packets are different sizes, and she has one tablet a day, and if you get a packet with thirty in that's all right, but the next packet's got forty-five in so you get complications. And that is a problem basically because "I only want this one, this one, and this one" she'll say, and then the next occasion it's some of the others, it's a different amount. And yes to me that is a little complex, specifically on those tablets. . . . So it's specifying which tablets are needed, then two days later, because it takes two days for the doctor to write the prescription, to return and collect the prescription.

Opening times of surgeries and pharmacies for some caregivers are inconvenient, especially for those who are working or have family commitments. At the surgery, the need for advance ordering, dealing with unexpected changes in prescriptions, spotting errors, delays in updating of computer systems with new prescription requirements, and different pack sizes for different products all lead to problems.

Difficulties in pharmacy services include frequent low stocks and nonavailability of products, which mean that return visits to the pharmacy are often necessary. Provision of medications from different manufacturers means that new supplies look different; caregivers and care recipients worry that the wrong product has been dispensed. Labeling also sometimes leads to uncertainty—for example, inadequate dose directions or dose changes about which the caregiver or care recipient has not been informed. These problems can increase the burden of caregiving because the caregiver has to take steps to obtain clarification or rectify errors.

Assisting with Administration

Assisting care recipients with the administration of medications, including reminding care recipients that it is time to take medications, is a common activity. Caregivers often devise systems, such as removing tablets from containers in advance and arranging them so that the care recipient knows exactly what has to be taken and when. Many older people use a large number of medications, and a number of different formulations.

> So all I do, she's got a bottle there, and I do about half a dozen tablets for her, just split them in half, they break badly. So what I've got is a Stan, a small Stanley knife, I do half a dozen for her. And they're in a bottle there for her.
>
> In the morning I give him his digoxin. Sometimes he's not all there, you see, so I actually put the tablet in there ready and he takes it with his morning cup of tea. The salbutamol and the Becloforte, he has an "Easibreathe" actuation unit, I just support it and he inhales. He can inhale quite easily, so that's how I do it. The Gaviscon I tend to put in a little jug, and just give it to him.

Caregivers have to understand the dosing regimen of each medication and devise a suitable schedule. Frequent dosing schedules can mean that caregivers have to be available to assist throughout the day. This may be difficult for caregivers with other commitments. Some caregivers, especially older caregivers, experience similar difficulties to the care recipients in remembering when to take medications, opening containers, and reading labels.

In reviewing medication for older people, the dose regimens and formulations should be discussed with caregivers and whenever possible should take into account their other commitments. Frequent and complex medication regimens can be very onerous for caregivers, significantly increasing both the burden and the stress of caregiving.

Clinical Roles of Caregivers

Advising on the use of medications, including interpreting information and making judgments about the need for, and appropriate use of, different products, is commonly undertaken by caregivers. Caregivers, like care recipients, inevitably have their own views and beliefs regarding the use of medications, which will be reflected in the advice they give and the decisions they make. Caregivers often take an active role in questioning the appropriateness of their care recipient's medication. They may have concerns regarding the quantity of different medications or the suitability of particular medicines, doubts about appropriate doses, and anxieties about side effects.

> I have questioned with the doctor, and the pharmacist, especially when she came out of hospital, certain medication I didn't think she needed, and they agreed, over prescribing in my opinion. She was on twenty-three tablets and nobody seemed concerned. It took two weeks to get them reviewed, and from twenty-three she went down to four.

The concerns of caregivers and their perceptions of their responsibilities to try to ensure that their care recipient receives appropriate medications can lead them to make independent decisions about doses.

> Well, yes. We, we were prescribed a quantity of phenytoin, and it made her so sleepy I reduced the amount.
>
> He has the nebuliser, as I say, the regular thing twice a day but I can tell by his breathing pattern whether he needs extra help so I say "Well, how about having an extra one?" So I set it up for him, and he can put it away.
>
> Well about a month ago, it was suggested that I increase the baclofen, which has a relaxing effect, but after two or three days I felt that he was too withdrawn so I went back to the dosage that he was on prior to that.

Caregivers may also take responsibility for deciding on the need for medications and the timing of doses. This may be dependent on the perceived clinical needs of the care recipients but can also be in relation to meal times or to fit in with the caregiver's own availability.

Communicating with the Care Recipient and Health Professionals

In providing wide-ranging assistance with medications, caregivers receive very limited systematic support. Although some health professionals may be aware that an informal caregiver assists the care recipient, the caregiver is not necessarily routinely involved in consultations.

> She used to go in and see her doctor on her own. But because of the short-term memory it's even that short she can go into the interview with the doctor and then come out and I say, "What did he say?" "I don't know.". . . So I now try to get into all her interviews and I pick up the information.

There is often very little assistance for caregivers in interpreting written information, such as printed leaflets in medication packages, especially in relation to recognizing side effects and assessing their importance. Caregivers need to understand how each product should be used and be able to assess whether it is being used effectively. They are also often in the position of having to answer care recipients' questions about their medications and to reassure them.

> Sometimes when you read side effects and things like that, a lot of drugs will say "if you have breathing difficulties consult your GP" and so on. Well yes, she does have breathing difficulties, but if the GP has prescribed them, then I have to assure her that he knows all about your breathing difficulties.

Presently, support for caregivers from health professionals, including pharmacists, is very limited.

Caregivers and care recipients work together in different ways in managing medications.[19] In many cases, caregivers and care recipients work as a team, sharing responsibilities and discussing needs and information.

> I also prepare the injections [insulin pen]. Well, she has to have a test, so we get everything out and we do her blood test. It's in a box, we can do that together, she'll get it all out and it's her blood test and then condition on the blood reading, . . . we've got a pen. So I dial the numbers into the pen and I give the pen to her and she injects herself.

It may not always be possible for caregivers to elicit the cooperation of the care recipient. They may feel a need to make unilateral decisions that they believe are in the best interests of the care recipient. For example, caregivers may withhold information in the belief that they are protecting care recipients from knowledge that they might find upsetting or that it would have a negative effect on the care recipients' adherence to their medication regimens.

> He knows that he's got glaucoma. He knows he has that medicine for the fluid in his legs. But the other[, phenytoin,] rather than upset him, I told him, he asked me, sometimes he asked me what that other medicine was for, and I just told him to keep his temperature down. Because he doesn't know he had fits.

Differing views between caregivers and care recipients commonly complicate the caregiving role and have implications for the clinical care of the care recipient. Dilemmas for caregivers can arise. These may be struggles by either the caregiver or care recipient to maintain some level of control over the use of medicines. Caregivers may wish to ensure that their care recipients receive appropriate drug therapy while also enabling them to maintain a level of independence and exercise autonomy in matters relating to their health care and medications. Care recipients may wish to retain some control over their use of medicines and to exercise their own judgments. The ability of caregivers to manage complex medication regimens, sometimes in the context of difficult partnerships, can be a source of great anxiety.

Health professionals often feel a duty to observe confidentiality, but also wish a patient to receive the most appropriate care. Autonomy has been defined as a person's ability and opportunity to make decisions relating to his or her own wishes.[22] In caring for older people, a balance needs to be found that respects the autonomy of the older person and ensures an appropriate level of confidentiality while making available the optimal information to enable caregivers to be effective in their roles.[19]

Caregiving is also dynamic. Health professionals can make no assumptions regarding the relative needs of caregivers and care recipients for support and information in relation to their medications based on a previous consultation or situation. A sudden or gradual change in the health of either caregiver or care recipient may trigger changes in the patterns of partnership and responsibility for medicines. Caregivers and care recipients also have concerns for the future. Many caregivers may worry about a possible deterioration in their own health or that of their care recipient such that they are no longer able to care for him or her. Health professionals require a range of strategies and approaches that may be implemented with caregivers and care recipients as each new situation presents itself.

CAREGIVERS OF CHILDREN AND YOUNG PEOPLE

Children and young people are a second major group of care recipients. For those caregivers looking after a child or young person with a chronic condition, managing medications can be an important part of caregiving. As children grow up, it is generally assumed that children will take on more responsibilities for their care and medications. However, there has been only limited research into how responsibilities are shared within the home, the roles of parents as caregivers in managing medications, and how this changes over time.

A study of young people aged 8 to 15 years with either asthma or diabetes examined medication management in the home from the point of view of the young people themselves and their parents (i.e., the caregivers).[20] Tables 12-2 and 12-3 describe which medication-related activities were undertaken by the young people, the parents, or shared between them.

In the case of young people with asthma, the responsibilities for obtaining supplies of medications, monitoring supplies in the home, liaising with health professionals for

TABLE 12-2   Children and Young People with Asthma: Sharing of Medication-Related Activities with Their Parents (n = 43)

Activity	Performed by Parent	Shared Between Young Person and Parent	Performed by Young Person	Not Applicable
Monitoring supplies and ordering prescriptions	38	1	2	2*
Collecting prescriptions	43	0	0	0
Remembering/reminding to take medications	40	0	3	0
Administration of medications	1	0	42	0
Decisions about the need for medications†	25	0	5	13‡

*Seasonal asthma, requiring only one prescription per year.
†Relates to medications prescribed for use as required or as needed.
‡Decisions reported as the responsibility of health professionals.
Adapted from Newbould J, Smith FJ, Francis S-A "I'm fine doing it on my own": partnerships between parents and young people in the management of medication for asthma and diabetes. J Child Health Care 2008;12:116-28.

TABLE 12-3   Children and Young People with Diabetes: Sharing of Medication-Related Activities with Their Parents (n = 26)

Activity	Performed by Parent	Shared Between Young Person and Parent	Performed by Young Person
Monitoring supplies and ordering prescriptions	23	1	2
Collecting prescriptions	25	1	0
Remembering/reminding to monitor blood glucose levels	15	3	8
Monitoring of blood glucose levels	2	4	20
Remembering/reminding to administer insulin	13	4	9
Administration of insulin	5	11	10

Adapted from Newbould J, Smith FJ, Francis S-A "I'm fine doing it on my own": partnerships between parents and young people in the management of medication for asthma and diabetes. J Child Health Care 2008;12:116-28.

further prescriptions, and collecting medications from a pharmacy were generally taken by parents. In contrast, the young people commonly took responsibility for the administration of their medications as well as some of the decision making regarding the need for medications. Similarly, the parents (caregivers) of young people with diabetes generally took responsibility for maintaining supplies, but the young people usually monitored their own blood glucose levels and administered insulin.

> I just do my prick [monitor blood glucose level] and if I am high or low I just dial up what [injection of insulin] I need . . . I don't bother Mum with it. (girl, 11 years)

Many studies have highlighted the limited involvement that children and young people have in consultations with health professionals. As a result, health professionals may well be unaware of the contrasting situation in the home, where young people are actively involved in medication-related activities and exercise some autonomy regarding the use of their medications.

Young people also have their own priorities and concerns, which they bring to decisions regarding the use of their medications. Thus, in supporting parents as caregivers, the perspectives of the young person should be sought.

> He [consultant] and my mum they both want me to go onto three jabs [injections of insulin] a day but I won't do it, I've told them I won't, I refuse to have to do one while I am at school, whatever they say. (boy, 10 years)

Some studies have also uncovered potential conflicts between parents and young people, perhaps wider struggles for autonomy within the parent–young person relationship, that are reflected in decision making about, and control regarding, the use of medications.[23] In the case of the need for medication to avert life-threatening situations, any conflict would lead to a high level of anxiety.

Again, the caregiving role is dynamic in that the patterns of responsibility for medications may change on a day-to-day basis. Circumstances that lead parents to increase their involvement include worsening of the condition or unsettled periods in home life. Situations that promote the transfer of responsibilities for medications to the young person include social and educational events, such as progressing to secondary or high school, staying overnight with friends, and going on school trips.[20]

A central aim of health policy is to find ways to encourage and empower young people to take a more active role in managing their health (which includes medications). Health professionals, including pharmacists, may also wish to consider how they can facilitate the longer-term transfer of responsibility for medications from parents to young people. Support for the transfer of responsibility for medications has been identified by caregivers as an issue for which advice and support is not necessarily available.

> I tried to mention it to her [diabetes nurse] once but she just sort of said "oh you can work it out at home." They are very nice and all that, but I think they are more concerned with the results, you know the HbA_{1c} rather than who does what. (mother of girl aged 12 years)
>
> She [asthma nurse] didn't really give us any advice or help. I didn't come away feeling very reassured, I mean I want Kate to be independent but I don't want to give her more responsibility than she can handle. (mother of girl aged 10 years)

Increasingly, in many countries, more sophisticated technological approaches to delivering pharmaceutical care are becoming feasible in the home. In many countries, because of the rising costs of institutional provision, governments are open to new and diverse ways of delivering care. Although many people with chronic health problems would prefer to be able to remain in their homes, this has implications for caregivers and their families. For example, in a study of young people with cystic fibrosis,[18] parents described having to be familiar with complex pharmaceutical delivery equipment, including intravenous lines, nebulizers, and inhalers. They also reported stress and anxiety in having to deal with the supply of incorrect products and equipment. To achieve policy goals of effective home-based care for people with complex health needs, the provision of pharmaceutical care that addresses the needs of caregivers as well as patients is essential.

In the case of young people, a common goal is to enable them to participate in normal everyday activities as far as possible. As regimens and equipment become more complex, the burden and strain on caregivers and the compromises in family life will increase. It is important for health professionals to take a holistic approach to the provision of pharmaceutical care in the home to achieve the best possible outcomes in relation to clinical care, wider health-related quality of life of patients, and the quality of life and burden on family and caregivers.

In a study of medication-related activities of parents (caregivers) of young people with cystic fibrosis, parents perceived themselves as "experts" in overseeing and making judgments about their child's therapy. Parents monitored the use of pancreatic enzymes, antibiotics, and inhalers. Although many parents felt confident in these activities, others preferred a health professional to be involved. Parents described their decision-making roles regarding the use of medicines, including actively making judgments about the need for therapy and doses. They experienced difficulties in fitting a complex medication regimen into daily life and maximizing the opportunities for their child to participate as fully as possible in educational and social activities. Parents mentioned the tensions that occur between dealing with the potential stigma of chronic conditions, the need to ensure adherence to regimens, the special requirements for medication management, and enabling integration into normal life.

Cystic fibrosis care in the United Kingdom involves health professionals in both the nonspecialist and specialist sectors. Many parents experienced limitations in the knowledge and experience of nonspecialists in providing appropriate advice and support. In particular, parents described disagreeing with recommendations and advice; these conflicts could be stressful. Also, an added problem when care is shared between specialist and nonspecialist centers is that the recommendations may differ. As caregivers in these situations, parents have the added role of acting as advocates for their child in persuading reluctant staff to follow the advice of the specialist center (in whom they usually have more confidence).

Effective communication pathways between specialist and nonspecialist pharmacy services may help to provide educational support to the community-based pharmacist, which in turn would provide a further avenue of local support for parents and young people dealing with these dilemmas.

IMPLICATIONS FOR PHARMACEUTICAL CARE

Effective pharmaceutical care for informal caregivers is dependent on the pharmacist identifying caregivers and taking time to understand their medication-related roles and associated problems. Many informal caregivers will not self-identify or even identify with the term *informal caregiver* because they see themselves as simply a family member, friend, or neighbor helping another family member, friend, or neighbor.

Studies among caregivers have identified a number of areas that may be improved to decrease the burden and anxiety associated with their medication-related activities. For example, effective systems for communication between prescribers and pharmacists to enable supplies to be ordered and prepared in advance are valued by caregivers. More streamlined ordering and collecting systems would reduce the burden of maintaining continuous supplies. Caregivers highlighted the benefits of a pharmacist who was familiar with their case and could be proactive in addressing potential problems such as clarifying prescription changes, providing reassurance, and being available for discussion.

Although the administering of medicines occurs in the home, the descriptions by caregivers of their roles and problems indicates ways in which pharmacists can support these activities—for example, ensuring full directions and explanations that are easy to read and understand for the use of all products. Review of medication should take into account the role of caregivers (e.g., considering the feasibility of dosing schedules that require frequent attendance, paying attention to the number of formulations, and simplifying dosing regimens to enable easy integration into daily routines). There is great value in pharmacists making themselves available to caregivers as a source of advice and support for the hidden "clinical" roles that are frequently undertaken by caregivers in the home. Pharmacists might advise caregivers on how to identify when care recipients need when-required or as-needed (and sometimes regular) medications, and on identifying and responding to side effects.

Fundamental to successful pharmaceutical care is effective communication between caregivers, care recipients, and pharmacists. As highlighted earlier, the first barrier to this communication may be the lack of awareness among pharmacists, and indeed of caregivers themselves, of each others' potential roles and the opportunities for working together to better address the medication needs of the care recipient and caregiver in the home. Pharmacists should ensure that they are available and accessible to discuss and review the administration and effectiveness of medicines and provide an opportunity for caregivers to express their views, observations, and concerns. Equally, the pharmacist must bear in mind the potential differing perspectives and agendas of caregivers and care recipients. Depending on the relationship, caution may be required regarding sharing confidential information. It may be necessary to involve the care recipient in discussions or to expressly obtain his or her consent. Pharmacists are often quite familiar with the barriers that third-party consultations pose for good pharmaceutical care. However, recognizing and addressing this as an important feature of pharmacy services may lead to ways to support and empower caregivers, who after all provide more health care than any group of professional caregivers.

Collecting prescriptions from a pharmacy is the medication-related activity that a young person is least likely to assume, partly because of legal constraints regarding the supply of medication to minors. However, pharmacists will often see young people in the pharmacy, and young people's lack of participation in any discussion should not be regarded as a reflection of a lack of wider involvement in the administration of their medications and decisions about their use. At an early age, and with parental consent, engaging with young people in a positive way to inform them of the potential source of advice and support that pharmacists can provide regarding medication use is an important aspect of developing a future constructive relationship. Supporting young people in making informed decisions may empower them to assume greater responsibility and appropriate management of their condition in the context of their daily lives.

One of the most difficult areas for the development of pharmacy services is the integration between nonspecialist and specialist services and the associated complex drug therapies and medication-related equipment. Greater communication between hospital-based and community-based pharmacists may be one way of improving the network of support for these patient/caregiver groups once they have left the specialist care providers. In the hospital setting, inpatients will often be able to identify others who will be assisting them with their medications when they return home. In most cases caregivers and care recipients will be happy to jointly discuss their medications.[15] The period following hospital discharge has been identified in a number of studies as being problematic because changes to medication regimens commonly occur. There is often a delay and confusion in transferring information to the community setting (e.g., uncertainty regarding which preadmission medicines are to be continued alongside any new ones). Upon discharge from the hospital, pharmacists could arrange their consultations for a time when the caregiver can be present. This will ensure that the caregiver has the opportunity to hear explanations about medications and their use and to ask questions.

It is also essential to recognize that some caregivers and care recipients are experts in the management of particular conditions. They are well informed and have high levels of knowledge regarding the use of their medications. They will also know what works for them in the context of their lives. It is important that pharmacists and other health professionals be ready to provide the support for these patients to enable them to maintain high-quality pharmaceutical care, and perhaps to individualize this according to their specific requests and agendas.

SUMMARY

This chapter has demonstrated the importance of identifying the perspectives and needs of caregivers in the provision of pharmaceutical care. The involvement of caregivers in medication management can be extensive and complex. Caregivers undertake a wide range of different activities and responsibilities in the context of their own perspectives, circumstances, and lives. The impact of pharmaceutical care will be seriously compromised until the medication-related needs and perspectives of caregivers are recognized as fundamental to its processes and outcomes.

REFERENCES

1. Office for National Statistics. Informal caregivers: results of an independent study carried out on behalf of the Department of Health as part of the 1995 General Household Survey. London: The Stationery Office, 1998.

2. Arno PS. Economic value of informal caregiving. Presented at the Care Coordination and Caregiving Forum, Department of Veterans Affairs, National Institutes of Health, Bethesda, MD, January 25–27, 2006.

3. Caregivers UK. Without us. . . ? Recalculating the value of caregivers support. London: Caregivers UK, 2002.

4. U.S. Department of Health and Human Services. Informal caregiving: compassion in action. Washington, DC: U.S. Department of Health and Human Services, 1998. Based on data from the National Survey of Families and Households (NSFH), 1998, and the National Family Caregivers Association, random sample survey of family caregivers, Summer 2000 (unpublished), and National Alliance for Caregiving and AARP, Caregiving in the U.S., 2004.

5. Office for National Statistics. Census 2001. London: HMSO, 2001.

6. Farfan-Portet MI, Deboosere P, van Oyen H, Lorant V. Informal health care in Belgium. Cah Sociol Demogr Med 2007;47:187-214.

7. National Alliance for Caregiving and AARP. Caregiving in the U.S., 2004.

8. Department of Health. Caring about caregivers: a national strategy for caregivers. London: Department of Health, 1999.

9. Ranelli PL. Exploratory study of caregivers' need and perceptions of pharmaceutical care for elder care-recipients. J Geriatr Drug Ther 1991;6:75-84.

10. Mallet L, King T. Evaluating family caregivers' knowledge of medication. J Geriatr Drug Ther 1993;7:47-58.

11. Ranelli PL, Aversa SL. Medication-related stressors among family caregivers. Am J Hosp Pharm 1994;51:75-9.

12. Ranelli PL, Hansen RW. Medication-related stressors and the family caregiver: a qualitative analysis. Res Sociol Health Care 1994;14:233-48.

13. Goldstein R, Rivers P. The medication role of informal caregivers. Health Soc Care Community 1996;4:150-8.

14. Boyle E, Chambers M. Medication compliance in older individuals with depression: gaining the views of family caregivers. J Psychiatr Ment Health Nurs 2000;7:512-22.

15. Gupta D, Smith FJ, Francis S-A. Supporting informal caregivers in their medication management activities: opportunities in the hospital setting. Hosp Pharm 2002;9:55-8.

16. Francis S-A, Smith F, Gray N, Graffy J. The roles of informal caregivers in the management of medication for older care-recipients. Int J Pharm Pract 2002;10:1-9.

17. Smith FJ, Francis S-A, Gray NJ, Denham MJ, Graffy JP. A multi-centre survey among informal caregivers who manage medication for older care-recipients: problems experienced and the development of services. Health Soc Care Community 2003;11:138-45.

18. Slatter AJ, Francis S-A, Smith FJ, Bush A. Medication use in children with cystic fibrosis: the caregivers' perspectives. Br J Nurs 2004;13:1135-9.

19. Francis SA, Smith FJ, Gray NJ, Denham M. Partnerships between older people and their caregivers in the management of medication. Int J Older People Nurs 2006;1:210-7.
20. Newbould J, Smith FJ, Francis S-A. "I'm fine doing it on my own": partnerships between young people and their parents in the management of medication for asthma and diabetes. J Child Health Care 2008;12:116-28.
21. National Family Caregivers Association. Survey of self-identified family caregivers. Kensington, MD: National Family Caregivers Association, 2001.
22. Rosin AJ, van Dijk Y. Subtle ethical dilemmas in geriatric management and clinical research. J Med Ethics 2005;31:355-9.
23. Atkin K, Ahmad WIU. Pumping iron: compliance with chelation therapy among young people who have thalassaemia major. Sociol Health Illness 2000;22:500-24.

Evaluating Patient Medication Use Behavior and Need for Change

CHAPTER 13

Psychosocial Aspects of Medication Adherence

Kevin C. Farmer, PhD

Advancements in pharmaceutical research and development have created highly effective pharmaceuticals designed to improve and extend patients' lives. However, patients need to take medication according to the proper dose and interval for the medication to have the intended therapeutic effect. A medication will be less effective or potentially have no benefit at all if not taken as intended. Conversely, the drug may be harmful to the patient if taken above and beyond the recommended therapeutic dosage. Healthcare professionals cannot simply assume the patient will use the medication as intended or directed by the prescriber. Patients can skip doses, forget to take doses, fail to refill a prescription on time, or stop therapy completely, often without the knowledge of the provider. Nonadherence with medications results in poor health outcomes and creates a significant economic cost. A consistent association has been found between medication adherence and mortality.[1] The estimated cost of nonadherence runs in the hundreds of billions of dollars each year.[2]

The extent to which patients take medications as prescribed by their healthcare providers has been termed medication compliance or adherence. *Compliance* and *adherence* have been used interchangeably to describe medication-taking behavior. For the purposes of simplicity and clarity, this chapter uses the term *medication adherence* or *nonadherence* as a general reference to the extent to which a patient adopts a prescribed medication regimen. This chapter explores the following topics: description of medication adherence, the nature and extent of medication nonadherence, the consequences of medication nonadherence, predictors of nonadherence, measurement of nonadherence, and interventions to improve medication adherence.

DESCRIPTION OF MEDICATION ADHERENCE

Several terms have been used to describe medication-taking behavior. Some of the first descriptions of aberrations in patients' medication-taking behavior occurred in conjunction with attempts to control tuberculosis with medications, in which individuals who deviated from instructions were labeled *ignorant*, *recalcitrant*, or *defaulters*.[3] The perception was that these patients were untrustworthy and unreliable, and were at fault for deviating from the physician's specific instructions. *Compliance* and *noncompliance* became the common terminology for medication-taking behavior in the 1970s.[4] Over time, *compliance* was viewed as too dictatorial or prescriptive, implying that the patient must do exactly as directed to achieve success. *Adherence* has become a more acceptable term because it implies a cooperative effort between the healthcare provider and the patient in the management of the patient's health. The term *concordance* evolved in a similar fashion as an attempt to define the medication-taking activity as part of a shared goal between the healthcare professional and patient.[5]

The evolution of these terms illustrates the joint responsibility and relationship between the patient and healthcare provider in managing the patient's health, and the recognition that ultimately the patient actively manages and controls his or her health. *Compliance*, *adherence*, and *concordance* have been used to describe the following medication behaviors: failure to fill a prescription, taking an incorrect dose, forgetting to take doses, skipping doses, committing errors in dose timing, and stopping the medication prematurely. A study of HIV-infected patients using antiretroviral therapies found nine different patterns of nonadherence behaviors.[6]

In 2007, a work group from the International Society for Pharmacoeconomics and Outcomes Research (ISPOR) published a paper to clarify and standardize the terminology and definitions related to adherence. According to this standard, medication-taking behavior or adherence consists of two components: medication adherence and medication persistence.[7] *Medication adherence* can be measured as the extent to which a patient follows the prescribed interval and dose of a medication regimen. This could be specific to the frequency, dosage, or timing of a medication regimen and represents dose taking in comparison with what was prescribed. In other words, how well did the patient take the medication compared with what was recommended? This is calculated by dividing the number of doses reported taken by the number of doses available during a specified time frame and is expressed as a percentage. A patient taking 26 tablets of a once-daily regimen in 30 days would have an adherence rate of 86.6% (26/30 × 100). *Medication persistence* refers to the length of time of taking a medication. Persistence is defined as the duration of time from start of therapy until discontinuation. This measure may be expressed as the number of days or months of therapy. It can also be represented as a yes/no variable if one is interested in determining whether a patient is still taking the medication at the end of a specified time.

NATURE AND EXTENT OF MEDICATION NONADHERENCE

The degree to which individuals adhere to their medication regimen differs by the person, the disease state, and the medication used. The rate of adherence with medications has been reported across a broad range of values, from averages in the single digits to over 90%. The variances in adherence figures are caused by a number of factors, including the various methods used to calculate adherence, the condition being treated, side effects of the drug used, and other factors related to the patient that can significantly influence adherence. Research has shown that differences in adherence depend on the disease state being treated and on the different therapeutic categories of drugs. Some patients simply stop taking their medication. A study of patients diagnosed with hyperlipidemia found that four of ten patients stopped taking their medication after 1 year of therapy.[5]

As a result of the extreme variations in rates of adherence reported in the literature, DiMatteo published a comprehensive study in 2004 examining 569 adherence studies published over the previous 50 years to better quantify nonadherence statistics.[8] The average rate of nonadherence was 24.8%. Adherence differed from one disease state to another, with the highest rates for HIV infections (88.3%) and arthritis (81.2%) and the lowest for pulmonary disease (68.8%) and diabetes (67.5%).[8] Adherence rates also differed by the method of measurement used in adherence studies. Pill counts reported the highest rates of adherence, followed by medical records or claims, patient self-report, and electronic monitoring. These methods and their use are discussed in the section on measurement of nonadherence later in this chapter.

PREDICTORS OF MEDICATION NONADHERENCE

The variability of adherence values in different disease states illustrates the difficulty in determining an individual's adherence with his or her medications. Healthcare providers often overestimate adherence and are not skilled in detecting poor adherence.[9] However, there are some common factors and predictors that can help to identify patients who may be at risk for medication nonadherence.[2,10,11] These indicators can then be used to target patients for further evaluation or for need of interventions to improve adherence.

Forgetfulness or the inability to remember the details of directions can be quite common. Memory issues are particularly a problem when the patient has a complex regimen involving receiving multiple medications or multiple doses per day, or one that requires devices for administration. In a similar fashion, a lack of understanding of specific instructions or details impedes the ability of patients to execute directions. Patients may be bombarded with a large amount of verbal instructions and tend to forget a large amount of it unless written instructions are provided as reinforcements. These latter concerns about understanding of medication information are particularly notable with patients with low health literacy.

Medication side effects can also lead to nonadherence, and can be particularly problematic when the medication is used for diseases in which the side effects of the medication are more troublesome than the condition being treated. The asymptomatic nature of a disease also represents a significant factor contributing to medication nonadherence because patients cannot readily identify the benefits of therapy.

The presence of depression or cognitive impairments has also been associated with nonadherence. Race, gender, or socioeconomic status have not generally predicted adherence. However, the cost of the medication or the insurance copayment can be a significant barrier for some individuals, depending on their current economic situation. Patient beliefs about medications, such as the potential for addiction and the value of medications, can affect their likelihood of starting or continuing medications. An often overlooked factor that contributes to medication nonadherence is patient satisfaction and relationship with the healthcare team.

CONSEQUENCES OF MEDICATION NONADHERENCE

Nonadherence with medications has significant consequences for the patient and the healthcare system. Nonadherence has been found to result in poorer health outcomes for the patient and greater costs and utilization of health resources. Estimates regarding the costs of nonadherence run in the hundreds of billions of dollars each year. This is particularly evident in chronic conditions such as heart disease, diabetes, hypertension, asthma, and depression.[1,12]

Table 13-1 illustrates differences in health outcomes and costs found with two prevalent chronic conditions in a study by Sokol and colleagues.[12] The costs of drug therapy were actually greater in the high-adherence groups (because they consumed more medication than poor adherers); however, this difference was offset by the increased medical costs associated with poor adherence. A meta-analysis study (in which data are compiled from numerous studies) examined the relationship between medication adherence and mortality. The results indicated that the risk of mortality

TABLE 13-1	Risk of Hospitalization and Total Healthcare Costs in Diabetes and Hyperlipidemia		
		Medication Adherence Less Than 20%	Medication Adherence 80% or Greater
Diabetes	Total health costs	$8,867	$4,570
	Risk of hospitalization	30%	13%
Hyperlipidemia	Total health costs	$6,810	$3,124
	Risk of hospitalization	15%	12%

Adapted from Sokol MC, McGuigan KA, Verbrugge RR, Epstein RS. Impact of medication adherence on hospitalization risk and healthcare cost. Med Care 2008;43(6):521-30.

for patients classified as having good adherence was one half that of those with poor adherence.[1] Similar results have been found in infectious diseases such as HIV. A study evaluating medication adherence with HIV antiviral drugs found that 62% of patients with adherence less than 70% failed to adequately suppress viral loads in the blood, compared with only 33.7% of patients with adherence of 95% or greater.[13]

Caution must be used when relating mean adherence values from studies to an individual patient. Mean values are calculated from groups or populations of individuals distributed around the mean. A specific individual's adherence value may not be close to the average. In a study evaluating adherence in diabetic patients using angiotensin-converting enzyme (ACE) inhibitors or angiotensin receptor blockers (ARBs), the mean adherence rate was 77%. However, upon closer examination of the data on an individual basis, only 60.4% of the patients had adherence rates considered "good" (80%), whereas 21.9% reported adherence categorized as "poor" (between 50% and 80%) and 17.7% had adherence categorized as "very poor" (<50%).[14] In essence, four of ten patients in the study were classified as having poor or very poor adherence. As a result, one cannot rely on the mean adherence rates reported in clinical studies to give one information about an individual patient. An individual assessment of each patient is needed to ascertain that patient's level of medication adherence.

A number of tools are available to the researcher and healthcare provider to assess medication adherence in their patients. Providers can then focus attention on intervention efforts to improve adherence for those patients experiencing difficulty using their medication correctly.

MEASUREMENT OF MEDICATION ADHERENCE _____

The data presented in the previous section on consequences of poor adherence illustrate how important it is to quantify an individual's medication-taking behavior to achieve optimal health and economic outcomes. It is important to know the methods that are available to assess the patient's medication-taking behavior, the benefits or drawbacks of each method, and which method would be the most appropriate for the provider's or researcher's needs. Table 13-2 identifies the key methods to measure adherence, whether they are used in research or clinical practice, whether they are useful for adherence or persistence measurement, and their primary advantages and disadvantages.

Historically, methods have been categorized as either direct or indirect. *Direct methods* are those which provide some type of evidence that the medication was taken by the patient. These methods include detection of the drug in a biological fluid (usually blood or urine), detection of a biological marker or tag attached to a medication, and directly observed administration. However, these direct methods have their own shortcomings because the level of drug or metabolite found may be poorly correlated with an objective assessment of adherence or persistence. The majority of methods used to detect or analyze medication-taking behavior are indirect methods. *Indirect methods* include medication use reported by the patient, pill counts of returned medications, prescription refill records, and electronic monitoring devices recording bottle opening or blister pack use. When indirect methods are used, the consumption or use of the medication by the patient is assumed.

DIRECT METHODS: BIOLOGICAL FLUID INDICATION _____

The use of a biological assay indicates the presence in the blood or urine of a drug, its metabolite, or possibly an indicator compound or tag administered with the drug of interest. A positive assay provides confirmation the patient received a dose of the medication within some limited time frame prior to analysis. Depending on the pharmacokinetic properties of the drug, it is possible for the patient to take just a few doses of the drug prior to the assay and achieve a detectable level of the drug, masking intentional nonadherence by the patient.[15,16] Many factors can also affect the therapeutic level of the drug, including food and drug interactions, which may make interpretation of the results very difficult. This type of adherence measure is generally impractical for several reasons. Biological assays are intrusive (e.g., requiring a blood draw), expensive, and basically provide a current snapshot with little information related to the individual's pattern of use.

TABLE 13-2   Methods for Measuring Medication Adherence

Measure	Use in Clinical Practice or Research Study	Adherence (A) or Persistence (P) Analysis	Advantages	Disadvantages
Blood/serum level	Research	P	Proof of use	Patient variability Invasive Expensive
Pill count	Practice Research	A	Inexpensive Ease of use	Obtrusive Pill dumping Accuracy
Electronic monitoring devices	Research	A P	Data on dosing intervals Accuracy	Expensive Patient may use other bottles
Prescription refill records (in same pharmacy or pharmacy system)	Practice	A P	Inexpensive Ease of use	All scripts must be filled in same pharmacy to see all records
Prescription refill records (large prescription databases)	Research	A P	Noninvasive Long-term data Population data	Quality of data
Patient diary	Practice Research	A	Inexpensive Can augment electronic monitoring	Patient must remember entries and return diary
Patient interview	Practice Research	A	Inexpensive Ease of use May provide reasons for behavior	Social desirability Skill of interviewer Qualitative Patient recall Can overestimate
Structured questionnaire(s)	Practice Research	A	Ease of use May provide reasons for behavior	Patient recall Can overestimate

Indirect Methods

Pill Counts

One of the most common and easiest methods of assessing patient adherence is the use of a pill count. Patients bring their prescription bottles (or blister packs) with them on their return visit to the clinic or pharmacy. The number of pills returned is counted and compared with the date the prescription was filled and the number of pills that should have been taken during this period of time. Excess pills indicate the patient has taken less than the prescribed amount of medication. (For nonoral dosage unit medications such as metered-dose inhalers, clinicians can weigh the devices and estimate the number of inhalations used by the weight change of the canister.[17])

Although easy to conduct and inexpensive, this method has a number of drawbacks that inhibit its reliability as an accurate measure of medication adherence. Because patients are aware that their medication is being counted, it is possible for patients to dump unused pills prior to the visit to hide their nonadherence. Pill counts can also be perceived as obtrusive and indicating a lack of trust, leading to an adversarial patient–provider relationship. The accuracy of pill counts can also be variable due to many other factors. Patients can simply forget to bring the container with them. The date of the prescription fill must be correct, and refills must be included. Studies have indicated that pill counts tend to overestimate adherence behavior compared with prescription claims databases and electronic monitoring.[18-21]

Electronic Monitoring Devices

Electronic drug monitoring devices have gained wide acceptance among researchers evaluating medication-taking behavior, and new devices are being developed to enhance adherence for patients. These devices are generally not used in clinical practice because of their costs. The devices contain a microprocessor chip in the bottle cap that records the date and time the bottle is opened to obtain a dose. Chips can also be contained in pill boxes, blister packaging, inhalation devices, eye droppers, and topical formulations to record an administration of the medication.[17,22,23] When the patient returns to the clinic or pharmacy, the bottle cap (or other packaging material) is simply passed over a receiver that downloads the captured data. The device can store a significant amount of data, so in the event a patient forgets to bring the container in on one visit, the data can be retrieved on the following visit.

This type of monitoring system has significant advantages over other adherence measures because it not only can provide continuous reliable data to capture medication adherence but also can provide information on dosing schedule adherence for medications requiring precise dosing regimens. In a study comparing the effectiveness of lovastatin administered in the morning versus in the evening for hypercholesterolemia, nearly one fourth of prescribed evening doses occurred before 5:00 PM, whereas researchers had assumed the doses would be taken by patients later in the evening.[24] Electronic monitoring has been especially useful in studying the relationship between medication adherence and viral suppression in HIV infection, in which significantly higher levels of adherence are required to maintain viral suppression. One of the most widely used electronic monitoring devices is the Medication Event Monitoring System (MEMS; Aprex Corp., Fremont, CA).

Electronic monitoring devices have several limitations. The recorded compliance activity (under- or overadherence) may be influenced if the bottle is opened by mistake or used incorrectly by the patient. Patients may remove more than one dose from the bottle at a time in situations in which they plan to take the dose or doses later, or may transfer several doses to a smaller, more convenient container. Adherence can be overestimated if the patient accidentally or purposefully opens the bottle without taking a dose of the medication. The use of a diary in conjunction with electronic monitoring allows the patient to document any opening of the device. There is also some evidence that, similar to pill counts, patients are acutely aware of the monitoring or surveillance. A limited "Hawthorne effect" has been noted for up to 40 days, in which adherence is initially higher due to known monitoring.[25] Some patients have also reported anxiety, depression, and somatic complaints because of the knowledge that their medication-taking behavior was being monitored.[26]

Pharmacy Refill Records

Pharmacy refill records have become a common tool to assess medication adherence and persistence. These records can be used by a pharmacist to review an individual patient's medication record in the pharmacy (if all medications were obtained there) or, more commonly, by researchers using large administrative prescription claims databases. At the individual pharmacy level, it is critical to know whether the patient obtained all medications through that pharmacy or associated pharmacies using the same computer system. Many pharmacies do not share common pharmacy records and therefore it is not possible to know whether what appears to be nonadherence is really a situation of a patient refilling a medication at a different pharmacy. In an HMO pharmacy system, researchers studied patients on antihyperlipidemic medications and found a 32% probability that patients would discontinue their medication after 1 year.[27] Large administrative prescription claims databases have been used extensively to analyze medication adherence and persistence.[28-30] Because these databases are generated by pharmacy claims to health insurers, employers, Medicaid, Medicare, or the Veterans Administration, all prescription activity by the patient is captured in the system regardless of the pharmacy used.

There are a number of different approaches for calculating medication adherence and persistence using pharmacy claims. Some involve the examination of individual claims and the gaps between refills, whereas others focus on multiple refills of the medication creating a continuous measure of adherence. A common approach for calculating medication adherence with prescription claims is the continuous measure of adherence (CMA), which provides a mean value of medication adherence (as a percentage) for a defined length of time.[31,32] Methods used in database research also include the following:[32]

- Continuous, single-interval measure of medication availability (CSA)
- Compliance rate (CR)
- Days between refills adherence rate (DBR)
- Continuous measure of medication gaps (CMG)
- Continuous multiple-interval measure of oversupply (CMOS)
- Medication possession ratio (MPR)
- Refill compliance rate (RCR)
- Medication possession ratio–modified (MPRm)
- Medication refill adherence (MRA)
- Proportion of days covered (PDC)

Research comparing each of these methods indicates that CMA, CMOS, MPR, and MRA are identical in measuring adherence.[32] The method selected depends on the research question of interest.

The use of pharmacy claims data has a number of advantages and limitations. The potential influence on patient behavior through direct observation via pill counts, electronic monitoring, or patient report does not occur with prescription records data. Databases create the opportunity to study medication-taking behavior at the population level, and generally do not have issues with small sample sizes, which can influence statistical significance. The researcher should be familiar with the source of the claims data and how the data were compiled. The data set should be complete and include patient eligibility information; otherwise, the researcher may not know whether the patient has simply stopped taking the medication, been switched to another drug, changed insurance, or may have even died.

Patient Self-Reported Behavior

Asking patients to self-report their medication-taking behavior is the simplest and most convenient method of evaluating medication adherence. This is frequently used in clinical practice by the healthcare provider to gauge a patient's medication-taking behavior. Patient self-reported adherence behavior may be collected in several ways. The clinician or researcher may conduct a patient interview, with specific questions regarding how (and whether) the patient is using his or her medication(s). Patients may also be asked to keep a diary of their medication use. Patients can be given (in person, by mail, or by other means) an adherence-specific questionnaire.

Advantages to self-report instruments are their simplicity and low cost. A limitation of self-report methods has been unreliability in reporting accurate adherence and persistence.[19-21,33-36] Patients are generally reluctant to reveal they have not taken their medication as instructed.[37] Patients may not recall that they forgot to take a dose. The lack of precision found with self-report methods is frequently a result of the manner and language used in the interview, or of poorly constructed questionnaires and surveys. Adherence-related patient interviews have sometimes been referred to as interrogations, which is likely how patients perceive them.[38] The nature and orientation of the questions can influence the patient's response. Questions that make the patient appear responsible for nonadherence and blame the patient for not complying with instructions can bias the response.[39] Patients frequently responded in what they perceived to be a more socially desirable manner and concealed their actual medication taking behavior when the adherence question was framed as "Did you take your medicine as your doctor told you?"[40] In some cases, patients were asked whether they had taken the prescribed number of doses, and if they had not, to estimate how many they had missed.[34]

The development and proliferation of validated structured adherence questionnaires has done much to address the unreliability issues noted with various patient self-report methods. Some of the more common instruments available for use are the following:

- Medication Adherence Survey (MAS)[41]
- Brief Medication Questionnaire (BMQ)[42]
- Medical Outcomes Study (MOS)[43]

In situations in which it is desirable to use a self-report instrument, a validated questionnaire provides an easy, reliable, ready-to-use instrument for either a practice or research setting.

SELECTION OF A METHOD FOR MEASURING ADHERENCE _____

The choice of a measurement method to assess medication adherence or persistence should match the strengths of a method to the goals and needs of the clinician or investigator. No single method will be the best choice for all purposes. For the healthcare provider, the measures of choice would ideally be inexpensive, practical, and easy to administer and interpret, and would not interfere with the patient–provider relationship. What is important to the clinician is the ability to identify patients with nonadherence issues and then employ interventions to optimize the patient's medication-taking behavior. Physicians and other healthcare providers often believe they can identify and estimate medication adherence in their patients. However, research has found that clinicians tend to overestimate medication adherence and do not adequately detect poor adherence.[9] The clinician may then alter or change therapy on the basis that the drug was ineffective, when the patient was actually nonadherent with initial therapy. This can lead to the addition of unnecessary drugs, side effects, and additional costs. In many cases, a structured questionnaire or patient interview (if the interviewer is skilled) is the most practical tool for the clinician. Prescription refill records can be very useful to identify potential adherence over the course of therapy and can provide pharmacists information before they see the patient again in a refill situation.

Measurement methods for adherence researchers and those conducting clinical trials require a reliable and accurate assessment of medication adherence or persistence. Electronic monitoring devices have become the standard measure of adherence in clinical trials. Detailed patient usage patterns can provide feedback to analyze the effectiveness of new drug products and to identify and correct misuse problems. One should not rely on a single method for adherence and persistence analysis, but rather use a combination of methods to compensate for the potential weaknesses of the methods used.

INTERVENTIONS TO IMPROVE MEDICATION ADHERENCE _____

What should the pharmacist do after a patient has been identified with poor or inadequate medication adherence? The pharmacist must work with such patients to help them understand their problem and improve their adherence. A number of strategies exist to assist healthcare providers in working with their patients to improve adherence with their medications.[10,44-46] These strategies fall into four categories: providing information, patient-centered counseling, behavioral reinforcement and support strategies, and medication regimen strategies.

Providing Additional Information

Because the inability to remember information may be a factor in the patient's nonadherence, education and the use of specific clear verbal and written information can be highly effective. This is of particular interest when the patient has complex regimens or requires information to deal with troublesome side effects. Information should be specific to the patient's condition and drug therapy. Information should be categorized and simplified to enhance patient understanding.

Patient-Centered Counseling

Counseling should focus on patient-specific needs and foster the patient–provider relationship. Patient concerns should be respected and not ignored. The importance of self-management and the patient's role in his or her own health should be discussed. It is important to assess the patient's barriers to nonadherence and develop interventions to address those barriers. Pharmacists can engage in a variety of techniques, such as motivational interviewing, to engage patients in seeing the need to improve their medication adherence.[47] Pharmacists should also encourage patient self-monitoring of their symptoms and how such changes in symptoms are related to the drug's effectiveness.

Behavioral Reinforcement and Support Strategies

Numerous strategies and tools exist to provide behavioral support for the patient. Adherence aids include pill boxes, calendars, automated phone messages, text messages, and email reminders. Reminder cues can also be developed based on patients' daily habits and activities to incorporate medication adherence into their daily lives.

Medication Regimen Strategies

The medication regimen should be tailored to the patient's lifestyle and needs whenever possible. Regimens that impinge on the patient's normal lifestyle will be difficult for the patient to adhere to. Dosing regimens should be simplified whenever possible, with once- or twice-daily regimens preferred or as the patient desires. Alternate drugs should be evaluated when adherence appears unlikely with a bothersome product.

Research has shown that multiple interventions and strategies are the most successful in improving adherence.[10] Additionally, provider support must continue on a regular basis; otherwise, adherence is likely to return to previous levels.[46] A number of resources are available to pharmacists and healthcare providers from health organizations, professional associations, and the pharmaceutical industry to assist with developing adherence intervention strategies. Sources of these resources include the National Council on Patient Information and Education (http://www.talkaboutrx.org/), the American Pharmacist Association (http://www.pharmacist.com), Adult Medication (http://adultmeducation.com), a joint project of the American Society on Aging and the American Society of Consultant Pharmacists Foundation, and websites supported by pharmaceutical companies and chain pharmacies.

SUMMARY

Nonadherence with medications presents both a health risk and an economic cost. The management of chronic diseases is primarily achieved through the use of prescription drug therapy. When medications are not used properly or are prematurely discontinued, they fail to provide optimum benefits, leading to poorer health outcomes and greater utilization of healthcare resources. The evolution of the term *adherence* illustrates how medication-taking behavior has come to be viewed more as a joint cooperative effort between healthcare providers and patients than as simply instructions that the patient is expected to follow.

Healthcare providers should be aware of common predictors that may identify patients who are more vulnerable to nonadherence. A number of methods exist to identify or quantify medication nonadherence. Self-report instruments or pharmacy prescription records are generally more appropriate for healthcare providers in their daily practice. Several self-report methods are easy to use and interpret. More sophisticated methods are available to researchers who require quantitative information and greater precision. Because no method is without some limitations, the use of multiple methods may be required to fully capture the dynamics of the specific medication-taking behavior being investigated.

When a patient has been identified or is suspected as having adherence issues, the pharmacist or other healthcare provider should design and employ a set of intervention strategies to work with the patient to improve medication adherence. The result is a richer patient–pharmacist relationship in which the patient views the pharmacist as a valuable partner in managing his or her health care. The future challenge to pharmacy is not getting medications to patients, but helping patients use medications in a manner to achieve the optimal benefit.

REFERENCES

1. Simpson SH, Eurich DT, Majumdar SR, Padwal RS, Tsuyuki RT, Varney J. A meta-analysis of the association between adherence to drug therapy and mortality. BMJ 2006;333:15.

2. Martin LR, Williams SR, Haskard KB, DiMatteo MR. The challenge of patient adherence. Ther Clin Risk Manage 2005;1(3):189-99.

3. Steiner JF, Earnest MA. Lingua medica: the language of medication-taking. Ann Intern Med 2000;132(11):926-30.

4. Sackett DL, Haynes RB. Compliance with therapeutic regimens. Baltimore, MD: Johns Hopkins University Press, 1976.

5. American Pharmacists Association. Medication compliance-adherence-persistence (CAP) digest. Washington, DC: American Pharmacists Association, 2008.

6. Hill Z, Kendall C, Fernandez M. Patterns of adherence to antiretrovirals: why adherence has no simple measure. AIDS Patient Care STDs 2003;17(10):519-25.

7. Cramer JA, Roy A, Burrell A, et al. Medication compliance and persistence: terminology and definitions. Value Health 2007;11(1):44-7.

8. DiMatteo MR. Variations in patients' adherence to medical recommendations. Med Care 2004; 42(3):200-9.

9. Miller LG, Liu H, Hays RD, et al. How well do clinicians estimate patients' adherence to combination antiretroviral therapy? J Gen Intern Med 2002;17(1):1-11.

10. Osterberg L, Blaschke T. Adherence to medication. N Engl J Med 2005;353(5):487-97.

11. Burra TA, Chen E, McIntyre RS, Grace SL, Robertson Blackmore E, Stewart DE. Predictors of self-reported antidepressant adherence. Behav Med 2007;32(4):127-34.

12. Sokol MC, McGuigan KA, Verbrugge RR, Epstein RS. Impact of medication adherence on hospitalization risk and healthcare cost. Med Care 2008;43(6):521-30.

13. Gross R, Yip B, Lo Re V III, et al. A simple, dynamic measure of antiretroviral therapy adherence predicts failure to maintain HIV-1 suppression. J Infect Dis 2006;194(8):1108-14.

14. Cooke CE, Fatodu H. Physician conformity and patient adherence to ACE inhibitors and ARBs in patients with diabetes, with and without renal disease and hypertension, in a Medicaid managed care organization. J Manag Care Pharm 2006;12(8):649-55.

15. Feinstein AR. On white-coat effects and the electronic monitoring of compliance. Arch Intern Med 1990;150(7):1377-8.

16. Cramer JA, Scheyer RD, Mattson RH. Compliance declines between clinic visits. Arch Intern Med 1990;150(7)1509-10.

17. Rand CS, Wise RA, Nides MA, et al. Metered-dose inhaler adherence in a clinical trial. Am Rev Respir Dis 1992;146(6):1559-64.

18. Liu H, Golin CE, Miller LG, et al. A comparison study of multiple measures of adherence to HIV protease inhibitors. Ann Intern Med 2001;134(10):968-77.

19. Grymonpre RE, Didur CD, Montgomery PR, Sitar DS. Pill count, self-report, and pharmacy claims data to measure medication adherence in the elderly. Ann Pharmacother 1998; 32(7-8):749-54.

20. Craig HM. Accuracy of indirect measures of medication compliance in hypertension. Res Nurs Health 1985;8:61-6.

21. Matsui D, Hermann C, Klein JJ, Berkovitch M, Olivieri N, Koren G. Critical comparison of novel and existing methods of compliance assessment during a clinical trial of an oral iron chelator. J Clin Pharmacol 1994;34(9):944-9.

22. Hermann MM, Diestelhorst M. Microprocessor controlled compliance monitor for eye drop medication. Br J Ophthalmol 2006;90(7):830-2.

23. Balkrishnan R, Carroll CL, Camacho FT, Feldman SR. Electronic monitoring of medication adherence in skin disease: results of a pilot study. J Am Acad Dermatol 2003;49(4):651-4.

24. Kruse W, Nikolaus T, Rampmaier J, Weber E, Schlierf G. Actual versus prescribed timing of lovastatin doses assessed by electronic compliance monitoring. Eur J Clin Pharmacol 1993; 45(3):211-5.

25. Berg KM, Arnsten JH. Practical and conceptual challenges in measuring antiretroviral adherence. Acquir Immune Defic Syndr 2006;43(suppl 1):S79-87.

26. Elixhauser A, Eisen SA, Romeis JC, Homan SM. The effects of monitoring and feedback on compliance. Med Care 1990;28(10):882-93.

27. Andrade SE, Walker AM, Gottlieb LK, et al. Discontinuation of antihyperlipidemic drugs—do rates reported in clinical trials reflect rates in primary care settings? New Engl J Med 1995;332(17):1125-31.

28. Steiner JF, Koepsell TD, Fihn SD, Inui TS. A general method of compliance assessment using centralized pharmacy records. Med Care 1988;26(8):814-23.

29. Hamilton RA, Briceland LL. Use of prescription-refill records to assess patient compliance. Am J Hosp Pharm 1992;49(7):1691-6.

30. Gurwitz JH, Glynn RJ, Monane M, et al. Treatment for glaucoma: adherence by the elderly. Am J Public Health 1993;83(5):711-6.

31. Peterson AM, Nau DP, Cramer JA, Benner J, Gwadry-Sridhar F, Nichol MB. A checklist for medication compliance and persistence studies using retrospective databases. Value Health 2007;10(1):3-12.

32. Hess LM, Raebel MA, Conner DA, Malone DC. Measurement of adherence in pharmacy administrative databases: a proposal for standard definitions and preferred measures. Ann Pharmacother 2006;40:1280-8.

33. Straka RJ, Fish JT, Benson SR, Suh JT. Patient self-reporting of compliance does not correspond with electronic monitoring: an evaluation using isosorbide dinitrate as a model drug. Pharmacotherapy 1997;17(1):126-32.

34. Park LC, Lipman RS. A comparison of patient dosage deviation reports with pill counts. Psychopharmacologia 1964;6:299-302.

35. Inui TS, Carter WB, Pecoraro RE. Screening for noncompliance among patients with hypertension: is self-report the best available measure? Med Care 1981;19:1061-4.

36. Gordis L, Markowitz M, Lilienfeld AM. The inaccuracy in using interviews to estimate patient reliability in taking medications at home. Med Care 1969;7:49-54.

37. Cramer JA, Mattson RH. Monitoring compliance with antiepileptic drug therapy. In: Cramer JA, Spilker B, eds. Patient compliance in medical practice and clinical trials. New York: Raven Press, 1991:123-37.

38. Myers ED, Branthwaite A. Out-patient compliance with antidepressant medication. Br J Psychiatry 1992;160:83-6.

39. Ross FM. Patient compliance—whose responsibility? Soc Sci Med 1991;32(1):89-94.

40. Sherbourne CD, Hays RD, Ordway L, DiMatteo MR, Kravitz RL. Antecedents of adherence to medical recommendations: results from the Medical Outcomes Study. J Behav Med 1992;15(2):447-68.

41. Morisky DE, Green LW, Levine DM. Concurrent and predictive validity of a self-reported measure of medication adherence. Med Care 1986;24(1):67-74.

42. Svarstad BL, Chewning BA, Sleath BL, Claesson C. The Brief Medication Questionnaire: a tool for screening patient adherence and barriers to adherence. Patient Educ Couns 1999;37: 113-24.

43. Kuller LH. The use of existing databases in morbidity and mortality studies [editorial]. Am J Public Health 1995;85(9):1198-9.

44. National Council on Patient Information and Education. Enhancing prescription medicine adherence: a national action plan. Bethesda, MD: National Council on Patient Information and Education, 2007.

45. Schneider PJ, Murphy JE, Pedersen CA. Impact of medication packaging on adherence and treatment outcomes in older ambulatory patients. J Am Pharm Assoc 2008;48(1):58-63.

46. Lee JK, Grace KA, Taylor AJ. Effect of a pharmacy care program on medication adherence and persistence, blood pressure, and low-density lipoprotein cholesterol. JAMA 2006;296(21): 2614-6.

47. Miller W, Rollnick S. Motivational interviewing: preparing people for change. 2nd ed. New York: Guilford Press, 2002.

CHAPTER 14

Facilitating Behavioral Change

Jan Kavookjian, PhD, MBA

The evaluation of interventions aimed at influencing medication-taking behavior is not a new topic. In fact, researchers and providers across most health professions have had an interest in studying medication adherence and nonadherence for the past several decades.[1,2] Because the expensive problem of nonadherence has not resolved itself or even improved remarkably, this field of interest continues to grow, incorporating new developments in what we know about patient and system barriers and about medication-taking behavior and motivation as well as incorporating new technological tools.

This chapter explores interventions that have been used to influence medication-taking behavior. These include the general categories of educational interventions, specific behavioral stimulus interventions, social or support network initiatives, organizational approaches, and structured communication or counseling strategies. It is important to point out that most behavior change initiatives use a combination of strategies.[3,4] For example, education alone is often not enough to maintain behavior change. In addition to knowledge barriers, patients often have motivational or practical barriers to adherence that must be addressed through counseling or initiatives at the healthcare-system level.

Many landmark interventions for medication adherence have been explored in healthcare settings outside pharmacy and are presented in this chapter along with interventions applied in pharmacy practice settings. In addition, although pharmacists engaging in disease management initiatives might intervene to help patients change a multitude of health behaviors (e.g., exercise, diet, monitoring), this chapter primarily focuses on interventions that influence medication-taking behavior.

EDUCATIONAL INTERVENTIONS FOR MEDICATION-TAKING BEHAVIOR CHANGE

Sometimes referred to as *informational* interventions,[3] educational interventions include cognitive strategies delivered through one or more avenues. These might include didactic instruction to an individual or a group or interactive, face-to-face approaches. In pharmacy practice settings, verbal delivery is often accompanied by the provision of written material for the patient to take home for future reference. This is also an important way to reinforce the decisions a patient might make while receiving the education. Written material is a tangible piece of "evidence" from the interaction that can serve as a resource and as a reminder. Other media for education delivery might include audio or video tapes, DVDs, take-home or on-site computer programs, books (and coloring books for children), and other technologically based information delivery tools,[3,4] including personal digital assistants (PDAs).[5]

When educating patients, whether verbally or by using other media, there are important considerations regarding the development and delivery of an educational intervention. Education is only a part of an effective intervention process, but it is essential. Patients must first understand their illness and their medication before they can decide to take a medication appropriately.[4] Because the patient's understanding is such a crucial part of medication-taking behavior, it is important to think about the target audience and characteristics that might pose barriers to understanding an educational intervention. Among many characteristics to take into account, two important considerations are literacy level and cultural differences. Although these topics are covered extensively elsewhere in this book, it is important to briefly discuss their implications for selecting or designing educational interventions to influence medication-taking behavior.

Literacy and Health Literacy

Healthcare providers are trained to communicate in a highly scientific manner throughout their studies and professional interactions. It can be challenging for providers delivering education to provide it at a literacy level that meets the comprehension needs of all of their patients. The functional reading level in the United States has been established as being at the eighth-grade level.[6] About 42 million U.S. adults are considered functionally illiterate, and it is estimated that over 20% of U.S. adults cannot read or comprehend at greater than the fifth-grade reading level.

The concern about general literacy extends to health literacy. Health literacy has been a topic of recent emphasis from national organizations such as the Institute of

Medicine, the Agency for Healthcare Research and Quality, and the American Medical Association. Reports from studies by these groups suggest that up to half of all U.S. adults may lack the skills needed to function optimally in a healthcare environment, including skills such as making appropriate decisions about dosing cold medicine for a child and understanding informed consent documents.[7]

Cultural Barriers

In addition to literacy concerns, pharmacists educating patients about medication taking should be aware of cultural issues that might contribute to misunderstandings or mistrust. There may be language or cultural barriers that will hinder patient adherence with medication as a result of misunderstanding what the provider meant when discussing the patient's medications. This may be related to traditions within a specific racial, ethnic, or religious group, or may be present among patients for whom English is not their primary language.

Regional customs may also pose barriers to understanding, even where language of origin is not a barrier. For example, fried foods are a mainstay in the dietary customs of the southeastern United States. Encouraging patients in this region to eat more vegetables to improve their health should be clarified to include a discussion about preparing them in a healthy way. In addition, other cultures may have medication-taking beliefs or restrictions that should be explored, including folk beliefs that may have little to no rational basis. Respectful discussion should take place in the face of such barriers in order to avoid offending the patient or risk having him or her become mistrustful and resistant to receiving education about medication taking.

Using Visual Aids to Overcome Barriers

It is important for pharmacists to become aware of the potential for literacy or cultural barriers among the patients they serve, particularly in the context of an educational intervention.[8] Some have focused on overcoming barriers to the delivery of education about medications by using visual aids that include pictures or universally recognized symbols to convey medication-taking instructions. For example, the warning labels that are placed on prescription vials often include symbols along with text in an attempt to address these very issues. The use of symbols, such as an ace of hearts to represent the class of medications known as angiotensin-converting enzyme (ACE) inhibitors, has resulted in improved adherence and patient outcomes for undereducated inner city heart failure patients for whom health literacy was a major concern.[8]

Reviews of the medication adherence intervention literature suggest that informational interventions alone sometimes contribute to improvements in self-reported adherence, but that most did not produce improved clinical outcomes.[3] Authors concluded that most educational interventions for medication taking are delivered in a single episode and that multiple or follow-up deliveries would be more effective.[4,8,9] In addition, educational interventions are more often effective when delivered in combination with other intervention methods discussed in the next several sections.[3,4,9-12]

BEHAVIOR STIMULUS INTERVENTIONS FOR MEDICATION-TAKING BEHAVIOR CHANGE

Behavior change interventions include strategies that can be generally organized into three stimulus categories: reminders (cues), tailoring of medication regimens, or reinforcement to encourage a patient to initiate and maintain change to a desired behavior.

Reminder Strategies

Reminder strategies for influencing medication-taking behavior have received a lot of attention in recent years. With the rise in society's technological sophistication, many simple and complex devices and services have been developed to help patients remember to take their medications. More complex developments include electronic reminder devices such as pill boxes or watches, automated medication dispensers, and even compliance reminder services. These services send a phone call or email message reminder at the time to take a dose, or will send a phone call, email, or postal mail card or letter reminder for refills. Some systems have had significant influence on medication-taking behavior when applied in controlled studies.[4,13]

In the everyday reality of many patients, cost, access, and lack of familiarity with technology often make these options unavailable. Simple, less expensive tools have also been developed. These include simple pillboxes, reminder packaging (blister), calendars, stickers, and pamphlets, among others. Krueger and colleagues' 2005 review of medication adherence interventions includes an extensive review of the medication memory aids available at the time of writing.[4]

The use of compliance aids alone has not been very effective, producing a median impact of about 3%; however, reminder systems by mail or telephone demonstrated consistent and significant improvements in adherence rates.[4] As with other intervention strategies presented in this chapter, compliance aids and reminder systems are more effective when used in combination with other strategies, particularly education.

In conditions such as schizophrenia and bipolar disorder, where nonadherence is prevalent and is affected by illness-produced lack of insight, reminder systems can be important. One such intervention has produced improvements in adherence and reduction in relapse and hospitalization by using a systematic approach with large calendars and attached pens to track appointments, signs, medication containers with alarms, bus passes to assist patients in getting to their appointments, and notebooks for recording side effects to assist in discussion with the provider at the next appointment.[14,15]

Tailoring the Medication Regimen

It is well known that the more complex the dosing schedule of a medication, the less adherent a patient is likely to be with the regimen. The review by Krueger and colleagues suggested that the characteristics of complexity of a regimen and the effects of the regimen itself negatively affect adherence, particularly when a patient is taking more than four medications, has more frequent daily doses, is confused about the regimen, believes that he or she cannot follow the regimen, and/or has a fear of side effects.[4] A review examining the impact of the complexity of the dosing regimen compared adherence rates between once-daily and four-times-daily regimens. The researchers concluded that the mean adherence rate was approximately 79% among 29 reviewed studies of once-daily dosing. This compares with a 69% adherence in 32 studies of twice-daily dosing, a 65% adherence rate in 13 studies of three-times-daily dosing, and a 51% adherence rate in 11 studies of four-times-daily dosing.[16]

Similar conclusions have been presented in other adherence intervention reviews,[3,4,10] and reducing the dosing regimen and complexity has been often recommended as a first-line strategy for gaining adherence. By tailoring the dosing regimen to the patient's daily routine, the negative impacts of the illness may be minimized and the patient's sense of control over the illness may be increased. This strategy includes not only simplifying the regimen but also tying the medication-taking process to other daily activities or routines to help the patient remember to take his or her medication. For example, suggesting that a coffee-drinking patient place his or her morning medication by the coffee pot will assist that patient in remembering to take the medication by tying it to another habitual behavior.

Reinforcement for Medication-Taking Behavior

Interventions aimed at reinforcing or rewarding medication taking have taken many forms across research studies and in practice. Providers who have given their patients skill-building types of training, or self-care training and planning or contracts, have demonstrated significant increases in medication adherence rates,[3,4,10] particularly when delivered over time and when combined with other intervention strategies.

According to Kripalani and colleagues in a 2007 review of the adherence intervention literature, the most effective strategy in the reinforcement category includes assessing/monitoring adherence and giving feedback to the patient.[3] Studies involving this process had patients monitor and report their medication use and/or blood pressure. They were then given tailored feedback by their providers, including reinforcing statements. Improvements in adherence and clinical outcomes were more significant than in a study that only provided blood pressure readings to the patient and his or her provider. Other reviews reported similar findings.[10,17]

In recent years, employers have used the monitoring and feedback method in the form of health risk assessments (HRAs) as part of a wellness initiative. HRAs use biometric assessment data to provide a report and feedback to employees, informing them of progress (or lack thereof), comparing their numbers to national standards, and encouraging them to engage in healthy behaviors, including medication adherence.[18]

Recent studies among pharmacist-delivered adherence interventions have included ongoing monitoring and feedback.[8,9,19,20] The positive influence on adherence supports the role of pharmacists as providers in a unique position to deliver a medication adherence intervention that includes ongoing monitoring and feedback, particularly given the ongoing interaction with patients on maintenance medications for chronic illnesses.

It is possible that this method of monitoring and feedback, which includes ongoing interaction, not only reinforces adherence but also actively involves the patient in the decision-making process. When a patient is involved in decision making about his or her care, more opportunity exists for the development of the internal motivation that is necessary to maintain change regarding a target behavior.[10,17] Studies using other external rewards for adherence behavior had limited long-term impact.[10,11] This is perhaps because external rewards generate extrinsic motivation, which is generally not sustained over time.[21,22] Patients tend to initially adopt either an approach or avoidance coping style when they find out they have a chronic illness, and will stick with the early coping style throughout treatment, even in the face of additional information or stressors.[23] Patients using an approach coping style actively deal with their illnesses and treatments by seeking information and problem-solving. Alternatively, patients using an avoidance coping style disengage or pull away from dealing with their illnesses and treatments. Getting patients involved early in the decision-making process in their care can help foster an approach coping style that may contribute to internal motivation and sustain behavioral movement toward medication adherence.

SOCIAL OR SUPPORT NETWORKS AND MEDICATION-TAKING BEHAVIOR CHANGE

For many patients, the support of family, friends, and/or caregivers provides the necessary coping mechanism to engage in health behaviors.[4] Whether structured (with facilitation or counseling and an agenda) or unstructured (informal support groups), in person or via chat rooms on the Internet, support can provide a sense of connection for individuals suffering with an illness or health condition.

Just as with the monitoring and feedback intervention described previously, ongoing support is important in sustaining a behavior change such as medication adherence. This is where a patient's healthcare provider can also have an important influence on medication adherence, particularly pharmacists, who have an opportunity to regularly see patients when it is time to refill maintenance medications. Interventions that occur more than once foster a caring, collaborative relationship between a pharmacist and a patient.[4,19] Support for a patient partners with the concept of reinforcement to not only help a patient feel understood and less alone in the face of his or her illness and its care, but also to enable the patient to continue engaging in target behaviors and avoid engaging in undesired behaviors.

It is often difficult for patients to make changes that are unsupported in their social networks. Smoking cessation, for example, is particularly difficult for a patient whose primary social networks involve going to bars and other settings where smoking is a prevalent social activity. Patients on medications that have an interaction with alcohol or certain foods may face the same challenge and may opt for nonadherence with the medication in order to maintain the social network and its contraindicated activities. It is important to explore these barriers with patients and help them to examine possible alternatives to the stimuli that may tempt them to be nonadherent.

Reviews of the literature on medication adherence include the notion of support as being important to successful intervention,[4,10] even to the extent that family therapy may be warranted in some difficult cases.[10] This is particularly true for patients with severe mental illnesses such as schizophrenia and bipolar disorder, where effects of the illness itself hinder a patient's cognitive processing ability (poor insight) and where nonadherence is prevalent, has very expensive consequences, and is particularly problematic. In severe cases of nonadherence with multiple relapses, a patient support intervention may even include a team of providers. Home visits from community services[12] are sometimes specified in the nature of outpatient commitment orders, even on a weekly basis, for patients newly discharged from inpatient psychiatric hospital stays.

The key to successful interventions for such patients is highly dependent on the level of support, including listening to the patient and customizing the regimen in accordance with the patient's needs regarding treatment effects and side effects,[12,24] focusing on the positive aspects of medication use, focusing on enhancing insight, and fostering a therapeutic relationship with patients and their caregivers.[25]

ORGANIZATIONAL OR HEALTHCARE SYSTEM APPROACHES TO MEDICATION-TAKING BEHAVIOR CHANGE

Patients often cite healthcare system–related barriers or facilitators that influence their decisions about taking their medication as prescribed. This section explores interventions at the system or organization level that have been employed to address issues under the patient's control as well as interactions between the patient and his or her provider and/or healthcare delivery system.

Several studies have agreed that a factor of significant influence on a patient's adherence with medication-taking and other health behaviors is the relationship with his or her healthcare provider.[3,4,10,12] The development of a therapeutic alliance between patient and healthcare provider is essential to this process. This includes an active effort on the part of the provider to listen and empathize with the patient in a nonjudgmental way, while empowering the patient to take a participative role in the decision making about his or her care. The goal is to gain the patient's trust while facilitating his or her autonomy, and then assessing and monitoring adherence with the medication regimen. These concepts are at the core of topics that are discussed in detail in the next section on counseling and communication interventions.

In addition to the therapeutic alliance with the healthcare provider, access to care (e.g., transportation, convenience and efficiency of follow-up visits, and parking) is important for getting patients back to the practice site to have prescriptions refilled.[12,17] Pharmacists should employ interventions aimed at reinforcing refills; running out of medication is an unfortunate opportunity for a patient to start a phase of nonadherence.

Interventions at this level might include refill reminder flags in the computer system or chart, with subsequent direct contact to remind the patient that a refill is due. Contracting with the patient for adherence, engaging health educators or patient advocates, scheduling appointments at a time and manner convenient to patients, facilitating collaboration among the patient's providers, and organizing the care in a disease-based clinic are also strategies that providers can use at the practice level to influence medication adherence.[4,10,12,17] Krueger and colleagues also reviewed organization-level technological initiatives, such as performing adherence drug utilization reviews at the point of care, reviewing patient charts, developing information/education kiosks or workstations, offering adherence incentives to providers, and engaging in public awareness campaigns.[4]

Patients engage in a variety of nonadherent behaviors to reduce medication dosing because of the financial burden of medications. It is often noted that elderly patients on a fixed income may be faced with the dilemma of spending money on food or on medications. Sometimes patients will take fewer pills than prescribed, will stretch out the interval between doses, will skip days, will use a pill splitter and take a portion of the dose, or will perform other activities that reduce the cost but also the therapeutic benefit.

Patients who are insured often have a co-insurance payment (copayment) ranging from $5 to the actual cost of the drug, depending on whether there is a formulary and whether the drug is a generic, a formulary-preferred brand, or a non-formulary-preferred brand. Pharmacists in particular can watch for patients with potential financial limitations and check to see that the prescribed drug is one that will require the lowest copayment for the patient; if this is not the case, the pharmacist should consider calling the prescriber to ask for a low-cost, therapeutically equivalent option.

Patients who are not insured or who are on federal assistance may find it very challenging to afford prescription drugs. Usually the copayment for patients on Medicaid is very low (a few dollars), but for those uninsured Americans who live just above the poverty line, the cost of prescription drugs can be prohibitive. Subsidized prescription drug programs exist and can influence adherence in a positive way.[26] Providers should become aware of programs that are available and how patients can qualify to use them. Many websites provide information about helping patients overcome financial barriers to acquiring medications. In addition, most of the pharmaceutical manufacturers have drug assistance programs; information can be found by visiting the manufacturers' home websites, or the website designated for a specific medication. The sites listed in Table 14-1 provide a few links to national initiatives; often, local resources are also available to assist in overcoming the financial barrier to taking medications.

TABLE 14-1	Web Addresses for Prescription Drug Assistance Programs or Resources
RxAssist	http://www.rxassist.org
Together Rx Access	http://www.TogetherRxAccess.com
Rx Outreach	http://www.rxoutreach.com
Drugstore.com	http://www.drugstore.com

COMMUNICATION OR COUNSELING STRATEGIES FOR MEDICATION-TAKING BEHAVIOR CHANGE

The process of patient counseling by pharmacists has been studied ever since it was noted that pharmacists communicating with patients had an impact on medication-taking behavior. With the previous emphasis on pharmaceutical care and the current emphasis on medication therapy management, pharmacists have been increasingly recognized as being in a unique position to intervene with medication-related problems. Many aspects of the interaction between patient and provider have been studied.

Research has suggested that providers can contribute to nonadherence when they have a poor therapeutic relationship with the patient.[12] This is particularly true with the complex and expensive adherence challenges for patients with schizophrenia and bipolar disorder.[24,25,27] Patients need to discuss and learn about their illnesses and medications in a safe, nonjudgmental interaction, regardless of their illness. When a patient feels listened to and understood, he or she will be more likely to trust the provider.

Not all providers understand how to build a therapeutic alliance with a patient and often do not realize how important it is. The traditional model of healthcare delivery and the biomedical model have been driven by a provider mentality known as the *righting reflex*.[28,29] Many who enter the health professions are motivated, at least in part, by a desire to help people. This often generates an overriding desire to fix what is "wrong" with patients, and a subsequent tendency to label patients by their illness or condition (e.g., "she is a diabetic," "he is an asthmatic") rather than recognizing patients for their individual barriers and motivators regarding the management of their illnesses (e.g., "Mrs. Jones is a patient with diabetes who takes her medication as prescribed most days but finds it challenging to follow the diet").

Miller and Rollnick's analogy for the biomedical model is wrestling.[28] The biomedical model assumes a provider-centered model of advising, persuading, arguing, demanding respect, and assuming that resistance to change is bad, among other characteristics. The biomedical model assumes that patients should be and are interested in their health once they are informed of their illness. However, knowing about an illness is only one aspect of patient motivation.

Most behavior change that occurs with an approach based on the biomedical model involves temporary extrinsic motivation, or the external push or pull of the provider while in his or her presence. As mentioned previously, external motivation is typically not sustained. In fact, resistant patients who encounter providers who push or pull by threatening and shaming may completely avoid change, thereby rendering the intervention more harmful than helpful.

The psychosocial model, on the other hand, is patient centered and takes into account an individual's motivators and barriers to change. The psychosocial model involves listening to the patient, collaborating to bring about change by facilitating the patient's own internal motivation, engaging the patient in decisions about his or her care, earning respect, and recognizing that resistance to change is important information to be explored. Miller and Rollnick's analogy for the psychosocial model is dancing.[28,29]

Many theories and models of behavior change have been used to explain and predict patient medication adherence. One theory or model that ties many other theories into a practical, brief method of intervention is the transtheoretical model of change (TTMC). The TTMC has been used to explain and predict behavior change across many health behaviors, such as smoking cessation, substance abuse, weight control, exercise, diabetes diet adherence, and medication adherence or discontinuation.[30-36] The TTMC suggests that people naturally change by moving across five sequential stages of motivation or readiness for change (precontemplation, contemplation, preparation, action, and maintenance), and that the primary objective of the intervention is to facilitate movement from the current stage to the next, not directly to action.

However, the TTMC is not only about stages of readiness for change. The model is applied in an intervention setting using the strategies of motivational interviewing (MI), which incorporate the TTMC concepts into brief (5- to 15-minute) encounters with patients. Most of the MI strategies involve efforts to influence another TTMC construct, the decisional balance, while also supporting self-efficacy. The decisional balance is the individual's internal motivation mechanism for driving movement along the stages toward change. Decisional balance represents the influence an individual's pros (motivators) and cons (barriers) have on the decision of whether or not to engage in a target behavior.[37,38] An individual who is more influenced by the cons will nearly always be in the pre-action stages of readiness for change and will be either resistant or ambivalent about change. Those individuals more influenced by the pros are typically in the preparation, action, or maintenance stages.[38]

Change in the influence or salience of the pros and cons creates movement along the stages of change. This is the process of development of internal motivation and is at the core of the MI strategies. Table 14-2 presents possible pros and cons that patients may state for their medication adherence behavior; patients may be more influenced by one or the other side of the balance, which will predict whether patients are adherent or nonadherent.[38]

One MI strategy for helping patients resolve ambivalence or resistance to a target behavior is to help them think about the differences in their own stated pros and cons. This MI strategy is labeled *developing discrepancy*.[28] It involves a nonjudgmental, non-shaming reflection back to the patient of the contrast between his or her own stated pros and cons toward the target behavior and is intended to create dissonance in the mind of the patient. Dissonance is motivating; the goal is to facilitate the patient's thinking about the discrepancy. Using the example in Table 14-2, a pharmacist using the developing discrepancy strategy might say something like this: "So on the one hand you want to have more energy and avoid being hospitalized, but on the other hand it's inconvenient to fit this drug regimen into your schedule."

Several MI strategies use decisional balance to facilitate patient motivation. The core of an MI intervention is allowing the patient to express his or her own pros and

TABLE 14-2 Example of a Patient's Decisional Balance Pros and Cons for Medication Adherence	
Pros	**Cons**
Control my own health	Inconvenient regimen
Prevent complications	The expense of copayments
Have more energy	Side effects are unpleasant
Avoid hospitalization	Food interaction with my favorites
Make my family happy	Embarrassing for people to know
Peace of mind	Don't want to be reminded I am ill

cons. If the pharmacist feels a need to add to the list of pros or cons, he or she should first ask permission ("Mrs. Jones, do you mind if I tell you some additional pros that other patients have said are important for them?"). It is important in an MI strategy to stay focused on patients' pros, rather than arguing against their cons. When a provider argues against their cons, it puts patients in a position of defending the cons, which only serves to reinforce the negative aspects of the target behavior and can erode the patient's trust for the provider.

MI strategies should consistently incorporate reflective listening and express empathy, explore a patient's goals and barriers to change, and provide support and reinforcement of self-efficacy for making the change or even talking about making the change. The process is a style of counseling that helps patients explore and resolve their ambivalence or resistance to making a change.

The spirit of MI incorporates all of these concepts in a nonjudgmental manner. This will assist patients in increasing their readiness for change by focusing on the perceived discrepancy between their actual behavior and ideal behavior.[28,29] The spirit of MI is empathy and respect. Rather than pushing an agenda on a patient, the provider asks the patient to set goals for the encounter (e.g., "Mrs. Jones, today we need to talk about the medication, the diet, and blood glucose monitoring. Which of these would you like to talk about first?"). In the spirit of MI, the provider also asks for permission to give information or advice (e.g., "May I share with you some things other patients have told me about what they do to remember to take their medications?").

The MI approach has been adopted or endorsed by U.S. entities such as the American Diabetes Association (ADA), the National Cancer Institute (NCI), and the Case Management Society of America (CMSA). An MI skills training initiative sponsored by the CMSA and the American Association of Colleges of Pharmacy includes pharmacists and pharmacy school faculty, along with nurse case managers, in an ongoing series of MI training institutes.[39]

Applications of MI intervention to the problem of medication adherence are fairly recent but have produced positive results. An intervention based on MI was successfully used among psychiatric patients to improve outpatient treatment adherence.[40] Another study by Liang and colleagues used MI-based decision support software to intervene over the telephone with multiple sclerosis patients who were at risk for discontinuation of drug therapy. The mean rate of discontinuation in the MI intervention group was reduced from 13% to 1.2%, a statistically significant reduction.[41]Additional research is needed to explore the impact of MI interventions on medication adherence for some of the challenging adherence topics presented in the next section.

CONSIDERATIONS OF PATIENT CHALLENGES REGARDING MEDICATION ADHERENCE

Getting to know a patient's response to his or her illness is an important first step in building rapport and in identifying potential barriers to adherence. Complex chronic illnesses may require change of multiple behaviors, which can be overwhelming. Consider the patient newly diagnosed with diabetes who is now being told to take medication or use insulin, to monitor blood glucose, and to change lifestyle habits regarding diet and exercise. The patient may also face other comorbid conditions, or the debilitating effects of the depression that often accompanies chronic illnesses such as diabetes and negatively affects medication adherence.

Considering all of these factors, a strategy of facilitating patients to make decisions about which behavior to address first contributes to building trust by offering patients the autonomy of deciding, rather than having an agenda forced on them. Often, if patients have successes with a behavior they are interested in working on, they will be more willing to address other related behaviors later. When targeting a multidimensional behavior such as medication taking (e.g., right number of pills, right times or interval per day, right dose) with particularly resistant patients, it may be helpful to choose one dimension to target first, if therapeutically possible, rather than to make several changes all at once.

This strategy is especially useful for lifestyle change behaviors such as diet and exercise, where a provider should encourage small, incremental steps toward change (e.g., switching from whole milk to skim milk this week instead of addressing the entire diet, or parking farther out in the parking lot and taking the stairs instead of the elevator this week instead of taking on an extensive walking or running regimen). For an overwhelmed or resistant patient, having success with one aspect of a target behavior may reinforce the patient to take on additional aspects of a target behavior.

It is also important to emphasize again that all of the strategies described in this chapter are particularly challenging to use with patients experiencing psychosis, mental illness, impaired insight, or dementia.[24,25] Little is known about improving medication adherence in patients with these illnesses and conditions, partly because many studies specifically exclude patients with psychosis or dementia.

Another area of challenge for medication adherence intervention is patients with HIV/AIDS. For patients with HIV/AIDS on highly active antiretroviral therapy (HAART), the target level of medication adherence must be greater than 95% in order to suppress replication of the virus and prevent resistance.[42] This requires multiple, expensive medications in a complex dosing regimen, with the potential for significant side effects and food interactions. Unlike other more forgiving medication regimens, missing even one dose can be substantially detrimental and, with repeats over time, can be fatal.

Little attention has been paid in this chapter to the problem of nonadherence among pediatric patients with chronic illnesses (e.g., diabetes, asthma, rheumatoid arthritis). The challenge in such cases lies not only in understanding the patient's decision making but also that of the parent or caregiver. Many of the psychosocial issues discussed throughout this book become more complex in the face of developmental and lifestyle changes that are a natural part of adolescence.

Most successful interventions in pediatric patients have involved a combination of interventions, including a behavioral intervention. The most common intervention used among pediatric patients is a token reinforcement process.[12] This reinforcement method provides pediatric patients the opportunity to earn tokens to use to "purchase" items of interest, privileges or activities, or other rewards. The involvement of family, school personnel, and other support networks has also been successful in reinforcing medication adherence behavior in pediatric patients.[12]

AREAS FOR FUTURE EXPLORATION

It is difficult to fully know the effectiveness of adherence interventions because of the challenges of study design and methods associated with adherence research. Many of the adherence interventions tested have been complex and labor intensive. Much of the adherence data is collected using self-report, and it is known that patients overestimate when self-reporting health behaviors (as a result of the social desirability of such reporting),[34,43] particularly in regard to medication taking.[44] In addition, the measures used and the ways they are implemented and interpreted varies considerably among studies, making comparisons of results difficult.[3,4] In fact, literature suggests that the studies on medication adherence exhibit substantial variability in design, measures, and methods, making it difficult to compare findings, particularly in studies that also have varied duration of follow-up.[3,44,45] The findings of several studies also suggest that once the intervention ends, the effect on adherence diminishes;[8] it is important to consider the implications of this in research and practice.

SUMMARY

Development of a therapeutic alliance between pharmacist and patient has been shown to significantly influence medication-taking behavior and should be established as the initial part of any intervention. As trust is established, it becomes the gateway to other behavior change strategies. Within the context of the therapeutic alliance or relationship, pharmacists should carefully listen, express empathy, and engage in nonjudgmental eliciting of patients' knowledge deficits, health goals, and barriers to adherence.

First-line strategies should attempt to facilitate patient decision making about how to simplify the regimen and how to tailor the regimen to other habitual activities in the patient's routine. This may include collaborating with the patient's other healthcare provider(s) or caregiver(s), while also helping the patient identify a support person or network to reinforce the commitment to medication adherence and other healthy behaviors. This may also include developing a therapeutic plan, which could include a contract between patient and provider and the use of compliance aids such as calendars, pill boxes, and so on, where needed.

Follow-up interactions with the patient are important to the reinforcement process and have clearly shown a sustained impact on medication adherence. A follow-up telephone call in the early stages of intervention is optimal to reinforce behavior change while also providing support; direct contact at refill visits should include assessment and feedback about medication-taking behaviors. This chapter further highlighted the importance of pharmacists helping patients see for themselves the need and value of improved medication use.

REFERENCES

1. Marston M. Compliance with medical regimens: a review of the literature. Nurs Res 1970;19: 312-23.
2. Sackett D, Snow J. Compliance in healthcare. Baltimore, MD: Johns Hopkins University Press, 1979.
3. Kripalani S, Xiaomei Y, Haynes R. Interventions to enhance medication adherence in chronic medical conditions: a systematic review. Arch Intern Med 2007;167:540-9.
4. Krueger K, Berger B, Felkey B. Medication adherence and persistence: a comprehensive review. Adv Ther 2005;22(4):319-62.
5. Smith S, Brock T, Howarth S. Use of personal digital assistants to deliver education about adherence to antiretroviral medications. J Am Pharm Assoc 2005;45(5):625-8.
6. National Institute for Literacy. Fact sheet: adult and family literacy. (Accessed August 27, 2006, at http://www.nifl.gov.)
7. Weiss B, Mays M, Martz W, et al. Quick assessment of literacy in primary care: the newest vital sign. Ann Fam Med 2005;3:514-22.
8. Murray M, Young J, Hoke S, et al. Pharmacist intervention to improve medication adherence in heart failure: a randomized trial. Ann Intern Med 2007;146(10):714-25.
9. Lee J, Grace K, Taylor A. Effect of a pharmacy care program on medication adherence and persistence, blood pressure, and low-density lipoprotein cholesterol: a randomized controlled trial. JAMA 2006;296(21):2563-71.

10. Haynes R, Yao X, Degani A, et al. Interventions for enhancing medication adherence. Cochrane Database Syst Rev 2007;(2):CD000011.

11. McDonald H, Garg A, Haynes R. Interventions to enhance patient adherence to medication prescriptions: scientific review. JAMA 2002;288(22):2868-79.

12. Osterberg L, Blaschke T. Adherence to medication. New Engl J Med 2005;353(5):487-97.

13. Sather B, Forbes J, Starck D, Rovers J. Effect of a personal automated dose-dispensing system on adherence: a case series. J Am Pharm Assoc 2007;47(1):82-5.

14. Maples N, Velligan D, Wang M, et al. Cognitive adaptation training and adherence to medication. Schizophr Bull 2005;31:528.

15. Bendle S, Velligan D, Mueller J, et al. The MedeMonitor for improving adherence to oral medication in schizophrenia. Schizophr Bull 2005;31:519.

16. Claxton A, Cramer J, Pierce C. A systematic review of the associations between dose regimens and medication compliance. Clin Ther 2001;23:1296-1310.

17. Jacobson T. The forgotten cardiac risk factor: noncompliance with lipid-lowering therapy. Medscape Cardiology 2004;8(2). (Accessed April 27, 2007, at http://www.medscape.com/viewarticle/496144.)

18. Gurley V. Leveraging health risk assessments for maximum effect. J Managed Care Med 2006;10(1):12-7.

19. Rickles N, Svarstad B, Statz-Paynter J, et al. Pharmacist telemonitoring of antidepressant use: effects on pharmacist-patient collaboration. J Am Pharm Assoc 2005;45(3):344-53.

20. Krass I, Taylor S, Smith C, Armour C. Impact on medication use and adherence of Australian pharmacists' diabetes care services. J Am Pharm Assoc 2005;45(1):33-40.

21. Murray E. Motivation and emotion. Englewood Cliffs, NJ: Prentice-Hall, 1964.

22. Deci E. Intrinsic motivation and self-determination in human behavior. New York: Plenum Press, 1985.

23. Lewis F, Daltroy L. How causal explanations influence health behavior: attribution theory. In: Glanz K, Lewis FM, Rimer BK, eds. Health behavior and health education: theory, research, and practice. 3rd ed. San Francisco: Jossey-Bass, 2002.

24. Lacro J, Dunn L, Dolder C, et al. Prevalence of and risk factors for medication nonadherence in patients with schizophrenia: a comprehensive review of recent literature. J Clin Psychiatry 2002;63:892-909.

25. Kikkert M, Schene A, Koeter M, et al. Medication adherence in schizophrenia: exploring patients', carers', and professionals' views. Schizophr Bull 2006;32(4):786-94.

26. Spiker E, Giannamore M, Nahata M. Medication use patterns and health outcomes among patients using a subsidized prescription drug program. J Am Pharm Assoc 2005;45(6):714-9.

27. Misdrahi D, Llorca P, Lancon C, Bayle F. Compliance in schizophrenia: predictive factors, therapeutic considerations, and research implications [in French]. Encephale 2002;28:266-72.

28. Miller W, Rollnick S. Motivational interviewing: preparing people for change. 2nd ed. New York: Guilford Press, 2002.

29. Rollnick S, Mason P, Butler C. Health behavior change: a guide for practitioners. New York: Churchill Livingstone, 2000.

30. DiClemente C, Prochaska J. Self-change and therapy change of smoking behavior: a comparison of processes of change in cessation and maintenance. Addict Behav 1982;7:133-42.

31. Prochaska J, DiClemente C. Common processes of self-change in smoking, weight control and psychological distress. In: Shiffman S, Wills T, eds. Coping and substance abuse. New York: Academic Press, 1986.

32. Moyers T, Miller W, Hendrickson M. How does motivational interviewing work? Therapist interpersonal skill predicts client involvement with motivational interviewing sessions. J Consult Clin Psych 2005;73(4):590-8.

33. Resnicow K, Davis R, Rollnick S. Motivational interviewing for pediatric obesity: conceptual issues and evidence review. J Am Diet Assoc 2006;106:2024-33.

34. Kavookjian J, Berger B, Grimley D, et al. Patient decision-making: strategies for diabetes diet adherence intervention. Res Soc Admin Pharm 2005;1:389-407.

35. Willey C, Redding C, Stafford J, et al. Stages of change for adherence with medication regimens for chronic disease: development and validation of a measure. Clin Ther 2000;22:858-71.

36. Berger B, Hudmon K, Liang H. Predicting treatment discontinuation among patients with multiple sclerosis: application of the transtheoretical model of change. J Am Pharm Assoc 2004;44:445-54.

37. Janis I, Mann L. Decision making: a psychological analysis of conflict, choice and commitment. New York: Free Press, 1977.

38. Prochaska J, Velicer W, Rossi J, et al. Stages of change and decisional balance for 12 problem behaviors. Health Psych 1994;13(1):39-46.

39. Berger B, Villaume W, Kavookjian J, Case Management Society of America, American Association of Colleges of Pharmacy. Auburn University Motivational Interviewing Training Institute. (Accessed May 15, 2007, at http://www.cmsa.org/PROGRAMSEVENTS/MotivationalInterviewingTrainingInstitute.)

40. Swanson A, Pantalon M, Cohen K. Motivational interviewing and treatment adherence among psychiatric and dually diagnosed patients. J Nerv Ment Dis 1997;187:630-5.

41. Liang H. Decreasing medication dropout: a study to develop and evaluate intervention software using the transtheoretical model of change and motivational interviewing [dissertation]. Auburn, AL: Auburn University, 2003.

42. Ickovics J, Cameron A, Zackin R, et al. Consequences and determinants of adherence to antiretroviral medication: results from Adult AIDS Clinical Trials Group protocol 370. Antivir Ther 2002;7:185-93.

43. Clark M, Abrams D, Niaura R, et al. Self-efficacy in weight management. J Consult Clin Psych 1991;59:739-44.

44. Smith S, Wahed A, Kelley S, et al. Assessing the validity of self-reported medication adherence in hepatitis C treatment. Ann Pharmacother 2007;41:1116-23.

45. Nichol M, Venturini F, Sung J. A critical evaluation of the methodology of the literature on medication compliance. Ann Pharmacother 1999;33:531-40.

CHAPTER 15

Patient-Reported Outcomes of Drug Therapy

Stephen Joel Coons, PhD, and Jeffrey A. Johnson, PhD

The United States spends more on health care than any other nation in the world. U.S. health spending per capita in 2004 ($6,102) was almost double that of Canada and was two and a half times greater than the median for the industrialized nations of the world.[1] In addition, it has been estimated that by 2015, health expenditures in the United States will account for 20% of the nation's gross domestic product, up from 16.5% in 2006.[2] Based on these statistics, there is no doubt that the United States consumes an abundance of health care. But does that level of health care actually produce better health?[3]

Even in countries where much less is spent on health, there is a need to maximize the health benefit derived from the consumption of healthcare resources. However, this is a far from simple task. A major barrier is the lack of information as to how the value or benefit obtained from healthcare expenditures is assessed. As Maynard stated, it is commonplace in health care "for policy to be designed and executed in a data free environment!"[4] This lack of critical information as to the outcomes produced by medical care is an obstacle to optimal health care decision making at all levels.

Although the implicit objective of medical care is to improve health outcomes, there is minimal evidence of the true effectiveness of many healthcare practices.[5] In addition, measures of the overall quality of the U.S. healthcare system, such as access to primary health care, health indicators (e.g., infant mortality and life expectancy), and public satisfaction in relation to costs, provide evidence that the United States trails other countries that spend significantly less on medical care.[6-11]

In 1988, Arnold Relman stated that the United States was entering the third era of modern medical care: the *era of assessment and accountability*.[12] This era followed the *era of expansion* (i.e., the late 1940s through the 1960s) and the *era of cost containment* (i.e., the 1970s and 1980s). During the era of expansion, in an effort to improve access to medical care, a great number of hospitals and healthcare facilities were built or better equipped through federal legislation such as the Hill-Burton Act of 1946 and the Hill-Harris Act of 1964. In addition, financial access was increased by the rapid growth of private health insurance and through the enactment of Medicare and Medicaid legislation in 1965. During the era of cost containment, containing costs was an explicit goal of most of the stakeholders in health care. Nevertheless, no significant cost containment appeared to have occurred, only cost shifting among payers. In fact, the United States experienced some of the largest annual increases in the rate of growth of healthcare expenditures during the era of cost containment. The excesses or failures of these earlier eras led to the era of assessment and accountability. An essential element of this third era was the growing consensus that health outcomes data are essential for the determination of the value of medical care interventions to individuals, systems, and societies.[12]

There is no doubt that the principal stakeholders in health care—payers, providers, regulators, accrediting bodies, manufacturers, and patients—have placed increasing emphasis on the outcomes that medical care products and services produce.[13] However, there is still a long way to go before the era of assessment and accountability can be said to have been successful in warranting Relman's label. Nevertheless, the collection of actionable outcomes data is a worthy goal. As stated by Ellwood, outcomes research is "designed to help patients, payers, and providers make rational medical care-related choices based on better insight into the effect of these choices on the patient's life."[14] More recently, Lipscomb and colleagues defined outcomes research as "the scientific field devoted to measuring and interpreting the impact of medical conditions and health care on individuals and populations."[15]

There are a number of ways of describing or categorizing the types of outcomes that result from medical care.[16,17] However, the health outcomes of most interest when evaluating the efficacy or effectiveness of medical interventions, particularly drug therapy, are those based on (1) biological parameters (e.g., blood pressure, tumor size), (2) reports by clinicians (e.g., Hamilton Depression Rating Scale), or (3) self-reports from patients (e.g., pain). Often, the first two are considered *clinical outcomes*, and the third, *patient-reported outcomes;* however, depending on the condition being treated, all three sources may provide key endpoint data for the evaluation of clinical interventions. This chapter focuses on patient-reported outcomes, with an emphasis on health-related quality of life as an outcome of pharmaceutical products and services.

PATIENT-REPORTED OUTCOMES

The term *patient-reported outcomes* (PROs) refers to "a spectrum of disease and treatment outcomes reported subjectively by the patient."[18] PROs include, but are not limited to, symptom experience, functioning, treatment satisfaction, health status, and health-related quality of life. PROs can enrich the evaluation of treatment effectiveness by providing the patient's perspective as a complement to traditional clinical endpoints.[19] In a review of efficacy endpoints reported in product labeling approved by the U.S. Food and Drug Administration (FDA) for new drugs approved from 1997 through 2002, Willke and colleagues found that PRO endpoints were included in reports on 64 (30%) of the 215 product labels examined.[18] For 23 of the products, PROs were the only endpoints reported. This latter finding reinforces the fact that, in some situations (e.g., pain), a PRO may be the only viable study endpoint when there are no observable or measurable physical or biological manifestations of the condition or its treatment.[20,21]

The U.S. FDA and the European Medicines Agency (EMEA) are increasingly being asked to review and approve clinical trial protocols that incorporate PRO measures as primary or secondary endpoints.[18,22] In an effort to describe how the appropriateness and adequacy of PRO measures proposed as effectiveness endpoints in clinical trials will be evaluated, the FDA released a draft guidance for industry entitled "Patient-Reported Outcome Measures: Use in Medical Product Development to Support Labeling Claims."[23] The draft guidance was created to make the process of developing and reviewing PRO measures more efficient for both the FDA and clinical trial sponsors. However, the process will remain challenging because of the multitude of potential PRO measures, the need for language and cross-cultural adaptations, and the numerous existing and emerging modes of questionnaire administration (e.g., ePRO).[24] The PRO that has commanded the most attention in regard to drug therapy is health-related quality of life.[25-29]

HEALTH-RELATED QUALITY OF LIFE

The term *quality of life* is used quite liberally in our society, particularly within medical care. In fact, the oft-quoted definition of pharmaceutical care (i.e., "the responsible provision of drug therapy for the purpose of achieving definite outcomes that improve a patient's quality of life") includes the term.[30] In addition, pharmaceutical manufacturers frequently use *quality of life* in their mission statements. For example, Merck's mission is, in part, "to provide society with superior products and services by developing innovations and solutions that improve the quality of life."[31] GlaxoSmithKline states that its mission is "to improve the quality of human life by enabling people to do more, feel better and live longer."[32] The mission of Novartis is, in part, "to discover, develop and successfully market innovative products to prevent and cure diseases, to ease suffering and to enhance the quality of life."[33] These are noble goals, but how do we know when the enhancement of quality of life has been achieved?

In the literature, the term *quality of life* has been used in a variety of ways.[34] It was proposed that studies of health outcomes use the term *health-related quality of life* to distinguish health effects from the effects of other factors (e.g., financial status, relationships, job satisfaction) that affect a person's perceived quality of life.[35] This is an important and appropriate distinction. Although there may be a general understanding of the meaning of the term, explicit definitions of health-related quality of life in the medical research literature are rare. The definition is often implicit, based on the manner in which its measurement was operationalized.

However, some authors have provided definitions. For example, Revicki and associates define health-related quality of life as "the subjective assessment of the impact of a disease and treatment across physical, psychological, social, and somatic domains of functioning and well-being."[27] Although the definitions of health-related quality of life may differ in certain respects, a characteristic they usually share is multidimensionality. The FDA states that a health-related quality of life measure should capture at least the following dimensions:[23]

- Physical functioning
- Psychological (emotional and cognitive) functioning
- Social functioning

In addition, perceptions of general well-being, disease-related or treatment-related symptomatology, and spiritual well-being are sometimes assessed. The latter is more likely to be included in measures developed for conditions that have the potential to shorten length of life (e.g., cancer).

Health-related quality of life is increasingly viewed as an important therapeutic endpoint by providers of medical care products and services. A factor leading to this has been the shift in the focus of primary medical care from limiting mortality to limiting morbidity and the patient-reported impact of that morbidity. This is a result of the shift in the pattern of illness in the United States and most of the industrialized world from mostly acute disease to one in which chronic conditions predominate. In the early part of the 20th century, many individuals died from infectious diseases for which cures (e.g., antibiotics) or effective preventive measures (e.g., sanitation, vaccines) were unavailable or underutilized. Although there are still diseases that lead to premature death, many chronic conditions have adverse health consequences leading to dysfunction and decreased well-being. For those conditions that shorten life expectancy and for which there are no cures, managing symptoms and maintaining function are the primary objectives of medical care. Medications are used extensively as a means of maintaining or enhancing patients' health-related quality of life.

Because therapeutic interventions such as medications have the potential to improve as well as diminish health-related quality of life, pharmacists and other medical care providers must strive to achieve enhanced health-related quality of life as an outcome of therapy. Although it must be assumed that health-related quality of life has always played an implicit role in the provision of health care, it has not always been viewed as equal in importance to the more biological outcome parameters (e.g., blood glucose level). The subjective nature of health-related quality of life assessment has made some people uneasy with it as a measure of the outcomes produced by medical treatment.[36] However, there is growing awareness that in certain diseases, health-related quality of life may be the most important health outcome to consider in assessing treatment.[37] The logic behind the increasing attention to health-related quality of life includes the following:[38]

- The goal of therapy is to make people feel better.
- Physiologic measures may change without people feeling better.
- People may feel better without measurable change in physiologic values.
- There may be tradeoffs between positive treatment effects and adverse events.
- There is an increased emphasis on patient-focused care.

TYPES OF HEALTH-RELATED QUALITY OF LIFE MEASURES

A multitude of instruments are available for measuring self-reported health status or health-related quality of life.[39-41] Although not all of them clearly fit into only one of the following categories, the following is a useful classification of the types of measures.[42]

- Disease-specific instruments
- Generic or general instruments
  - Health profiles
  - Preference-based index instruments

Disease-Specific Instruments

Disease-specific instruments are intended to provide greater detail concerning particular outcomes, in terms of functioning and well-being, that may be uniquely associated with a condition or its treatment. Guyatt and colleagues provide a further distinction in the types of specific instruments available: disease specific (e.g., arthritis, diabetes), population specific (e.g., frail older adult), function specific (e.g., sexual functioning), and condition or problem specific (e.g., pain).[42] Table 15-1 lists selected examples of disease-specific instruments.

Generic or General Instruments

Some investigators believe that all conditions have a general effect on health and that the purpose of health-related quality of life assessment should be not only to identify clinical information relevant to a specific disease but also to determine the impact of the condition on general function and well-being. A concern is that by focusing too specifically on clinical correlates of a disease or condition, the general or overall impact is overlooked. In studies involving pharmacotherapy, the combined use of a generic and a specific instrument may be the best approach. The generic instrument will provide a more holistic outcome score and allow comparability across other populations and disease states in which it has been used. An appropriately selected specific instrument will provide more detailed clinical information regarding expected changes in the particular patient population. The Kidney Disease Quality of Life (KDQOL) instrument is an example of an instrument that contains a generic core (namely, the RAND 36-Item Health Survey 1.0) plus disease-targeted items.[43]

Health Profiles

Health profiles provide an array of scores representing individual dimensions or domains of health-related quality of life or health status. An advantage of a health profile is that it provides multiple outcome scores, which may be useful to clinicians

TABLE 15-1   Selected Disease-Specific Instruments
Asthma Quality of Life Questionnaire (AQLQ)[85]
Migraine-Specific Quality of Life Questionnaire version 2.1 (MSQ v2.1)[86]
Functional Assessment of Cancer Therapy–General (FACT-G)[87]
Quality of Life in Epilepsy (QOLIE)[88]
Kidney Disease Quality of Life (KDQOL) instrument[89]
Adult Attention-Deficit/Hyperactivity Disorder Quality of Life scale (AAQoL)[90]

or researchers who are attempting to measure differential effects of a condition or its treatment on various health-related quality of life domains. A commonly used profile instrument is the Medical Outcomes Study 36-Item Short-Form Health Survey (SF-36). The SF-36 is also known and distributed as the RAND 36-Item Health Survey 1.0. The SF-36 grew out of the Medical Outcomes Study (MOS) conducted by researchers from the RAND Corporation.[44,45] The instrument includes eight multi-item dimensions or scales (Table 15-2). The SF-36 can be self-administered (via paper, telephone, or computer) or interviewer administered (face to face or by telephone). Further information regarding available administration modes can be obtained at www.SF-36.org. The SF-36 is brief (taking approximately 5 to 10 minutes to complete), and there is substantial evidence supporting its reliability and validity. The original SF-36 instrument (version 1) has been translated and adapted into many country-specific instruments and has been modified by its developers (SF-36 version 2) to improve its measurement properties.[46]

Preference-Based Health-Related Quality of Life Instruments

Preference-based instruments, also known as *multiattribute health status classification systems*, enable the application of a population-based preference weight to the health status reported by the respondent. The preference weights are an adjustment for the perceived

TABLE 15-2   SF-36 Scales
General health perceptions
Physical functioning
Social functioning
Role limitations attributed to physical problems
Role limitations attributed to emotional problems
Bodily pain
General mental health
Energy/fatigue (vitality)
From Ware JE Jr, Sherbourne CD. The MOS 36-Item Short-Form Health Survey (SF-36): I. Conceptual framework and item selection. Med Care 1992;30:473-83; and Hays RD, Sherbourne CD, Mazel RM. The RAND 36-Item Health Survey 1.0. Health Econ 1993;2:217-27.

relative quality of the health states, based on expected utility theory, from the fields of decision science and economics.[47] The preference weights are empirically derived through a variety of direct preference elicitation procedures, including visual analogue scales, the time tradeoff technique, and standard gamble.[48] The outcome score, or health index, is on a scale where 0.0 and 1.0 represent the health-related quality of life associated with death and perfect health, respectively. This makes preference-based instruments useful in pharmacoeconomic research, particularly cost-utility analysis.[49] Cost-utility analysis involves comparing the costs of an intervention (e.g., a medication) to its outcomes, with outcomes usually expressed in terms of *quality-adjusted life years (QALYs) gained.*

QALYs gained is an outcome measure that incorporates both quantity and quality of life. This can be a key outcome measure, especially in diseases such as cancer where the treatment itself can have a significant impact on patient functioning and well-being. A study by Smith and colleagues illustrates the importance of adjusting length of life or survival for quality of life.[50] The authors compared the incremental costs and outcomes associated with surgery plus adjuvant chemotherapy versus surgery alone in colon cancer patients. Their results indicated that 2.4 unadjusted years of life were gained from the addition of the chemotherapeutic regimen. However, after adjusting for quality of life, only 0.4 QALYs were gained. The calculated cost per life year gained was $2,916, whereas the cost per QALY gained was $17,500. Maximizing the potential of pharmaceutical care will require that pharmacists understand and be able to adequately address the economic and health-related quality of life implications of therapeutic decisions, such as those made in regard to adjuvant chemotherapy.

Examples of preference-based instruments include the Quality of Well-Being Scale (QWB),[51] the Health Utilities Index (HUI),[52] the EQ-5D,[53] and the SF-6D.[54]

MEASUREMENT AND ADMINISTRATION ISSUES

Patient-reported outcomes are closely linked to individual attitudes and beliefs relating to health and health care. As such, the measurement of these outcomes is inherently subjective. A number of methodologic issues must be considered when evaluating existing PRO measures or deciding on the appropriate instrument to use when designing a study or assessment. A thorough review of these issues is not within the scope or objectives of this chapter. More in-depth reviews of methodologic considerations are available in the literature.[55,56] Of particular concern, however, are the psychometric properties of a chosen instrument. The discussion in this section focuses on psychometric properties of instruments that are essential for the successful measurement of health-related quality of life and practical issues regarding administration of the instruments.

Psychometric Properties

Psychometrics refers to the measurement of psychological constructs, such as health-related quality of life. It is concerned with the development and testing of instruments in such a way that we can have confidence in the measurement made. Psychometric properties include the reliability and validity of measurements.[57] This chapter discusses different instruments that have been used to measure health-related quality of life and addresses their use in terms of these psychometric properties. This section reviews reliability and validity as they pertain to the measurement of most PROs.

Reliability of the Measure

Reliability refers to the consistency, stability, or reproducibility of scores obtained on different administrations of a measure when all pertinent conditions remain relatively unchanged. The two reliability assessment methods most often discussed in the health-status literature are test-retest and internal consistency. *Test-retest methods* correlate the results of multiple measurements, spread over time. However, as opposed to a measure of a trait that is assumed to be constant over the course of time, there can be a problem in attempting to use test-retest methods to assess the reliability of measures of PROs. For example, health-related quality of life is not assumed to be constant over the course of time. In fact, most clinical studies attempt to assess how health status or health-related quality of life changes. Nonetheless, assurance that measures provide consistent scores when health status has not changed provides greater confidence in an instrument's measurement properties. *Internal consistency*, which indicates the extent to which an instrument is free of random error, is an aspect of reliability assessment that can be very important to outcome measures. It has been recommended that internal consistency reliability coefficients should be at least 0.70 for group comparisons and 0.85 to 0.95 for individual comparisons.[58,59] *Interrater agreement*, although not as critical with self-administered instruments, is a consideration when obtaining data through interviews or direct observation. The assessment of reliability is a complex topic that is reviewed in detail in the psychometrics literature.[60,61]

Validity of the Measure

Validity defines the range of inferences that are justifiable on the basis of a score or measure—that is, whether the instrument is really measuring what it is supposed to be measuring. Validity is not absolute, but is relative to the domain under study. Three basic types of validity commonly considered are criterion, content, and construct. *Criterion validity* is achieved when a new measure corresponds to an established measure or observation that accurately reflects the phenomenon of interest. By definition, the criterion must be a superior measure of the phenomenon if it is to serve as a comparative norm.[62] However, in health-related quality of life assessment, gold standards or criteria rarely exist against which a new measure can be compared. *Content validity*, which is infrequently tested statistically, refers to how adequately the sampling of items reflects the aims of the measure. *Construct validity* refers to the relationship between measures purporting to measure the same underlying theoretical construct (i.e., convergent evidence) and those purporting to measure a different construct (i.e., discriminant evidence). For example, convergent evidence for the validity of role performance items is established by showing associations between the responses to the items and observed verifiable functioning. Evidence for the construct validity of other aspects of the measure might be established through comparisons with physiologic measures, organ pathology, or clinical signs. Construct validity is not absolute. We do not say that a measure is "valid," but rather support its validity through accumulated research findings.

Another aspect of a measure that supports its validity is responsiveness or sensitivity to change. *Responsiveness* is the ability or power of the measure to detect clinically important change when it occurs.[63] Although some authors have suggested that responsiveness is a psychometric property of a measure that is distinct from validity,[64] others argue that responsiveness is an aspect of validity rather than a separate property.[65] This chapter includes it as an indication of a measure's validity.

Administration

Practical aspects of the measurement of health-related quality of life include the length of the instrument and the administration time involved. Instruments should be as brief as possible without significantly compromising the validity and reliability of the measurement. The longer an instrument is, the greater the respondent burden, which can lead to unwillingness or refusal to complete the instrument or to incomplete responses.

Another issue is the mode of administration. Although most health-related quality of life measures were developed in a self-administered, paper-based format, it is likely that they can be administered in multiple ways. The primary means of administration are self-administered and interviewer administered (e.g., in person, over the telephone); however, the emergence of new electronic platforms (e.g., web based, handheld computers, interactive voice response systems) has significantly changed the questionnaire administration landscape. The measurement equivalence between the various administration modes for a PRO measure must still be demonstrated, however.

In some situations, it may be necessary to use surrogate or proxy responders (i.e., using a healthcare provider, family member, or friend to respond for the subject when the subject is unable to complete the instrument himself or herself). Because patient-reported outcomes are personal and subjective, it is essential that patients have the opportunity to provide their perspective on the impact of the disease or its treatment on their life. Their perspective is likely to be quite different from that of an outside observer. For example, Jachuck and colleagues, in an assessment of the quality of life of hypertensive patients, found noteworthy differences between the assessments provided by the patients, their spouses (or close companions), and their physicians.[66] In other situations, however, proxy assessments may provide data that would otherwise be missing or may provide a unique and important perspective on health outcomes for certain populations (e.g., pediatrics) or conditions (e.g., dementia).

PATIENT-REPORTED OUTCOMES AND PHARMACEUTICAL CARE _____

Information on the impact of pharmaceutical products and services on health-related quality of life can provide additional data for making healthcare policy and clinical decisions. The inclusion of health-related quality of life data in economic analyses of alternative interventions is becoming increasingly prevalent and involves the comparison of the costs and outcomes of the interventions. It is no longer acceptable to make a selection between two medications of equal clinical efficacy based on the acquisition costs alone. One of the medications may be more appropriate because it produces better outcomes relative to its cost than does the alternative.

Health-related quality of life assessment can assist by providing documentation of differential patient outcomes. Pharmacists on pharmacy and therapeutics committees should be prepared to assist other committee members in incorporating existing health-related quality of life data into the formulary or practice guideline decision-making process. A study by Croog and colleagues was one of the first in a growing body of literature reporting the health-related quality of life impact of antihypertensive agents.[67-71] This is just one area of pharmacotherapy that is receiving a considerable amount of attention in regard to health-related quality of life implications.

Health-related quality of life as an input to clinical decision making at the patient level is also very important. For example, alternative treatments may have equal efficacy based on traditional clinical parameters (e.g., blood pressure reduction) but produce very different effects on the PROs. Thus, a provider's selection among competing alternatives may hinge upon documented differential impact on quality of life. A perceived decrease in health-related quality of life attributed by the patient to an adverse effect of the drug may lead to a decrease in adherence to the medication regimen.[72] However, empirical evidence regarding the relationship between health-related quality of life and patient adherence is lacking.

In an attempt to explore that relationship, Hays and colleagues examined the association between self-reported adherence to medical recommendations and health outcomes over time for patients in the Medical Outcomes Study with one or more chronic conditions (i.e., diabetes, hypertension, congestive heart failure, recent myocardial infarction, and/or depressive symptoms).[43] The PROs measured were physical, role, and social functioning; energy/fatigue; pain; emotional well-being; and general health perceptions. For this analysis, two composite indices of functioning and well-being (i.e., physical health and mental health) were produced from these scales or dimensions. The findings were mixed; specifically, adherence to medication recommendations was associated with negative effects on physical health for both insulin-using diabetic patients and depressed patients. The authors suggest that the perceptions of impaired physical health among those who complied with the medications may have been due to side effects. Adherence with medication regimens is a complex issue. For example, several studies have found higher levels of adherence to be related to better outcomes regardless of whether the drug was active or a placebo.[73,74] Adherence is discussed in much greater detail in Chapter 13 of this book.

As described by Smith, when a patient takes a medication, there are four possible health-related quality of life outcomes: (1) improved, (2) maintained as a direct result of the medication, (3) decreased, or (4) remains unchanged.[75] When health-related quality of life data are available in the literature from pharmaceutical trials or other studies, the pharmacist should be aware of the data and communicate this information to the prescriber and patient. When the information is not available, the pharmacist should take an active role in monitoring the health-related quality of life impact at the individual patient level.

Published research regarding the impact of pharmaceutical care on health-related quality of life has been equivocal,[76] with only a few reports of significant improvements using published health-related quality of life assessment approaches.[77,78] Pickard and associates, in a review of pharmacy-based studies that included health-related quality of life as an outcome measure, found little evidence of a positive impact of pharmacist interventions.[79] The authors of the review discussed the potential reasons for the lack of a significant effect, including insufficient sample size and power, selection bias, length of study period, choice of PRO measure, labeling effects, and a lack of true impact. However, the fact that pharmacist-managed interventions can have a positive impact on clinical outcomes suggests that improvements in PROs may follow.[80-84] One problem may be that overall health-related quality of life is being assessed when a less complex outcome, such as symptom experience or physical functioning, is the more direct outcome of the pharmaceutical care intervention. In addition, the most positive and profound health-related quality of life benefits are likely to manifest themselves when the prevention of the long-term consequences of uncontrolled diabetes, hypertension, or lipid levels leads to longer and healthier lives. Hence, pharmacists should not be discouraged when clinically effective programs do not directly translate into concurrent health-related quality of life improvements.

Pharmacists have a tremendous opportunity to play a significant role in optimizing patient-reported outcomes of medication therapy. Smith and colleagues provide a list of action items aimed at empowering pharmacists to routinely consider health or medication-related quality of life as an outcome of pharmaceutical care.[84] The action items reflect the importance of pharmacists proactively increasing their awareness of how medications may interfere with important aspects of their patients' lives and the steps that can be taken to prevent or alleviate the negative consequences.

SUMMARY

As described by Relman, the U.S. healthcare system is in the era of assessment and accountability.[12] Based on the shortcomings of the earlier eras of modern medical care, there is a pressing need for the appropriate measurement of health outcomes and the assignment or acceptance of responsibility for those outcomes by the people and organizations charged with producing them. Within this context, patient-reported outcomes are gaining increasing attention and significance in the evaluation of health care, including pharmaceutical products and services. In fact, for certain diseases, PROs may be the most important outcome to consider in assessing the effectiveness of healthcare interventions.

Health-related quality of life has emerged as a particularly salient PRO. Although it has not always been clearly defined, the concept of health-related quality of life resonates with patients, their families, and medical care providers. With continuing advances in medical technology, it is particularly important to remember that efforts to increase length of life must not be allowed to outstrip the ability to maintain an acceptable level of quality of life.

Pharmacists have an opportunity to play a significant role in optimizing drug therapy in an effort to enhance patient outcomes. However, it must be recognized that the ultimate impact of drug therapy, particularly in regard to health-related quality of life, may not be manifested in patients' lives for many years. Hence, there may be more proximal PROs (e.g., pain relief, enhanced sleep quality) that could be measured to document the value of pharmaceutical care services.

Although there are a number of unresolved theoretic and methodologic issues in regard to the measurement of PROs, there are some general concepts that should be carefully considered when designing a study, reviewing existing research, or evaluating new programs or services. This chapter has provided only a brief overview of the concepts in an effort to sensitize current or potential pharmaceutical care practitioners to the complexity of the topic as well as to provide insight into how these concepts can and should be incorporated into their practice.

REFERENCES

1. Anderson GF, Frogner BK, Reinhardt UE. Health spending in OECD countries in 2004: an update. Health Aff 2007;26:1481-9.
2. Borger C, Smith S, Truffer C, et al. Health spending projections through 2015: changes on the horizon. Health Aff 2006;25:w61-73.
3. Farley T, Cohen DA. Prescription for a healthy nation: a new approach to improving our lives by fixing our everyday world. Boston: Beacon Press, 2005.
4. Maynard A. Developing the healthcare market. Econ J 1991;(September):1277-86.
5. Roper WL, Winkenwerder W, Hackbarth GM, Krakauer H. Effectiveness in healthcare: an initiative to evaluate and improve medical practice. N Engl J Med 1988;319:1197-202.
6. Starfield B. Primary care and health: a cross-national comparison. JAMA 1991;266:2268-71.
7. Glied S, Little SE. The uninsured and the benefits of medical progress. Health Aff 2003;22:210-9.
8. Zuvekas SH, Taliaferro GS. Pathways to access: health insurance, the healthcare delivery system, and racial/ethnic disparities, 1996–1999. Health Aff 2003;22(2):139-53.
9. Schoen C, Osborn R, Huynh PT, et al. Taking the pulse of healthcare systems: experiences of patients with health problems in six countries. Health Aff 2005;24:w5-509-w5-35.
10. Schoen C, Doty MM, Collins SR, Holmgren AL. Insured but not protected: how many adults are underinsured? Health Aff 2005;24:w5-289-w5-302.
11. Schoen C, Davis K, How SKH, Schoenbaum SC. U.S. health system performance: a national scorecard. Health Aff 2006;25:w457-75.
12. Relman AS. Assessment and accountability. New Engl J Med 1988;319:1220-1.
13. Zitter M. Outcomes assessment: true customer focus comes to healthcare. Med Interface 1992;(May):32-7.
14. Ellwood PM. Outcomes management: a technology of patient experience. N Engl J Med 1988;318:1549-56.
15. Lipscomb J, Gotay CC, Snyder C, eds. Outcomes assessment in cancer: measures, methods, and applications. Cambridge: Cambridge University Press, 2005.
16. Lohr KN. Outcome measurement: concepts and questions. Inquiry 1988;25:37-50.
17. Kozma CM, Reeder CE, Schulz RM. Economic, clinical, and humanistic outcomes: a planning model for pharmacoeconomic research. Clin Ther 1993;15:1121-32.
18. Willke RJ, Burke LB, Erickson P. Measuring treatment impact: a review of patient-reported outcomes and other efficacy endpoints in approved product labels. Controlled Clin Trials 2004;25:535-52.

19. McHorney CA. Generic health measurement: past accomplishments and a measurement paradigm for the 21st century. Ann Intern Med 1997;127:743-50.

20. Wiklund I. Assessment of patient-reported outcomes in clinical trials: the example of health-related quality of life. Fund Clin Pharmacol 2004;18:351-63.

21. Shiffman S, Hufford MR, Paty J. Subject experience diaries in clinical research, part 1: the patient experience movement. Appl Clin Trials 2001;10(2):46-56.

22. Szende A, Leidy NK, Revicki D. Health-related quality of life and other patient-reported outcomes in the European centralized drug regulatory process: a review of guidance documents and performed authorizations of medicinal products 1995 to 2003. Value Health 2005;8:534-48.

23. Food and Drug Administration. Guidance for industry (draft). Patient-reported outcome measures: use in medical product development to support labeling claims. February 2006. (Accessed at http://www.fda.gov/cder/guidance/5460dft.htm.)

24. Shields A, Gwaltney C, Tiplady B, Paty J, Shiffman S. Grasping the FDA's PRO guidance. Appl Clin Trials 2006;15(8):69-72, 83.

25. European Medicines Agency. Reflection paper on the regulatory guidance for the use of health-related quality of life (HRQL) measures in the evaluation of medicinal products. July 27, 2005. (Accessed at http://www.emea.eu.int/pdfs/human/ewp/13939104en.pdf.)

26. Leidy NK, Revicki DA, Geneste B. Recommendations for evaluating the validity of quality of life claims for labeling and promotion. Value Health 1999;2:113-27.

27. Revicki DA, Osoba D, Fairclough D, et al. Recommendations on health-related quality of life research to support labeling and promotional claims in the United States. Qual Life Res 2000; 9:887-900.

28. Santanello NC, Baker D, Cappelleri JC. Regulatory issues for health-related quality of life—PhRMA Health Outcomes Committee Workshop, 1999. Value Health 2002;5:14-25.

29. Shah SN, Sesti A-M, Copley-Merriman K, Plante M. Quality of life terminology included in package inserts for US approved medications. Qual Life Res 2003;12:1107-17.

30. Hepler CD, Strand LM. Opportunities and responsibilities in pharmaceutical care. Am J Hosp Pharmacy 1990;47:533-43.

31. Merck & Company. Our mission. (Accessed November 5, 2007, at http://www.merck.com/about/mission.html.)

32. GlaxoSmithKline. About us. (Accessed November 5, 2007, at http://www.gsk.com/about/index.htm.)

33. Novartis. About Novartis: mission. (Accessed November 5, 2007, at http://www.novartis.com/about-novartis/our-mission/index.shtml.)

34. Sirgy MJ, Michalos AC, Ferriss AL, et al. The quality-of-life (QOL) research movement: past, present, and future. Soc Indicators Res 2006;76:343-466.

35. Kaplan RM, Bush JW. Health-related quality of life measurement for evaluation research and policy analysis. Health Psychol 1982;1:6l-80.

36. Schipper H, Clinch JJ, Olweny CLM. Quality of life studies: definitions and conceptual issues. In: Spilker B, ed. Quality of life and pharmacoeconomics in clinical trials. 2nd ed. Philadelphia: Lippincott-Raven, 1996:11-23.

37. Staquet M, Aaronson NK, Ahmedzai S, et al. Health-related quality of life research [editorial]. Qual Life Res 1992;1:3.

38. Torrance GW, Feeny DH. Cost-utility workshop. Presented at Eli Lilly and Company, Indianapolis, IN, December 6, 1993.

39. Bowling A. Measuring health: a review of quality of life measurement scales. 2nd ed. Buckingham, England: Open University Press, 1997.

40. Bowling A. Measuring disease: a review of disease-specific quality of life measurement scales. 2nd ed. Buckingham, England: Open University Press, 2001.

41. McDowell I. Measuring health: a guide to rating scales and questionnaires. 3rd ed. Oxford: Oxford University Press, 2006.

42. Guyatt GH, Feeny DH, Patrick DL. Measuring health-related quality of life. Ann Intern Med 1993;118:622-9.

43. Hays RD, Kravitz RL, Mazel RM, et al. The impact of patient adherence on health outcomes for patients with chronic disease in the Medical Outcomes Study. J Behav Med 1994;17:347-60.

44. Ware JE Jr, Sherbourne CD. The MOS 36-Item Short-Form Health Survey (SF-36): I. Conceptual framework and item selection. Med Care 1992;30:473-83.

45. Hays RD, Sherbourne CD, Mazel RM. The RAND 36-Item Health Survey 1.0. Health Econ 1993;2:217-27.

46. Ware JE Jr. SF-36 health survey update. Spine 2000;25(24):3130-9.

47. Revicki DA. Relationships between health utility and psychometric health status measures. Med Care 1992;30:MS274-82.

48. Drummond MF, Sculpher MJ, Torrance GW, et al. Methods for the economic evaluation of healthcare programmes. 3d ed. Oxford: Oxford University Press, 2005.

49. Coons SJ, Kaplan RM. Cost-utility analysis. In: Bootman JL, Townsend RJ, McGhan WF, eds. Principles of pharmacoeconomics. 3rd ed. Cincinnati, OH: Harvey Whitney Books, 2005.

50. Smith RD, Hall J, Gurney H, Harnett PR. A cost-utility approach to the use of 5-fluorouracil and levamisole as adjuvant chemotherapy for Dukes' C colonic carcinoma. Med J Aust 1993;158:319-22.

51. Kaplan RM, Anderson JP. The general health policy model: an integrated approach. In: Spilker B, ed. Quality of life and pharmacoeconomics in clinical trials. 2nd ed. Philadelphia: Lippincott-Raven, 1996:309-22.

52. Furlong WJ, Feeny DH, Torrance GW, Barr RD. The Health Utilities Index (HUI) system for assessing health-related quality of life in clinical studies. Ann Med 2001;33:375-84.

53. Rabin R, de Charro F. EQ-5D: a measure of health status from the EuroQol Group. Ann Med 2001:33;337-43.

54. Brazier J, Roberts J, Deverill M. The estimation of a preference-based measure of health from SF-36. J Health Econ 2002;21:271-92.

55. Fayers P, Hays RD, eds. Quality of life assessment in clinical trials. 2nd ed. Oxford: Oxford University Press, 2005.

56. Streiner DL, Norman GR. Health measurement scales: a practical guide to their development and use. 3rd edition. New York: Oxford University Press, 2003.

57. Frost MH, Reeve BB, Liepa AM, et al. What is sufficient evidence for the reliability and validity of patient-reported outcome measures? Value Health 2007;10(suppl 2):S94-105.

58. Nunnally JC, Bernstein IH. Psychometric theory. 3rd ed. New York: McGraw-Hill, 1994.

59. Weiner EA, Stewart BJ. Assessing individuals. Boston: Little Brown, 1984.

60. Hays RD, Anderson R, Revicki D. Psychometric considerations in evaluating health-related quality of life measures. Qual Life Res 1993;2:441-9.

61. Kaplan RM, Saccuzzo DP. Psychological testing: principles, applications, and issues. 3rd ed. Pacific Grove, CA: Brooks/Cole, 1993.

62. Kaplan RM, Bush JW, Berry CC. Health status: Types of validity and the index of well-being. Health Services Res 1976;11:478-507.

63. Juniper EF, Guyatt GH, Jaeschke R. How to develop and evaluate a new quality of life instrument. In: Spilker B, ed. Quality of life and pharmacoeconomics in clinical trials. 2nd ed. Philadelphia: Lippincott-Raven, 1996:49-56.

64. Guyatt G, Walter S, Norman G. Measuring change over time: assessing the usefulness of evaluative instruments. J Chronic Dis 1987;40:171-8.

65. Hays RD, Hadorn D. Responsiveness to change: an aspect of validity, not a separate dimension. Qual Life Res 1992;1:73-5.

66. Jachuck SJ, Brierly H, Jachuck S, Wilcox PM. The effect of hypotensive drugs on the quality of life. J R Coll Gen Pract 1982;32:103-5.

67. Croog SH, Levine S, Testa MA, et al. The effects of antihypertensive therapy on quality of life. New Engl J Med 1986;319:1220-1.

68. Hollenberg NK, Testa M, Williams GH. Quality-of-life as a therapeutic end-point: an analysis of therapeutic trials in hypertension. Pharmacoeconomics 1991;6:83-93.

69. Beto JA, Bansal VK. Quality of life in the treatment of hypertension: a metaanalysis of clinical trials. Am J Hypertens 1992;5:125-33.

70. Bulpitt CJ, Fletcher AE. Quality-of-life instruments in hypertension. Pharmacoeconomics 1994;6:523-35.

71. Côté I, Grégoire J-P, Moisan J. Health-related quality-of-life measurement in hypertension: a review of randomised controlled drug trials. Pharmacoeconomics 2000;18:435-50.

72. Curb JD, Borhani NO, Blaszkanski RTP, et al. Long-term surveillance for adverse effects of antihypertensive drugs. JAMA 1985;253:3263-8.

73. Horowitz RI, Viscoli CM, Berkamn L, et al. Treatment adherence and risk of death after a myocardial infarction. Lancet 1990;336:542-5.

74. Gallagher EJ, Viscoli CM, Horwitz RI. The relationship of treatment adherence to risk of death after myocardial infarction in women. JAMA 1993;270:742-4.

75. Smith M. Medication, quality of life and compliance: the role of the pharmacist. Pharmacoeconomics 1992:1;225-30.

76. Côté I, Moisan J, Chabot I, Grégoire J-P. Health-related quality of life in hypertension: impact of a pharmacy intervention program. J Clin Pharm Ther 2005;30:355-62.

77. Carter BL, Barnette DJ, Chrischilles E, Mazzotti GJ, Asali ZJ. Evaluation of hypertension patients after care provided by community pharmacists in a rural setting. Pharmacotherapy 1997;17:1274-85.

78. Armour CL, Taylor SJ, Hourihan F, Smith C, Krass I. Implementation and evaluation of Australian pharmacists' diabetes care services. J Am Pharm Assoc 2004;44:455-66.

79. Pickard AS, Johnson JA, Farris KB. The impact of pharmacist interventions on health-related quality of life. Ann Pharmacother 1999;33e:1167-72.

80. Tsuyuki RT, Johnson JA, Teo KK, et al. A randomized trial of the effect of a community pharmacist intervention on cholesterol risk management: the Study of Cardiovascular Risk Intervention by Pharmacists (SCRIP). Arch Intern Med 2002;162:1149-55.

81. Weinberger M, Murray MD, Marrero DG, et al. Effectiveness of pharmacist care for patients with reactive airways disease: a randomized controlled trial. JAMA 2002;288:1594-1602.

82. Cranor CW, Christensen DB. The Asheville Project: short-term outcomes of a community pharmacy diabetes care program. J Am Pharm Assoc 2003;43:149-59.

83. Bunting BA, Cranor CW. The Asheville Project: long-term clinical, humanistic, and economic outcomes of a community-based medication therapy management program for asthma. J Am Pharm Assoc 2006;46:133-47.

84. Smith M, Juergens J, Jack W. Medication and the quality of life. Am Pharmacy 1991;NS31:275-81.

85. Juniper EF, Guyatt GH, Epstein RS, et al. Evaluation of impairment of health-related quality of life in asthma. Development of a questionnaire for use in clinical trials. Thorax 1992;47:76-83.

86. Cole JC, Lin P, Rupnow MFT. Validation of the Migraine-Specific Quality of Life Questionnaire version 2.1 (MSQ v. 2.1) for patients undergoing prophylactic migraine treatment. Qual Life Res 2007;16:1231-7.

87. Cella DF, Tulsky DS, Gray G, et al. The Functional Assessment of Cancer Therapy Scale: development and validation of the general measure. J Clin Oncol 1993;11:570-9.

88. Perrine KR. A new quality of life inventory for epilepsy patients: interim results. Epilepsia 1993;34(suppl 4):S28-33.

89. Hays RD, Kallich JD, Mapes DL, Coons SJ, Carter WB. Development of the Kidney Disease Quality of Life (KDQOL) instrument. Qual Life Res 1994;3:329-38.

90. Brod M, Johnston J, Able S, Swindle R. Validation of the Adult Attention-Deficit/Hyperactivity Disorder Quality of Life scale (AAQoL): a disease specific quality of life measure. Qual Life Res 2006;15:117-29.

PART III

Targeting Care of Specific Patients

The first two parts of the book discussed the general way of viewing how most patients act in response to illness and treatment. However, as social scientists, we know that these responses to illness and treatment are affected by various factors, including people's background characteristics and the nature and severity of their illness. Chapters 16 and 17 present the specific issues involved with medication use at different ends of the age spectrum. Chapter 18 explores the processes that individuals and their families experience at the end of life. Chapter 19 provides a historical perspective on the psychosocial challenges of receiving diagnoses and treatments for mental illnesses in the U.S. healthcare system. Chapter 20 reviews the growing cultural diversity of the U.S. healthcare system and how pharmacists can best prepare to meet the needs of diverse cultural groups. Understanding the content of these five chapters will help pharmacists acquire a greater awareness and sensitivity toward the specific needs of various populations and how to tailor drug therapy to best meet such diverse needs.

PART III

Targeting Care of Specific Patients

CHAPTER 16

Children, Adolescents, and Medicines

Patricia J. Bush, PhD, and Katri Hämeen-Anttila, PhD

Traditionally, relative to health and illness behavior, children have been viewed as passive, with adults making decisions for them and providing information about them to health professionals. However, children take medicines themselves, are aware that medicines are stored at home, observe medicine use by family members, and view medicine promotion by the media on a regular basis. In addition, every trip to the pharmacy and grocery store exposes children to the sight of medicines and sometimes to the sight of a pharmacist. In view of this exposure, it is very likely that children form beliefs and attitudes about medicines. Moreover, these beliefs and attitudes should change as children gain more experience and develop more skills at interpreting what they observe.

During the past few decades there has been a gradual shift from viewing children as passive recipients of health information and health care to viewing them as active partners whose competence and information needs should be considered by healthcare professionals.[1,2] Some pharmacy organizations, such as the United States Pharmacopeia (USP) and the International Pharmaceutical Federation (FIP), have adopted statements emphasizing that children should be educated about their own medicines and also about medicine use in general during school health education.[2,3] Such education is crucial if we want to have a new generation of active and empowered medicine users who are competent in discussions with healthcare professionals. This is also the aim of the change in the healthcare approach from compliance to concordance.[4]

Interviews with mothers in Washington, DC, revealed that the average mother believed that 12 years is the age at which a child should be able to take a medicine for common health problems, such as a headache or sore throat, without asking an adult.[5] This raises several questions. What should that average child know about medicines before assuming this responsibility? Do children know enough to take medicines on their own? How do children learn about medicines? Who should teach them?

No consensus exists among health professionals or health educators about the need for children to be educated about medicines, who should assume the responsibility for education, or what forms such education should take. Certainly no one profession is solely responsible. It is a matter of cooperation, in which the role of the parents and the active involvement of the child should not be undermined.

The fact that children are not simply little adults is important. Not only do children have less experience than adults, but also children's thinking progresses through stages and is *qualitatively* different from that of adults. For reasons of differences relating to knowledge, experience, autonomy, and developmental levels, children may view and understand health, illness, and treatment differently than adults. Thus, children should be treated differently with regard to pharmaceutical care, and programs intended for teaching children about medicines should take into account what children already know, do, and want to know.

The goal of this chapter is to review what is known about children and medicines and to produce some pragmatic suggestions for health professionals and health educators. The remainder of this chapter presents information on how children learn, children's autonomy, knowledge, and attitudes relative to medicine use, and factors associated with children's medicine-related beliefs and behaviors. A section deals with how health professionals and health educators can help children learn to use medicines wisely before the children bear some responsibility for doing so. A separate section deals with the special situation of adolescents and medicines.

HOW CHILDREN LEARN

Cognitive Development Stages

Adults not only know more than children, but also are capable of processing what they know in a more complex way. Children progress through four stages as they develop more complex cognitive skills. The theory of cognitive development stages is credited to Jean Piaget.[6] Although the sequence of progression through the stages is the same, there is individual variation in the rate of progression, and the progression has been shown to vary with the specific topic area. For health in particular, even some adults do not operate at the highest stage.

A value in being aware of the cognitive development stages of children is appreciating that adults cannot provide children with information about health and illness and expect them to infer appropriate behavior. Moreover, in any given situation of health education addressed at a particular behavior, an adult may not be able to predict what a child will perceive.[7] Knowledge of cognitive development theory may not help you to predict what a child thinks, but at least you should not be surprised to hear a 7-year-old child who, when asked to name some "bad" drugs, correctly does so, but then says that you get them at the "drug" store. That is perfectly logical. Another lovely example occurred when a 6-year-old was asked how likely she would be to take something special if she had trouble falling asleep. Her response, indicated by pointing to the largest bar on a graph: "Very likely." She was then asked, "What would you take?" Her response: "A teddy bear."

Stage 1: Sensory Motor

The first stage, lasting from birth to about 2 years, is known as the sensory motor stage. In this stage, the child learns through interacting with the environment, and cannot recall or imagine an object or person that is not present. Thus, learning about medicines does not (cannot) occur during this stage.

Stage 2: Preoperational

The second stage, roughly from 2 to 7 years, is known as the preoperational stage. During this stage, children begin to be able to recall past events, to understand symbols, and to use mental imaging. However, links from cause to effect are not understood, and magical thinking is often used to explain events. For example, an asthmatic child at this stage may not understand the connection between exercise and difficulties in breathing—that is, the link from cause to effect. Children in this stage are often "yea sayers." Here is an example from an interview with a 4-year-old child, illustrating both "yea saying" and magical thinking: "Did you ride an elephant to school today?" "Yes." "Do you have wings?" "Yes." "How do you know you have wings?" "The elephant told me."

Clearly, it is wise to avoid questions that call for a yes/no response when trying to get information from children in the preoperational stage. In addition, children at this stage are sensitive to what they perceive the interviewer wants to hear and will respond to please the interviewer. Thus, the interviewer must take great care not to provide either verbal or physical indicators of approval or disapproval of a young child's answers.

Stage 3: Concrete Operational

From age 7 to 12 years, children's thinking becomes more logical and systematic. Children become problem solvers and are able to focus on several aspects of the same situation. They understand the difference between change and permanency.

Compared with the previous stage, an asthmatic child at this stage will understand the connection between exercise and difficulties in breathing. Furthermore, if told, a child at the concrete operational stage is able to understand why two asthma medicines may need to be used.

Children use whatever is at hand within their sphere of knowledge and experience to explain an event, however illogical it may seem to an adult. For example, a 7-year-old urban boy, when asked, "Is that good, being on drugs?" responded, "No, you can mess up your mind and then you die." But, when asked next, "So what happens . . .?" the boy said, "[A]nd then the police catch you and then they take you to the hospital and they gonna have to break your head open to get all the drugs out."[7] This 7-year-old represents a child entering the concrete operational stage and just beginning to apply logic and reasoning to events in his life. A sensitive adult, understanding this developmental process, can understand the child's logic. In this case, if drugs "mess up the mind," the child reasons that the mind is in the head and that hospitals fix people. Thus, it follows, with compelling logic, that the head must be broken open and the drugs removed to unburden the mind from its "messed up" state.

Stage 4: Formal Operational

The fourth stage is considered to exist from 12 years on. Children become more capable of hypothetical and abstract thought as they enter adolescence, but for formal operational thinking to occur in a particular area, attention and motivation are required. Thus, although individuals develop the capacity for this type of thinking—a capacity fully developed by late adolescence—the associated skills are not always applied. Understanding causal processes in health and illness is one of those content areas that seems to lag in some individuals through lack of interest or motivation, but certainly a better understanding of related processes and the relationships between internal and external factors is acquired. Someone trying to get information about health and illness from an adolescent (or an adult, for that matter) or to educate the adolescent cannot simply assume that the adolescent (or adult) is operating at this most advanced stage.

Theories and Models

Three conceptual systems predominate in explaining how children learn. One of these, cognitive development theory (CDT), as explained earlier, emphasizes the role of developmental processes that influence children's understanding. CDT has influenced studies of children's health beliefs and understanding of illness-related processes.[8-10] Behavioral intention theory (BIT)[11] is more often used for adults but is attractive for children because it emphasizes the influence of reference group norms and focuses on specific behaviors rather than inferences and abstractions for which children are often not cognitively prepared. Moreover, BIT posits that a behavior intention is the best predictor of an actual behavior. Social cognitive theory (SCT), a revision of social learning theory (SLT), predominates.[12] According to SCT, behaviors are acquired and shaped through attention, retention, production, and motivation operating in three domains: personal, behavioral, and environmental. Personal factors include the child's own value system and his or her expectations derived from observation and experience; behavioral factors include performance skills; and environmental factors include modeling and expressed opinions of peers, family, and media.

The children's health belief model (CHBM) was adapted from the classic health belief model (HBM) to explain children's expectations of taking medicines (Fig. 16-1).[13] The CHBM is consistent with Gochman's recommendation to place children's health behavior within their personal and social context,[14] recognizing that their personal attributes are influenced by peers, families, and other social groups. This view of children's health behaviors supports the inclusion of the influence of the child's primary caregiver, as well as cognitive and psychological attributes that change with age and experience, such as knowledge, risk taking, and perception of control over health status (health locus of control).

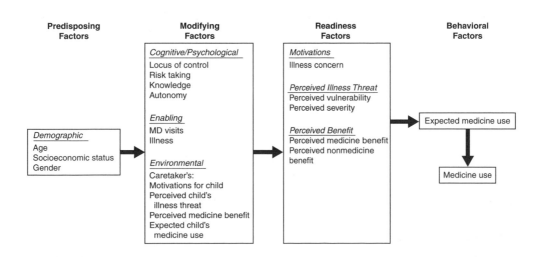

FIGURE 16-1   A Children's Health Belief Model
Source: Adapted from Bush PJ, Iannotti RJ. A children's health belief model. Med Care 1990;28:69–86.

The CHBM was very successful in predicting urban elementary schoolchildren's expectations regarding taking medicines for five common health problems: cold, fever, upset stomach, trouble sleeping, and nervousness.[13,15] The children's perceptions of illness severity and the benefit of taking medicines were the two strongest predictors, with illness concern and perceived vulnerability having weaker relationships.

From a developmental perspective, two findings are particularly noteworthy. Older children's variables were not more highly correlated with those of their mothers than younger children's. Also, the children's own cognitions and attitudes appeared to develop independently of their mothers. The primary message is that mothers' health beliefs are correlated with those of their children, but this effect is relatively small when compared with other developmental influences associated with the child. In fact, expected medicine use is not correlated between mothers and their children. Children's own motivational variables, influenced by their cognitive and affective processes, are more important in determining their expectations to take medicines than their mother's values, beliefs, and expectations. For example, perceived vulnerability, a strong predictor in adult models, is a weak predictor in the CHBM. The explanation is likely to be that children are not as cognitively prepared to predict events as are adults, because of lack of experience.

The variables in the CHBM are surprisingly stable.[15] Not only were most of the variables correlated over 3 years, but also expected medicine use among children aged about 8 to 12 years was predicted from variables measured 3 years earlier. These findings support educating children about medicines from an early age.

MEDICINE-RELATED BELIEFS AND BEHAVIORS

Factors likely to influence a child's beliefs, attitudes, and expectations regarding medicines include the child's frequency of medicine use and environmental exposure. Some or all of these factors may interact.

Frequency of Medicine Use

Medicine use is common among children. In the United States, one survey found that one half of the children younger than 3 years had been given an over-the-counter (OTC) medicine in the previous 30 days.[16] Similar and higher rates have been found in other countries for older children.[17-21] However, comparison of these studies is difficult because medicine use may be reported by parents,[16] by children themselves,[18-21] or by both the children and the parents.[13] Furthermore, the time during which medicines were used may differ considerably, from 2 days[13] to 1 or 2 weeks,[19] 1 month,[18,20] or even 3 months.[22] Although rates of medicine use, both OTC and prescription, tend to decrease after infancy and to begin to rise for females as they reach reproductive age, all surveys lead to the conclusion that medicine use is a common activity for children and adolescents.[13-23] Mothers' reports of their children's use tend to be higher than the children's reports, with the primary discrepancy attributable to vitamin and mineral use.[15] The higher incidence reported by the mothers may reflect their reporting what the child was supposed to have done rather than what the child actually did.

Girls use more medicines than boys, and this trend increases with age.[18,19,21] Socioeconomic class and ethnicity have also been shown to have some influence on children's medicine use. Children in lower social classes and ethnic minorities reported using medicines more often than other children.[23,24] When mothers of 3-year-old children were asked about OTC medicine use, women with higher education and incomes were more likely than other women to report they gave their child OTC medications.[16]

Medicines in the Child's Household

The number of medicines in the household is also likely to influence children's medicine-related expectations and behaviors. In addition to health status, differences are most likely accounted for by culture and economic status.

The number of medicines and the ratio of OTC to prescription medicines varies widely among countries and subpopulations. In "medicine cabinet" surveys in homes where children live in the United States and seven European countries, the average number of medicines varied from 7 (Washington, DC) to 24 (Yugoslavia and Chapel Hill, USA).[25] The number of medicines per person in the households varied from 2 (Finland) to 6 (Madrid and Yugoslavia). The average number of medicines per person in Chapel Hill was 7, compared with only 1.4 in Washington, DC. In addition, the percentage of OTC medicines varied from 36% (Athens, Greece) to 74% (Chapel Hill).

Most or all household medicines are easily accessible to most children of school age, a situation found in several European countries and the United States.[5,25-28] Medicines are rarely locked up and are kept in more than one place in the average household.

Children's Medicine Knowledge

A medicine knowledge index containing ten items believed to include those fundamental to appropriate use of medicines was administered to urban elementary schoolchildren.[5,17]

Table 16-1 shows the results from children in the third, fifth, and seventh grades. Only in seventh grade did the average child answer more than half of the questions correctly. In general, the children scored best on questions relating to prescriptions and poorest on questions relating to the relationship between efficacy (i.e., how well a medicine works)

TABLE 16-1   Children's Medicine Knowledge Index (percentage of children responding correctly)

Items	Grade 3 (%)	5 (%)	7 (%)
If you were sick, which would help you more . . . a big pill or a little pill? *No difference/it depends*	23	14	35
a good- or a bad-tasting medicine? *No difference/it depends*	28	22	46
medicine from the drug store or the same thing from the grocery store? *No difference/it depends*	16	7	40
Could the same medicine be different colors? *Yes*	50	54	78
Would medicine a doctor told you to take always make you feel better? *No*	66	63	76
What is a doctor's prescription? *Correct response*	38	58	82
Can the same medicine be good for people and also bad for people? *Correct response*	64	63	75
Are drugs the same as medicines? *Yes/sometimes*	36	45	56
Mean score on sum of correct items	3.8	4.2	5.9

Average age of children in grade 3 = 8 years, grade 5 = 10 years, grade 7 = 12 years.

Adapted from Bush PJ, Iannotti RJ, Davidson FR. A longitudinal study of children and medicines. In: Breimer DD, Speiser P, eds. Topics in pharmaceutical sciences. Amsterdam/New York: Elsevier Science Publishers, 1985:391-403.

and medicine characteristics such as size, color, taste, and place acquired. Almarsdottir and Zimmer[29] used a similar knowledge scale (eight items) to test 7- and 10-year-old children's knowledge of medicines, including their efficacy, and found that the average score was 4.0, with a range from 0 to 7.

Furthermore, children have limited ideas of how medicines work.[30-32] For example, no Finnish child was able to explain how antibiotics work.[32] Finnish children (7–14 years) had a better understanding of why some medicines needed to be taken with a special diet or on a given dosage schedule than they did of how medicines work.

Children in various countries recognize the possibility that medicines may have harmful effects.[31-33] For example, children in Germany (15–17 years) and in Finland (10–11 and 13–14 years) were aware that medicines can cause adverse reactions.[19,32,33] However, younger Finnish children (7–8 years) did not mention this possibility. Furthermore, in the study of Almarsdottir and colleagues, American children did not freely mention adverse reactions as possibly harmful.[34]

On average, children view medicines cautiously. According to several studies, children have said that medicines should be taken only for sickness and when really needed.[31-35] Some studies have reported that some children have fears about getting the wrong medicine, especially an adult's medicine.[31] In other studies children have viewed medicines quite positively and have attributed recovery to them.[32]

Young children often talk about medicines by referring to their appearance (e.g., color, form, or taste), name, or therapeutic purpose.[17,26,31,34] Older children are more likely to refer to medicines by their brand names.[31,34,36] However, even 5- to 6-year-old children are aware of brand names. When 20 kindergarten children were asked to name the medicine they would take for a cold, their responses included 18 different brand names plus vitamins and other medicines described by form, taste, or color (e.g., cherry-tasting medicine).[17]

Children's Autonomy With Medicines

Self-administration of medicines is quite common among children. In two American studies, 36% of 5- to 12-year-old children[17] and 36% of 10- to 14-year-old children[27] indicated they had taken medicine independently the last time they had taken medicine. Rudolf and coworkers discovered that 44% of 9- to 16-year-old campers at a residential summer camp brought medicines with them.[37] During the camp session, 25% of the younger (9–12 years) and 58% of the older (13–16 years) children self-medicated without consulting or informing an adult.

A 14-item medicine autonomy scale was administered to American children and their mothers (Table 16-2).[5,17] As expected, for every item, the oldest students indicated the most autonomy. The item receiving the most positive responses was household accessibility of medicines. As noted earlier, the average mother said that 12 years was the age when the average child could take a medicine for a headache independently; however, about one fifth of third and fifth graders indicated they would do so, although most of them were younger than 12 years.

In the same study, from 14% to 29% of the children in the third, fifth, and seventh grades indicated they had purchased a medicine independently, and 34% to 44% of the children said they had picked up a prescription.[5,17] In the summer camp study of Rudolf and colleagues, 8% of the younger children (9–12 years) and 28% of the

TABLE 16-2   Children's Autonomy in Medicine Use

Autonomy Items	Grade		
	3 (%)	5 (%)	7 (%)
Has access to household medicines	77	83	100
All household medicines are accessible	45	75	78
Asked for the last medicine taken	67	72	78
Got household medicines for self	73	83	89
Got household medicines for self independently	22	33	45
Got household medicines for others	62	62	71
Got household medicines for others independently	9	24	36
Took medicine independently	23	28	51
Took medicine independently for headache	20	21	45
Took medicine independently for sore throat	17	28	33
Gave medicine to another child independently	9	9	25
Purchased medicine independently	14	29	29
Picked up prescription independently	38	34	44
Had medicine at school on day of interview	6	5	9

Average age of children in grade 3 = 8 years, grade 5 = 10 years, grade 7 = 12 years.

Adapted from Iannotti RJ, Bush PJ. The development of autonomy in children's health behaviors. In: Susman EJ, Feagans LV, Ray W, eds. Emotion, cognition, health, and development in children and adolescents: a two-way street. Hillsdale, NJ: Lawrence Erlbaum, 1992:53-74; and Bush PJ, Iannotti RJ, Davidson FR. A longitudinal study of children and medicines. In: Breimer DD, Speiser P, eds. Topics in pharmaceutical sciences. Amsterdam/New York: Elsevier Science Publishers, 1985:391-403.

older children (13–16 years) shared medicines with others.[37] In a more recent American study, 20% of the girls (9–18 years) had borrowed or shared prescription medicines, as did 13% of the boys.[38] Pain medicine is shared most often and, furthermore, used independently more often than other medicines. Chambers and associates found that 58% to 76% of Canadian children (12–15 years) reported having taken OTC pain medication without first checking with an adult.[22] In the same study, 29% to 48% of the children reported that they had shared or borrowed medicines for different types of pain.

Children also take medicines to school. In Washington, DC, more than 8% of the children had one or more medicines at school on the day they were interviewed.[5,17] Children believe themselves to be involved in their treatment. In the Washington, DC, study, fewer than 16% of school-aged children thought they did not have a role in treatment of their last episode of injury or illness. As another example, Danish children (6–11 years) reported that they took medicines by themselves, even if the mother actually gave the medicine to the child.[39]

Media Exposure

Medicine advertising on television is permitted in some countries but not in others. The long-term impact of such exposure appears to be unknown. Much of the debate has concerned the impact on abusable substance use rather than on medicine-related beliefs, attitudes, and behaviors.[40]

Several U.S. studies, from the mid-1970s to the early 1990s, reported on children's exposure to medicine advertising on television.[41-44] In the mid-1970s, it was documented that the average U.S. child saw 1,139 drug commercials on television annually.[41] However, exposure has likely increased because prescription and OTC medicines are now widely advertised. In 2005, a Belgium study reported on relationships between adolescents' exposure to television advertising and OTC medicine use.[45]

To assess the impact of television commercials on children, fifth- and sixth-grade U.S. students (about 10–11 years old) were asked to watch commercials in two schools, one with and one without a program in which children participated in decisions involving their own health care.[42] The students were asked to record information about six messages involving health. The students in the school without the program were more likely to report they believed the messages in the commercials and took more vitamins and tonics.

In another study, conducted in the mid-1970s among 673 children aged 8 to 12 years, exposure to television was moderately related to children's proprietary medicine-related beliefs, intentions, and request behavior.[43] In a later study involving children the same age, the children were found to have negative attitudes toward OTC drug advertising in general, but this general attitude was found to be unrelated to their attitudes toward specific brand-name drugs, about which most children seemed uncertain.[44]

Children's recognition of OTCs was investigated in the early 1990s by showing 7- and 10-year-old children 23 medicines that had been advertised frequently on television during the previous month.[40] Children were asked if they had ever seen the medicine before, and if yes, where. Generic drugs and drugs in the same category, but not advertised, were also shown to the children. The average number of medicines recognized was 5.5 for the younger children and 7.9 for the older children. The source mentioned most often was television or advertising (mean, 2.9 drugs for younger children and 4.1 drugs for older children), followed by "the store" for the younger children (1.7) and "at home" for the older children (2.1). There were very few instances of a child claiming to recognize one of the unadvertised drugs.

In the Belgium study, a relationship was found between adolescents' TV exposure and OTC analgesic use, even after controlling for gender and lifestyle.[45]

Although cross-sectional studies have shown correlations, unfortunately there are no longitudinal studies tracking children's exposure to medicine advertising and later beliefs, attitudes, and behaviors.

Interrelationships

In the longitudinal study in Washington, DC, testing the CHBM (Fig. 16-1), children who knew the most about medicines and who felt the most in control of their health (health locus of control) were less likely than other children to perceive that medicines would help them for five common health problems and were less likely to expect to take medicines for them.[13] These relationships were also found in other populations of children in Spain and in the United States.[30,46] Studies have consistently found that the more internal a child's health locus of control, the more knowledgeable the child is about medicines. Moreover, the parent's level of education contributes to the child's knowledge.

The mother's medicine use and the child's prior use of medicines have also been shown to be significant predictors of children's expectations of using medicines.[15,17] Children in kindergarten to sixth grade (5–11 years) who were using medicines in the first phase of this study were more likely to be using medicines 3 years later. Furthermore, if the mothers reported taking medicines, 41% of their children indicated taking medicines, compared with 22% of the children of non-medicine-taking mothers. This stresses the importance of parental modeling and advice concerning medicines during the early school years.

HELPING CHILDREN LEARN ABOUT MEDICINES _____

Children rarely learn about medicines in school and rarely learn about them from their healthcare providers either. This leaves families and the media as the current main medicine "educators" of children.

Pediatricians, and likely other healthcare professionals as well, usually seek some information from children about their illness and symptoms. However, when giving information about diagnosis and treatment, physicians tend to address the parent.[47,48] The age of the child influences the situation, with older children given more information than younger children.[47,48] However, even young children are interested in and often anxious about their medical condition, and they retain some information better than adults. It is important to talk to children, if for no other reason than that the quality of communications to children affects adherence and treatment outcomes, probably through reducing anxiety.[49,50]

It is not enough simply to have good intentions and to decide to educate children about medicines. Most healthcare professionals are poor judges of what children at various levels can comprehend.[51] However, most can be taught to recognize the child's developmental level and to communicate at that level effectively.[52] Moreover, if a healthcare professional communicates with children at an appropriate level, a bonus is that the children's parents are more likely to understand.

For communication with children, the first step is to make a commitment to do it, and the second step is to learn how to communicate with children at their cognitive developmental levels,[52] to do it consistently, and to not give up if not every child responds. The third step is to decide where communication should take place. The fourth step is to prepare developmentally appropriate materials to augment communication.

One-on-One Communication

The following guidelines provide advice on how to communicate with children regarding medicine.

Immediately Focus on the Child

Engaging the child immediately will reduce the probability that a parent will respond for the child and will help the child recognize that you are interested in her or him. Bring yourself to the child's eye level and make eye contact. A good way to start communicating is to ask what kind of experiences the child has had with medicines. If you get a positive response and the child starts a discussion, first address the topics that the child raises. For example, for a preschool child, the taste and the way the medicine is taken (e.g., swallowing difficulties) may be the most important things. You should respect that and address the child's concerns even if at the end of the meeting that has been the only thing that you discussed.

Remember that the child can also be asked to find solutions. For example, in a Finnish study, one child said that she learned to swallow tablets by swallowing blueberries.[32] If you get any response from the child it is a *must* to react to it, to answer the child's questions, and to encourage the child to be active in future communications with healthcare professionals.

Attempt to Communicate at the Child's Developmental Level

The following are developmentally different responses to the same question, "What makes a cold go away?" from three children, aged 6, 8, and 10 years.[52] The 6-year-old and 8-year-old both replied, "A medicine." The 10-year-old said, "By taking the right medication from your doctor." When asked, "What kind of medicine?" the 6-year-old replied, "Medicine that helps you." The 8-year-old replied, "Tylenol, Dimetapp." The next question was, "How does that help?" The 6-year-old responded, "It takes the coughing away so you won't have a cold anymore." The 8-year-old said, "It helps fight the germs away." The 10-year-old replied, "If you take it and it goes in your system and it clears away the fluids and stuff that is in your body, like the mucus in your nose or something when it is stuffed up."

Although there is a general correlation with age, children develop at different rates that vary with the subject. The skills may be present but not applied within a content area, or a child may appear more advanced during a transitional phase. For example, another 8-year-old exhibited formal operational thinking when asked how a medicine would help cancer: "Well, the medicine kind of helps your immune system and white blood cells and from what I've heard kind of sterilizes the germs."

For a child in the preoperational stage with otitis media, you might say, "This medicine will go into your body to make your ear feel better. It will only work if you take it three times every day. Your mom will help you to know when to take the medicine. Be sure to use up all the medicine, even if your ear feels better."

For a child in the concrete operational stage, you might say, "This medicine will go into your body to help fight off the germs that are causing the infection in your ear. The medicine will only work if you take it three times a day until (date). If you don't take it that way, your ear infection is likely to come back. So keep taking it even if you feel better. Work with your mom so you both know you have taken the medicine at the right time."

For a child in the formal operational stage, you might say, "This medicine goes into your system to help your immune system fight off the bacteria that are causing your ear infection. The medical name for your ear infection is otitis media. The medicine used to fight the bacteria is an antibiotic. Its name is (name). What time do you usually get up? You must take this antibiotic every eight hours, that is, three times a day at (times) for the next ten days. If you don't, the bacteria may not all be killed and your ear infection can return. Keep taking it until it is all gone, even if you think your ear infection is cured. Let's look at the label together. What does it say? What time will you be taking it? What would you do if you miss a dose?"

Ask Open-Ended Questions Rather Than Those Requiring Only a Yes-or-No Response

Ask follow-up questions to make sure the child understands, and have the child repeat what you said. A child may parrot a correct response or read the label correctly without real understanding.

Use Simple Declarative Sentences for All Children

This is good advice when talking to adults as well. The goal is not to empower the child with total responsibility but to build a partnership between parent and child, that is, to work with the parent to begin to grant autonomy coupled with proper patient education and information. Modeling an appropriate communication style will help the parent continue communicating with the child about medicines and other health issues and to grant appropriate autonomy.

Ask Children to Ask You Questions

Be a medication educator. Try to empower the child to feel comfortable asking you questions about his or her health problem, the particular medicine, or medicines in general.

Augment Oral Communications with Written Material

Average adults only recall about 30% of what they are told by a doctor. You should not expect more from children. Written materials can be reviewed at home after the hospital, clinic, or pharmacy visit.

Give Children Tasks

Have the child put a colored sticker on the medicine so the child will know it is hers or his at home. For antibiotics, a calendar can be given to the child with times and dates to be taken noted. The child can be asked to cross off each dose and to bring the calendar to the next visit. The date for a follow-up visit can also be on the calendar. The child could be given the task of reminding a parent in the morning and in the evening to give the child the medicine. The child might be told to eat something (e.g., some bread) before taking the tablet. By committing children to such tasks and giving them a feeling of ownership, potential problems (e.g., a bad taste) may be overcome.

Children with Special Needs

Chronically ill children need special attention. Many (e.g., children with asthma) are responsible for taking their own medicines.[5] Older children in large families and urban children also may have more autonomy at an earlier age than other children. Illustrated materials are particularly important for those chronically ill children who use devices such as inhalers, patches, or syringes to take their medicines. The children can demonstrate their proper use.

Medication Education in Schools

Considering the pervasiveness of medicines in society, it is surprising that school health education relative to medicines has been almost completely restricted to prevention of poisoning among young children and prevention of abusable substance use among older children. It is most certainly possible to begin to educate children about medicines as early as preschool, as recommended by the United States Pharmacopeia and American School Health Association.[53]

To become active participants in their own medication use, children need to learn knowledge and skills about rational medicine use. The underlying ideology of empowerment is thus present. In the context of medication education, the empowerment approach would mean, first, giving sufficient information about medicines (e.g., what should be known before taking medicines); second, teaching the skills needed to use medicines (e.g., the steps needed for taking medicines rationally, or what to do to avoid possible adverse reactions); and third, facilitating active involvement in discussions concerning the child's own medicines with healthcare professionals. This kind of approach would build up the skills and competencies needed for children to gradually take more responsibility regarding their own medicines

In practice, after selecting a target grade, your first task is to learn what these children already know, do, and want to know about medicines. The second task is to set out learning objectives, a task that involves clarifying what you think these children should know. Children's interest in medicines at different ages has been studied. It was found that children are quite similar in various countries in their desires for information about medicines, and that children are eager to learn about medicines.[26,31,32]

As for what to teach children of different ages, the USP *Guide to Developing and Evaluating Medicine Education Programs for Children and Adolescents* is helpful.[53] It presents ten key behaviors for taking medicines and links them to specific behaviors for children by their ages, from 3 to 12 years. It also includes lists of what children said they want to know about medicines at different ages.

After deciding what to teach, the third task is to prepare a teaching plan. For example, for third-grade children (about 8 years old), you might decide that you want to address attributes of medicines that are unrelated to medication efficacy, such as color, taste, size, dose form, cost, and name. Examples can be brought to the class. To illustrate that the same medicine can be different colors, two tablets of different colors that are bioequivalent can be shown along with two M&Ms that are different colors. The children understand that the M&Ms have the same "active" ingredient inside, and the analogy can be made with the tablets. Labels can be read to teach that the same medicine can have different names and may also vary in cost.

For older children, you may want to develop a lesson about antibiotics and the importance of completing the course, with the lesson including the differences between viruses and bacteria. Or read patient information leaflets with the children and try to find ways to avoid side effects that children could try at home. This could be as easy as taking an antibiotic with food; however, the main point is that the children themselves find such ideas and have an opportunity to try them in practice. Children from the early grades can practice going to a pharmacy by role playing in which they first decide on some important questions that can be asked from a pharmacist, and then act as both pharmacist and customer.

Some particular points that you may want to make include how to understand and counteract media promotion of medicines and to understand that legal drugs may be as dangerous as illegal drugs and should not be taken without restraint. However, it is important that children understand that even though every medicine has its side effects, everyone must sometimes use medicines and that they are almost always safe to use when used as instructed. Studies have found that most school-aged children have a healthy respect for (and sometimes fear of) medicines. To induce fear of using them is definitely not a goal of medication education.

In practice, the empowerment approach is reflected in the way the educator addresses children. If you genuinely want to involve children, you should appreciate their competence and give them power even during classes. You will find that children have more autonomy and competence than adults usually expect. Find out what the children know, do, and want to know regarding medicines before you start telling them what you think they should know.

A medication curriculum is now available in English for use with different-aged children anywhere in the world. All you have to do is give appropriate attribution to the developer (see www.uku.fi/medicinescurriculum).

Adolescents

Some recommendations regarding communicating with adolescents can be made. Adolescents need privacy, and they need to know that their communications are confidential. Adolescents need to talk with adults who are absolutely comfortable talking with them about *any* subject, including abortion, acne, birth control, sexuality, steroids, and sexually transmitted infections (including HIV and AIDS). This must be done in a completely nonjudgmental way and without letting the adolescent perceive that you find his or her beliefs foolish, irrational, or amusing. Adolescents have a great deal of misinformation about how their bodies work and how they should be maintained. Many adolescents are distrustful of information provided by older persons. If you cannot be completely comfortable when talking with adolescents, you can at least provide appropriate written materials and referrals.

When communicating with adolescents, you should remember that they may be embarrassed very easily, even when discussing very common medicines such as painkillers. This is why you should explain carefully that the questions you ask are necessary to help you choose the correct medicine. Furthermore, remember that the adolescent might be alone in the pharmacy for the first time and might not know how to behave.

Some typical features of cognitive development may affect the counseling situation: the invincibility fable, the personal fable, and the imaginary audience.[54] The *invincibility fable* refers to an adolescent's feeling that he or she never will be harmed; consequently, adolescents may take all kinds of risks, falsely secure in the belief in their own immunity. This belief explains a lot of teen risk taking. Such risk taking may include, for example, taking medicines with alcohol. The *personal fable* refers to an adolescent's belief that his or her own life and feelings are unique. For example, a teen may complain to his or her mother that the mother does not know what it is like to be in love. The *imaginary audience* refers to adolescents' typical fantasies about how others react to their appearance and behavior. Adolescents may feel that everyone around them is just as concerned with, and as critical of, their actions and appearance as the adolescents themselves. This belief explains why a small pimple may seem catastrophic to a teenager.

Another concern is medication sharing and taking medicines belonging to a parent or other relative without their permission. If adolescents have had a solid foundation on various issues affecting medication use, they will understand when sharing is dangerous (e.g., sharing a tranquilizer) and when it is probably not (e.g., sharing an acetaminophen tablet). As for taking someone's medicine without permission (i.e., stealing), such behavior should be addressed in medication education long before the child reaches adolescence.

SUMMARY

This chapter has sought to provide health professionals and health educators with the tools necessary to both plan medication education programs for children and to communicate with children when counseling them about their own medicines.

REFERENCES

1. Kalnins I, McQueen D, Backett K, Curtice L, Currie C. Children, empowerment and health promotion: some new directions in research and practice. Health Promot Int 1992;7:53-9.
2. Bush PJ, Ozias JM, Walson PD, Ward RM. Ten guiding principles for teaching children and adolescents about medicines. US Pharmacopeia. Clin Ther 1999;21:1280-4.
3. International Pharmaceutical Federation. FIP statement of policy on the pharmacist's responsibility and role in teaching children and adolescents about medicines. Singapore: International Pharmaceutical Federation, 2001. (Accessed at http://www.fip.org/www2/uploads/database_file.php?id=180&table_id=.)
4. Britten N, Weiss M. What is concordance? In: Bond C, ed. Concordance. London: Pharmaceutical Press, 2004:9-28.
5. Iannotti RJ, Bush PJ. The development of autonomy in children's health behaviors. In: Susman EJ, Feagans LV, Ray W, eds. Emotion, cognition, health, and development in children and adolescents: a two-way street. Hillsdale, NJ: Lawrence Erlbaum, 1992:53-74.
6. Piaget J. The moral judgement of the child. Gabain M, trans. New York: Harcourt, Brace, World, 1932.
7. Bush PJ, Davidson FR. Medicines and "drugs": what do children think? Health Educ Q 1982: 9:113-28.
8. Bibace R, Walsh ME. Development of children's concepts of illness. Pediatrics 1980;66:913-7.
9. Burbach DJ, Peterson L. Children's concepts of physical illness: a review and critique of the cognitive developmental literature. Health Psychol 1986;5:307-25.
10. Perrin E, Gerrity S. There's a demon in your belly. Pediatrics 1981;57:841-9.
11. Fishbein M, Ajzen I. Belief, attitude, intention, and behavior: an introduction to theory and research. Reading, MA: Addison-Wesley, 1975.
12. Bandura A. Social foundations of thought and action: a social cognitive theory. Englewood Cliffs, NJ: Prentice-Hall, 1986.

13. Bush PJ, Iannotti RJ. A children's health belief model. Med Care 1990;28:69-86.

14. Gochman DS. Labels, systems and motives: some perspectives for future research and programs. Health Educ Q 1982;9:167-74.

15. Bush PJ, Iannotti RJ. The origins and stability of children's health beliefs relative to medicine use. Soc Sci Med 1988;27:345-55.

16. Kogan MD, Pappas G, Yu SM, Kotelchuk M. Over-the-counter medication use among U.S. preschool-age children. JAMA 1994;272:1025-30.

17. Bush PJ, Iannotti RJ, Davidson FR. A longitudinal study of children and medicines. In: Breimer DD, Speiser P, eds. Topics in pharmaceutical sciences. Amsterdam/New York: Elsevier Science Publishers, 1985:391-403.

18. Hansen EH, Holstein BE, Due P, Currie CE. International survey of self-reported medicine use among adolescents. Ann Pharmacother 2003;37:361-6.

19. Stoelben S, Krappweis J, Rossler G, Kirch W. Adolescents' drug use and drug knowledge. Eur J Pediatr 2000;159:608-14.

20. Holstein BE, Hansen EH, Due P, Almarsdottir AB. Self-reported medicine use among 11- to 15-year-old girls and boys in Denmark 1988–1998. Scand J Public Health 2003;31:334-41.

21. Dengler R, Roberts H. Adolescents' use of prescribed and over-the-counter preparations. J Public Health Med 1996;18:437-42.

22. Chambers CT, Reid GJ, McGrath PJ, Finley A. Self-administration of over-the-counter medication for pain among adolescents. Arch Pediatr Adolesc Med 1997;151:449-55.

23. Holstein BE, Hansen EH. Self-reported medicine use among adolescents from ethnic minority groups. Eur J Clin Pharmacol 2005;61:69-70.

24. Holstein BE, Hansen EH, Due P. Social class variation in medicine use among adolescents. Eur J Public Health 2004;14:49-52.

25. Sanz EJ, Bush PJ, Garcia M. Medicines at home: the contents of medicine cabinets in eight countries. In: Bush PJ, Trakas OJ, Sanz EJ, Wirsing R, Vaskilampi T, Prout A, eds. Children, medicines, and culture. Binghamton, NY: Pharmaceutical Products Press, 1996:77-104.

26. Trakas DJ, Sanz E, eds. Childhood and medicine use in a cross-cultural perspective: a European concerted action. Brussels: European Commission Directorate, 1996. (Report EUR 16646 EN.)

27. Sloane ED, Vessey JA. Self-medication with common household medicines by young adolescents. Issues Compr Pediatr Nurs 2001;24:57-67.

28. Bozoni K, Kalmanti M, Koukouli S. Perception and knowledge of medicines of primary schoolchildren: the influence of age and socioeconomic status. Eur J Pediatr 2006;165:42-9.

29. Almarsdottir AB, Zimmer C. Children's knowledge about medicines. Child Glob J Child Res 1998;5:265-81.

30. Aramburuzabala P, Garcia M, Polaino A, Sanz E. Medicine use, behaviour and children's perceptions of medicines and healthcare in Madrid and Tenerife (Spain). In: Trakas D, Sanz E, eds. Childhood and medicine use in a cross-cultural perspective: a European concerted action. Brussels: European Commission Directorate, 1996:245-68. (Report EUR 16646 EN.)

31. Menacker F, Aramburuzabala P, Minian N, Bush PJ, Bibace R. Children and medicines: what they want to know and how they want to learn. J Soc Adm Pharm 1999;16:38-52.

32. Hämeen-Anttila K, Juvonen M, Ahonen R, Bush PJ, Airaksinen M. How well can children understand medicine related topics? Patient Educ Couns 2006;60:171-8.

33. Garcia M, Sanz E, Aramburuzabala P, Almarsdottir AB. Concepts of adverse drug reactions among children in eight countries. In: Bush PJ, Trakas DJ, Sanz E, Wirsing RL, Vaskilampi T, Prout A, eds. Children, medicines, and culture. New York: Pharmaceutical Products Press, 1996:193-208.

34. Almarsdottir AB, Hartzema AG, Bush PJ, Simpson KN, Zimmer C. Children's attitudes and beliefs about illness and medicines: triangulation of open-ended and semi-structured interviews. J Soc Adm Pharm 1997;14:26-41.

35. Vaskilampi T, Kalpio O, Ahonen R, Hallia O. Finnish study on medicine use, health behaviour and perceptions of medicines and healthcare. In: Trakas D, Sanz E, eds. Childhood and medicine use in a cross-cultural perspective: a European concerted action. Brussels: European Commission Directorate, 1996:191-219. (Report EUR 16646 EN.)

36. Christensen P. The Danish participation in the COMAC medicines and childhood project. In: Trakas D, Sanz E, eds. Childhood and medicine use in a cross-cultural perspective: a European concerted action. Brussels: European Commission Directorate, 1996:103-21. (Report EUR 16646 EN.)

37. Rudolf MC, Alario AJ, Youth B, Riggs S. Self-medication in childhood: observations at a residential summer camp. Pediatrics 1993;91:1182-4.

38. Daniel KL, Honein MA, Moore CA. Sharing prescription medication among teenage girls: potential danger to unplanned/undiagnosed pregnancies. Pediatrics 2003;111:1167-70.

39. Christensen P. Difference and similarity: how children's competence is constituted in illness and its treatment. In: Hutchby I, Moran-Ellis J, eds. Children and social competence: arenas of action. London: Falmer Press, 1998:187-201.

40. Almarsdottir AB, Bush PJ. The influence of drug advertising on children's drug use attitudes, and behaviors. J Drug Issues 1992;22:361-76.

41. Choate R, Debevoise N. Caution! Keep this commercial out of reach of children! J Drug Issues 1976;6:91-8.

42. Lewis CE, Lewis MA. Children's health-related decision making. Health Educ Q 1982;9:225-37.

43. Robertson TS, Rossiter JR, Gleason RE. Children's conception of medicine: the role of advertising. Adv Consumer Res 1978;515-21.

44. Riecken G, Yavas U. Children's general, product and brand-specific attitudes toward television commercials—implications for public policy and advertising strategy. Int J Advertis 1990; 9:136-48.

45. Van den Bulck J, Leemans L, Laekeman GM. Television and adolescent use of over-the-counter analgesic agents. Ann Pharmacotherapy 2005;39:58-62.

46. Almarsdottir AB, Aramburuzabala P, Garcia M, Sanz EJ. Children's perceived benefit of medicines in Chapel Hill, Madrid, and Tenerife. In: Bush PJ, Trakas DJ, Sanz EJ, Wirsing R, Vaskilampi T, Prout A, eds. Children, medicines, and culture. Binghamton, NY: Pharmaceutical Products Press, 1996:127-153.

47. Pantell RH, Lewis CC. Physician communication with pediatric patients: a theoretical and empirical analysis. Adv Develop Behav Pediatrics 1986;7:65-119.

48. Tates K, Meeuwesen L, Bensing J, Elbers E. Joking or decision-making? Affective and instrumental behaviour in doctor-parent-child communication. Psychol Health 2002;17:281-95.

49. Iannotti RJ, Bush PJ. Toward a developmental theory of compliance. In: Krasnegor N, Epstein S, Johnson S, Yaffe S, eds. Developmental aspects of health compliance behavior. Hillsdale, NJ: Lawrence Erlbaum, 1992:59-76.

50. Sanz E. Concordance and children's use of medicines. BMJ 2003;327:858-60.

51. Perrin EC, Perrin JM. Clinicians' assessments of children's understanding of illness. Am J Dis Child 1983;137:874-8.

52. O'Brien RW, Bush PJ. Helping children learn how to use medicines. Office Nurse 1993;6(3): 14-9.

53. United States Pharmacopeia. Guide to developing and evaluating medicine education programs and materials for children and adolescents. Naples, FL: United States Pharmacopeia, 1999. (Accessed at http://www.usp.org/pdf/EN/consumers/guide.pdf.)

54. Stassen BK. The developing person through the life span. New York: Worth, 1998.

CHAPTER 17

Social, Behavioral, and Economic Aspects of Medication Use in Older Adults

Denise L. Orwig, PhD, Linda Gore Martin, PharmD, MBA, BCPS, and Nicole J. Brandt, PharmD, CGP, BCPP, FASCP

The topic of human aging has become increasingly important, especially as the number of older adults continues to increase. By 2030, the number of Americans aged 65 and older will more than double to 71 million, composing roughly 20% of the U.S. population.[1,2] In addition to the increase in both the number and proportion of people older than 65, people older than 85 (and especially those older than 100) will compose the fastest-growing group. In 1900, the average life expectancy was 47 years, and it had increased to a little more than 68 in 1950. By 1980, humans could expect to live 74 years. Extraordinary breakthroughs in health care were largely responsible for the increase in average life expectancy, which included decreased death rates of infants and children and the eradication of infectious diseases through better sanitation, vaccinations, and antibiotics. Although the changes in prevention of death from chronic diseases have not had such a large numeric impact, it is anticipated that the average life expectancy will reach 80 years by 2050.

With a larger proportion of the population living longer, the issue of health in older adults becomes more relevant. The last years of life are often accompanied by illness. At least 85% to 90% of persons aged 65 and older have at least one chronic illness, 60% have two or more, a third have three or more, and 25% have four or more.[3,4] The cost of providing health care for an older adult is three to five times greater than the cost for someone younger than 65.[1] By 2030, projected U.S. health-care spending will increase by 25% because of the aging of the population unless improving and preserving the health of older adults is more actively addressed.[5]

Great variability exists among people as they age (individually, and by gender and ethnicity), both with respect to the age at which age-related changes are noticed and the rate at which these changes occur. Each individual is subject to a unique combination of factors that affect aging. It is subsequently difficult to define an age at which a person becomes "elderly." There are different types of aging, including chronological age, functional age, cosmetic age, and economic age. Many of the biological age changes that occur do not become significant until after age 50, although age 65 is commonly used to define older adults since the Social Security Administration began using it in 1935 to denote retirement age.[6] Further classifications of older adults have been made, referring to those aged 65 to 74 as the "young old," those aged 75 to 84 as the "middle old" or "old old," and those 85 or older as the "oldest old."[7]

The shift in demographics—namely, a maturing society living longer, with more heterogeneity—is creating an undeniable imperative regarding the healthcare provider's knowledge of medication therapy in the older patient. This knowledge is especially important because older adults have a higher rate of medication use compared with the general population. The healthcare delivery system will be challenged to meet the needs of the growing and aging population who will incur problems of comorbid diseases, dependency, and functional loss. The healthcare delivery system needs to focus on preventing hospitalizations and premature mortality, reducing disease morbidity, minimizing institutionalization and inappropriate utilization of services, and maximizing the appropriate use of medications. Because medications are a significant part of health care for older adults, the unique aspects of medication use among older adults is the topic of the remainder of this chapter. Pharmacists need to be proactive in improving the use of medications through reducing adverse drug events, identifying adherence issues, and ensuring appropriate therapeutic use and effect. To be successful in these endeavors, pharmacists and other healthcare providers should be aware of the biological, social, economic, and behavioral factors that can affect medication use.

MEDICATION USE

Prescription and Over-the-Counter Medications

The most common health problems affecting older adults are often treated with medications, which provide valuable, if not lifesaving, therapy but also carry the risk of an adverse response. Persons 65 and older are the leading consumers of drugs, accounting for 34% of prescription medications and 50% of over-the-counter (OTC) medications.[3,8,9] This is most likely due to increasing levels of chronic disease conditions with age, such that 85% of persons in this age group have at least one chronic illness, and a third have three or more.[3] A survey has shown that more than 40% of individuals over the age of 65 use five or more medications per week, with approximately 12% using ten or more different medications, making polypharmacy a common problem among older adults.[10] The average older adult living in the community takes four medications concurrently.[11,12] Medication use is even more pronounced in the nursing home setting, where, on average, residents are taking approximately nine medications on a daily basis.[13] As the average life expectancy increases, so does the incidence of chronic diseases and the number of persons receiving long-term drug therapy. The continued growth of the older adult population means the burden on the healthcare system and society will also increase. A greater number of people with multiple chronic conditions who have reduced physiologic functioning are likely to be treated with medications.

The medications that are used most commonly by older adults are not surprising. The top three categories represent cardiovascular medications (e.g., antihypertensives), central nervous system (CNS) agents (e.g., antidepressants), and treatments for musculoskeletal and joint diseases (e.g., nonsteroidal anti-inflammatory agents). Overall, there is no real difference in the number of prescription medications taken by elderly men and women; however, men and women do differ in the therapeutic categories of medications they take.[14] In addition to using more diuretics and CNS medications (hypnotics, anxiolytics, and antidepressants), women take more thyroid medication, immunosuppression medications, and treatments for nutrition and blood disorders.[14]

The pharmacist needs to obtain a medication history and make sure that the older adult is asked about all medications, including OTC products as well as herbal remedies. In addition to tobacco use, it is important to look for alcohol abuse and illicit drug use, which can confound diagnoses as well as the risks and benefits of medications. Targeted questions concerning medication use, and "brown bag" assessments, in which the patient brings in all his or her medications, may help to identify potential problems.

Alcohol

Alcohol use, misuse, and abuse among older adults are growing healthcare concerns. As the baby boomers reach 65 and older, there will be an increase in the number of older adults with a history of heavier drinking habits.[15] Currently, it is estimated that approximately 25% of individuals over the age of 65 in the community consume alcohol daily and that 10% of this population "binge drink."[16] Alcohol use in older adults has a more pronounced effect due to physiologic changes. This predisposes an older adult to a greater risk for confusion or falls. Chronic abuse of alcohol can lead to numerous effects on the body, such as liver damage, gastrointestinal bleeds, anemia, and dementia.

Alcohol has the potential to adversely interact with numerous prescribed medications, OTC medications, and herbal remedies. Although some of the interactions occur mostly among people who drink heavily, many of the interactions can occur with smaller amounts of alcohol (e.g., in light-to-moderate drinkers). The prevalence of alcohol and medication interactions among older adults who consume alcohol ranges from 19% to 38%.[17-19] A survey that noted that there are numerous medications that interact with alcohol indicated that 48% of patients did not receive any advice regarding an interaction of their medication with alcohol.[20] All of these facts stress the importance of pharmacists educating patients not only about the harmful effects of alcohol but also about its potential interactions with medications. It is vital for pharmacists to educate, screen, and empower all patients, especially older adults who are at greater risk for adverse events.

Other Drugs of Abuse

Drug misuse and abuse is less common in the older adult. The fact that many older adults see more than one prescriber and often have family members who have prescriptions for abusable drugs means that obtaining these medications can be relatively easy. Commonly, these medications are used (and prescribed) for grief, depression, anxiety, and stress. Frequently, the older adult does not understand the proper use of the medications and begins using more than prescribed; this is followed by escalation of the use until abuse occurs.[21]

Researchers using the National Household Surveys on Drug Abuse (NHSDA) data from 1999 to 2001 found two prominent types of drug abuse in older adults: marijuana use (1.1%) and nonmedical use of prescription psychotropic drugs (1.3%); a small percentage (0.1%) used both. They then projected the drug abuse prevalence to 2020, when the baby boomer generation (1946–1964) will be older than 55. The projection for any use of illicit drugs during the year will increase by 113% (based on a larger older population and more common drug use in this generation), from 1.6 million to 3.5 million users.[22] The implications of this drug abuse, including increased health-related problems as the body ages and increased drug interactions with prescribed medications, are enormous.

Studies have found that older patients are more motivated and likely to continue in treatment for substance abuse than younger patients, but treatment is often complicated by multiple chronic illnesses. Pharmacists can be the central healthcare professional to help manage these patients and their medication use.[21]

Complementary and Alternative Medicine

Statistics indicate that Americans are increasingly replacing prescription medications with not only vitamin and mineral supplements but also with herbal and other natural products or treatments referred to as complementary and alternative medicine (CAM); thus, the use of CAM is receiving increasing attention in the medical community. It is estimated that 30% to 40% of older adults in the United States use a variety of CAM.[23,24] The rising popularity of alternative therapies may reflect attempts to augment formal medical care as well as the belief that "natural" preparations are safe.[25,26] Quite the contrary, the number of adverse events, drug interactions, and deaths involving these products has been on the rise.[27-31] In a recent survey on the use of herbal products among older adults, 21% were currently taking at least one herbal product or dietary supplement, and the potential for adverse drug reactions was apparent in 19% of the users. A supplemental questionnaire to the 2002 National Health Interview Survey showed that the most commonly used herbal products reported by older adults were echinacea, garlic, ginkgo biloba, ginseng, and saw palmetto.[32] Most patients are reluctant to share their use of CAM with their healthcare providers; thus, it is imperative for providers and pharmacists to create a supportive environment for open communication to learn about CAM use and advise on possible interactions.[33,34]

BIOLOGICAL ISSUES

Age-Related Physiologic Changes

An important aspect of medication use among older adults is their increased physiologic vulnerability to medications and impaired ability to recover from drug-induced side effects. Even though humans age at different rates, all people have decreasing physiologic reserves over time. The series of physiologic alterations in the aging body affects how drugs produce their effects on the body (pharmacodynamics) and how a drug is absorbed, distributed, metabolized, and excreted from the body (pharmacokinetics). These changes affect renal, hepatic, gastrointestinal, pulmonary, cardiovascular, and neurologic function.[35] This loss of function and reserve leads to both an increase in drug utilization (to treat disease and dysfunction) and the potential for increased adverse effects and intolerance. The inadequacy of homeostatic control mechanisms in older adults greatly increases the likelihood that an exaggerated response or drug interaction will assume clinical importance or require lower doses.

Additional biological changes with age can also affect the appropriate use of medications, including hearing and vision changes as well as cognitive decline.

Hearing and Vision Loss

In 1990, approximately 4 million people in the United States had severe vision impairment. Vision impairment is the most common sensory issue in the older population. The prevalence of vision impairment increases significantly with age: persons aged 0 to 54 have a rate of 6.1; 55 and older, 104; and 85 and older, 216 (rates are from 1990 and per 1,000). Watson states that vision loss is the third major reason older adults need assistance with activities of daily living (after arthritis and cardiac disease).[36] Most of these persons are not blind, and therefore can use devices and techniques to help them with medication use.

The normal aging of the eye becomes apparent about age 45, when near and far vision is affected by the decreased ability to focus (presbyopia). Most older adults have similar acuity to younger adults under high-contrast conditions, but have major decreases when illumination or contrast is decreased; this is especially important in glare conditions. Color discrimination, adaptation to dark, and field of vision (which depends on higher-order processing) decline with age. The major diseases that increase loss of vision include cataracts, glaucoma, macular degeneration, and diabetic retinopathy. Persons with low vision need more spacing between words than those with normal vision, which may have important implications for providing medication literature.[37] Vision loss may eliminate the use of written material altogether and make medication labels difficult to read, particularly on a glossy surface.

Helzner and colleagues[38] found an overall prevalence of hearing loss of 59.9% in their cohort aged 73 to 84. White men had the highest rate (64.9%), followed by white women (59.3%), black men (58.1%), and black women (55.0%). Men, white and black, had the highest rate of high-frequency loss, experiencing a loss of 91.8% and 76.1%, respectively. Also, for each 5-year increase in age, the prevalence rate of hearing loss doubled. Hearing loss has been associated with several systemic diseases, including cardiovascular and diabetes mellitus, as well as ototoxic drugs used for other disorders.[38] Hearing impairment can greatly affect the medication counseling process.

Because both hearing and vision loss involve changes at both the organ system level and within the nervous system, the association between hearing and vision loss and cognition has been investigated. A study by Anstey and coworkers found that decrease in vision over 2 years was positively associated with memory decline (but not verbal ability or processing speed), whereas hearing decline was not associated with any cognitive domain.[39]

Cognition and Memory

Medication management skills decrease with advancing age regardless of whether measurable cognitive decline exists. However, the concurrent existence of cognitive decline exacerbates the problem.[40] Aging causes a decline in short-term memory, particularly for information that is presented quickly and verbally. On average, the decline is gradual and slow until approximately age 60 to 70. Information about completely unfamiliar things also becomes much harder to remember with age. Declines in working memory, especially when the tasks have high levels of executive control, are also seen with aging. However, Kramer and associates found that older adults have a better memory for previously identified objects, indicating that some memory processes are preserved or improved with age.[41] Decreased cognitive levels have been associated with an increased risk of hearing loss (23% for each standard deviation decrease in the modified Mini-Mental State Examination). A decline in hearing may affect older adults' understanding of information. These decreases in cognitive and hearing functioning may have a common vascular cause.[38]

Dramatic increases in the number of people with cognitive impairment will have a tremendous impact on the healthcare system and the need for supportive services, particularly when it comes to medication management.[42] With an increase in age also comes an increase in the incidence and prevalence of Alzheimer's disease (AD) and other dementias, so that by 2050 there will be more than 14 million patients with AD.[43] In addition, depending on the definition, the prevalence of mild cognitive impairment is 3% to 53%, with a reasonable estimate of 19% in persons older than 75 years.[44] In 2000, AD and other dementias (of which AD is the most frequent) constituted the third most expensive health condition in the United States, after heart disease and cancer.[45,46] The Alzheimer's Association and the National Institute on Aging estimate that current direct and indirect costs of caring for AD patients are at least $100 billion annually. Medicare costs for beneficiaries with AD, at $91 billion in 2005, are expected to increase 75%, to $160 billion in 2010. Medicaid expenditures on residential dementia care will increase 14%, from $21 billion in 2005 to $24 billion in 2010.[47]

A study by Maioli and colleagues found that although mild cognitive impairment has been considered prodromal to dementias, in a mean follow-up of 1.2 years (range 0.23–3.1), only 28.6% of the 52 patients studied converted to dementia, and 17.3% reverted to normal. Of those who converted, AD was diagnosed in 53.3%, with the remaining percentage of cases due to other causes.[48] The differentiation between mild cognitive impairment related to pseudodementia (or reversible forms) and that related to dementia is critical because many of these patients are experiencing medication-related impairment or disorders that can be treated (such as depression).

Chronic and Comorbid Disease

As mentioned earlier, as people age they are more likely to experience acute illnesses and suffer from chronic conditions. The existence of more than one condition, or comorbidity, is common. Joyce and colleagues examined the Medicare Current Beneficiary Surveys (MCBS) from 1992 to 1999 and Medicare claims for individuals aged 65 years and found that only a small percentage had no comorbidities.[49] Fewer than 20% of 65-year-olds with hypertension or cancer did not have another comorbidity. Ninety percent of older adults with chronic obstructive pulmonary disease or diabetes had at least one additional comorbid condition. Patients with coronary heart disease or stroke have comorbidities over 95% of the time. Hypertension, osteoarthritis, and heart disease are the most common comorbid diseases among older adults; of those older adults with hypertension, at least 20% also have diabetes.

Many older adults do not remember all of their disorders unless prompted with a checklist or other method.[50] Wetzels and coworkers found that underreporting of health problems is frequent, particularly in people without pain.[51] This underreporting may increase the chance that medications are also underreported (especially OTC or herbal products) or that patients with treatable conditions are not receiving medications. Knowledge and understanding of diseases has been associated with increased adherence. Beliefs, especially about the severity of disease (or when symptoms exist), are also important. The number of comorbidities is highly correlated with the number of medications and the complexity of the drug regimen.

SOCIAL ISSUES

Cultural

The United States has always been a melting pot of cultures. For centuries the population was primarily of European descent, but today's culture represents a diversity of people from around the world. Increasing diversity brings possible disparities in health care that include lack of access to quality health care, inappropriate or suboptimal treatments, and underutilization of preventive and specialty services. The Institute of Medicine (IOM) in 2002 issued a nearly 800-page report on disparities in health care related to cultural characteristics.[52] The report covered all aspects of cultural differences, showing that disparities can occur between age groups, racial or ethnic groups, genders, socioeconomic groups, geographic locations (north versus south), and between urban and rural groups.

Despite recent progress, disparities persist in access to health care in the United States.[53-55] In particular, blacks are less likely to have regular sources of health care.

They receive less preventive care, see physicians less often, visit fewer specialists, and receive services later in the course of many diseases than whites.[54,56-58] Minority older adults may be more likely to consider health conditions to be part of the normal aging process, which may inhibit appropriate health service utilization.[59-61] Disparities in medication use have been reported for some conditions (e.g., depression, diabetes, hypertension, hypercholesterolemia), with whites being more likely to receive treatment.[62] Even when similarities exist in rates of medication use among racial groups, the issue of appropriateness or quality of treatment is still not clear.

Recent emphasis in the research on older adults has been on the differences between rural and urban residents. Rural older adults, however, are not homogeneous; local cultures are often based on ethnicity.[63] Gesler and colleagues, in summarizing three rural studies, stated that regardless of what belief is prevalent, health professionals must be aware of it in order to be culturally sensitive.[63] For example, in a cultural context, rural residents have been shown to allow their religious beliefs to play a greater role in their health behavior. Pharmacists who are aware of these differences may be better equipped to establish rapport with patients and to determine whether they are telling the provider what they think that person wants to hear as opposed to expressing their true feelings, beliefs, and symptoms.[64]

Health Literacy

An estimated 90 million Americans have low health literacy, defined by the IOM as "the degree to which individuals can obtain, process, and understand the basic health information and services they need to make appropriate health decisions."[65]

A systematic review of health literacy in the United States found an overall low health literacy rate of 26% and a marginal literacy rate of an additional 20%. Lower health literacy levels are associated with increasing age, ethnicity, and lower levels of education. Studies with subjects who had an average age older than 50 showed a low literacy prevalence of 37.9%.[66] Wolf and associates found that older adults with significant deficits in health literacy had higher rates of hypertension, diabetes mellitus, heart failure, and arthritis. They also had significantly lower physical and mental health functioning, with increased limitations on activities.[67]

Changes in cognition and memory in older adults may be factors in the low literacy levels and the resultant low adherence to medication regimens. Older adults have reduced processing resources (attention and working memory).[68] This change means that extra time should be spent on counseling to allow older adults to comprehend the messages being presented about their medications. To maximize working memory capacity in older adults, unique education efforts should be designed to provide repeated information.

Other factors that may be associated with reduced health literacy in the older adult are changes in vision and hearing. Decreased visual acuity reduces the ability to read prescription labels and to tell colors apart (especially yellows and greens). The decreased ability to see, in association with decreased hearing, can lead to errors in interpreting printed instructions, even if verbal instructions are also given.

Medication counseling may be affected by the cultural aspects of hearing loss. A small study that interviewed groups of hard-of-hearing (some elderly) and deaf patients found that deaf patients believe that physicians do not appreciate their full lives and have misconceptions about how to communicate with them. Because of the grammatical differences between American Sign Language and spoken English, the patients feel that healthcare providers think they are stupid. The providers often also fail to maintain eye contact. This is especially a problem if the patient is trying to lip read, but the patient also feels left out if the contact is with an interpreter. The deaf would like more time and accommodations other than writing notes; this may be significant in older adults, who often have problems writing because of vision loss or arthritis.

The hard of hearing did not have as strong feelings as the deaf, but they are often ashamed, frustrated, and in denial. Older adults with impaired hearing felt that providers did not understand how hard it was to communicate and thought that speaking louder would be helpful. However, the providers usually do not slow down or take any more time to determine whether the patient understood. The hard of hearing frequently have problems with staff and with automated phone systems.[69] Jacobson gave some advice on how to counsel hearing impaired patients: (1) respect their intelligence, sensitivity, and confidentiality; (2) rephrase and clarify if the patient does not appear to understand; (3) ask the patient about preferences using any assistive devices or interpreters; and (4) arrange for a quiet area to decrease competing sounds.[70]

Communication

With the aging population in the United States becoming more ethnically diverse, communication is going to become even more of a concern. Not only are there physical limitations such as decreased hearing and impaired vision that can impede effective communication, but also there is the potential for language and cultural barriers. Communication issues in addition to all of the other issues discussed can ultimately decrease adherence to interventions such as medications. Increasing attention has been given to concordance, which is "an agreement reached after negotiation between a patient and a healthcare professional that respects the beliefs and wishes of the patient in determining whether, when and how medications are to be taken"; essentially, concordance hinges on the ability of a provider to effectively communicate with his or her patient.[71] Miscommunication and unresolved patient concerns result from information gaps in the patient education process and the inability of the patient to express and resolve personal concerns. Studies suggest that effective communication between patients and healthcare providers improves self-management of medications.[72]

Communication is critical not only between the patient and healthcare provider but also with the caregiver. Often, an inability to manage medications is not identified until a crisis happens, such as a hospitalization. The principle of empowering and supporting the caregiver is evident from individuals caring for people with Alzheimer's disease. Evidence has shown that providing support to the caregiver through education ultimately results in the patient remaining in the community longer.[73]

ECONOMIC ISSUES

Healthcare System

Ability to pay is a major factor in being able to obtain necessary treatment and services, including medications. In general, older adults pay for their medications either through insurance or self-pay; insurance usually has a patient contribution for services (a copayment or deductible) in addition to a premium. Three major types of insurance coverage are available to older adults: Medicare, Medicaid, and private insurance. The Medicare program (Social Security Act Title XVIII, a federal program) has several parts. The three parts that are relevant to nearly all U.S. citizens aged 65 and older are Part A (hospital insurance coverage), Part B (supplemental insurance coverage for items such as physician visits and other outpatient services), and Part D (prescription drug program). The Medicaid program is health insurance coverage for the poor; Medicaid is a joint program that is managed by the individual states, with additional funding from the federal government. Older adults who have Medicaid benefits to cover medical costs not covered by Medicare are called "dual eligibles."[74]

Medicare Part D was enacted with the implementation of the Medicare Prescription Drug, Improvement and Modernization Act of 2003 (MMA).[75] In addition to the prescription plan, new regulations require pharmacists as well as other healthcare providers to provide medication therapy management (MTM) services to targeted beneficiaries. Targeted beneficiaries are defined as individuals with Medicare Part D who have multiple Part D medications or multiple chronic disease states and are likely to incur annual costs for Part D medications that exceed a level set by the Department of Health and Human Services ($4,000 in 2007). Although the spectrum of services is extremely broad, the aim of this program is to optimize therapeutic outcomes related to medications, improve medication use, reduce the risk of adverse events and drug interactions, and increase patient compliance with prescribed regimens. This initiative has increased the role of the pharmacist as an active member of the interdisciplinary team.

Types of Environments

The elderly in the United States may be living in one of a variety of arrangements (Table 17-1). Most older adults continue to live in the community (either in their own home or with a caregiver; who may or may not be a relative) until they need significant supervision that warrants being in a nursing home. As older adults live longer, they move out of their homes later in their life. With the growing availability of assisted living facilities and increased services for home care, the current residents of nursing homes commonly have more progressed illness than residents of the 1970s and 1980s. Much of this shift in living arrangements is due to the implementation of

TABLE 17-1 Types of Long-Term Care				
Type of Long-Term Care	Help with Activities of Daily Living	Help with Additional Services	Help with Care Needs	Range of Costs
Community-based services	Yes	Yes	No	Low to medium
Home health care	Yes	Yes	Yes	Low to high
In-law apartments	Yes	Yes	Yes	Low to high
Housing for aging and disabled individuals	Yes	Yes	No	Low to high
Board and care homes	Yes	Yes	Yes	Low to high
Assisted living	Yes	Yes	Yes	Medium to high
Continuing care retirement communities	Yes	Yes	Yes	High
Nursing homes	Yes	Yes	Yes	High

From Centers for Medicare and Medicaid Services. Types of long-term care. April 10, 2007. (Accessed August 14, 2007, at http://www.medicare.gov/LongTermCare/Static/TypesOverview.asp.)

the Medicaid home and community-based waiver programs that provide funding for some types of care so that older adults can stay at home.[74] Approximately 95% of the elderly population resides in the community at any one time.[76] Therefore, only a small number of older adults live in an environment (e.g., a nursing home) where medication use is federally regulated; a much larger number of elderly are managing their own medications with varying degrees of oversight in the community.

Long-Term Care

Long-term care encompasses a variety of services, including medical and nonmedical care, to people who have a chronic illness or disability. The services address the health, personal care, and social needs of the older adult. Long-term care services can be provided in a variety of locations, with the ultimate goal of restoring or maintaining the health and function of the individual. The level and type of services required depend on the extent of the person's disability and comorbidity profile. A majority of long-term care services are provided in community settings, and a smaller percentage is provided in nursing homes. By 2020, 12 million older Americans will need long-term care.[77]

Generally, Medicare does not pay for long-term care. Medicare pays only for medically necessary skilled nursing facilities or home health care. Most long-term care assists people with support services such as activities of daily living, and Medicare does not pay for this "custodial care" or nonskilled care, including care that most people do for themselves—for example, diabetes monitoring. Medicaid may pay for certain health services and nursing home care for older people with low incomes and limited assets. In most states, Medicaid also pays for some long-term care services at home and in the community. Eligibility criteria and what services are covered vary from state to state.[74]

Approximately 14% of those older than 65 and 50% of those 85 and older need help with one or more activities of daily living or instrumental activities of daily living (long-term care needs).[78] However, at least 75% of these people live in the community (61% for those 85 and older).[78] Of these community-based older adults, as many as 28% receive no needed care, while 47% receive care only from nonpaid caregivers.[78] Of the older adults living at home, about 10% of the 65- to 74-year-olds and about 35% of those older than 85 require help from a caregiver.[76] Children and other relatives of older adults provide about 80% of all care; these informal caregivers provide three times as much direct care for older adults as do all nursing homes, hospitals, and other institutions combined.[79]

Formal long-term care may be given through community or home care, adult day care, assisted living, or nursing homes. Those with terminal illnesses may be under the care of hospice organizations; most hospice care (80%) for those 65 and older is paid for by Medicare.[74] Acute situations that require more medical services may involve hospitals, inpatient rehabilitation facilities, skilled nursing units, and long-term acute care hospitals; the latter three may involve months of care. The Research Triangle Institute has tried to define the types of long-term acute care facilities.[80] The long-term care hospital is similar to the step-down unit of an intensive care unit in a hospital for medically complex patients. The inpatient rehabilitation facility cares for less medically complex, but acutely functionally impaired, patients. The skilled nursing facility is reserved for the least medically complex patients. These facilities are all covered under Medicare Part A.[80]

Many communities provide services and programs to help older adults and people with disabilities with a variety of personal activities. These services include Meals-on-Wheels, transportation services, personal care, chore or errand services, adult day care, and a variety of activities in senior centers (including case management). These services are usually free or provided at low cost to individuals who qualify. Local organizations, called Area Agencies on Aging, coordinate these services to promote the independence and dignity of older adults.[77]

Often, older adults get help with personal activities (e.g., help with the laundry, bathing, dressing, cooking, and cleaning) at home from family members, friends, or volunteers. Some home care can only be given by licensed health workers, such as skilled nursing care and certain other healthcare services that are provided in the home for the treatment of an illness or injury. Medicare only pays for home care if the individual meets certain conditions. The state Medicaid program may pay for home health services, including skilled nursing care, home health care, personal care, chore and errand services, and medical equipment. Home care costs can vary depending on where the person lives, the type of care needed, and how often care is needed. Usually, home care payment is based on hourly charges.[77]

Independent Housing

Independent housing arrangements may include staying in the former home, moving into an in-law apartment, or obtaining housing through programs for low-income housing for the elderly and disabled. An in-law apartment is a separate housing arrangement within a single-family home or on the same lot; it may also be referred to as a second unit, accessory apartment, or accessory dwelling unit. An in-law apartment is a complete living space and includes a private kitchen and bath. The federal government and most states have programs that help pay for housing for older people with low or moderate incomes. Residents usually live in their own apartments in the complex; waiting lists for units are common. Some of these housing programs also offer help with meals and other activities, such as housekeeping, shopping, and doing the laundry.

Board and Care Homes

Board and care homes are group living arrangements that provide help with activities of daily living for those who cannot live on their own but do not need nursing home services. Such a home is sometimes referred to as a *group home*, having one to five residents. In some cases, private long-term care insurance and other types of assistance programs may help pay for this type of living arrangement. Many of these homes do not receive payment from Medicare or Medicaid, exist with regulations varying by state, and are often not strictly monitored.

Assisted Living

Assisted living facilities are state-regulated group living arrangements that provide help with activities of daily living, including taking medicine and getting to appointments. Residents often live in their own room or apartment within a building or group of buildings and have some or all of their meals together. Social and recreational activities are usually provided. Some assisted living facilities have health services on site. Nearly a million individual assisted living units now exist in the United States. Funding is nearly always private pay. Medicare does not pay for assisted living, and Medicaid (in the 41 states where authorized) pays only for the services and not for room and board.[81] Residents usually pay a monthly rent and then pay additional fees for the services that they receive.

Continuing Care Retirement Communities

Continuing care retirement communities (CCRCs) are housing communities that have different levels of care based on the individual needs of residents. In the same community, there may be individual homes or apartments for residents who still live on their own, an assisted living facility for people who need some help with daily care, and a nursing home for those who require higher levels of care. Residents move from one level of care to another based on their needs, but still stay in the CCRC. The contract usually requires the individual to use the community's assisted living facility or nursing home. CCRCs generally charge a large payment before an individual moves in (called an entry fee) and then charge monthly fees.

Nursing Homes

Nursing homes are facilities that provide care to people who cannot be cared for at home or in the community. Because of the decrease in disabilities and the increase in alternative living arrangements, the total number of nursing home residents has decreased; the percentage of adults aged 85 and older in nursing homes was 13.9% in

2004, compared with 21.1% in 1985.[81] A study by the U.S. Department of Health and Human Services reports that people who reach age 65 will likely have a 40% chance of entering a nursing home. About 10% of the people who enter a nursing home will stay there 5 years or more. Payment is through private funds or Medicaid. Medicare will pay for skilled rehabilitative care for limited periods (100 days total, most of which have a copayment).[81] Nursing homes provide a wide range of personal care and health services. In most cases, this care generally is to assist people with custodial care services. Medicare does not pay for these types of services; approximately 48% of nursing home care is paid by Medicaid.[81] Some nursing homes may provide skilled care after an injury or hospital stay; Medicare pays for such skilled nursing facility care for a limited period of time and for those who meet certain conditions.

Residents of nursing facilities are mandated by regulations to have a medication regimen review (MRR) done at least monthly by a licensed pharmacist. Residents may also be eligible for MTM services, but the provision of such services is complicated by the fact that the MRR is required for all residents and that compensation for the MRR is the responsibility of the facility. The American Society of Consultant Pharmacists has published guidelines on how to provide both services legitimately.[82] Provision of MTM services to residents of assisted living or other facilities is no different than for those living in their own homes.

MEDICATION MANAGEMENT ISSUES

Medication Adherence

Nonadherence or errors in taking medications correctly are disturbingly common, with over half of the 1.6 billion prescriptions written annually in the United States taken incorrectly.[83] Studies have reported nonadherence rates in older adults that range from 26% to 59%.[84] The medical and economic consequences of older patients' nonadherence to drug therapy may include lack of drug efficacy, treatment failure, disease progression, emergence of resistant bacteria, medication overdose, otherwise avoidable hospitalizations, and unnecessary medical expenses.[85] It is estimated that 30% to 50% of prescribed medications fail to produce their intended results.[83] Medication management is a complicated process, involving selecting the right drug, ensuring that the patient can obtain it and take it correctly, and evaluating its action on the patient.[86] One study by Ruscin and Semla showed that in a sample of elders (average age 80), 22% of those physically dependent and a third of those with cognitive impairment were still responsible for taking their own medications.[11] Compounding this situation, a study by Royall and colleagues showed that half of persons in the community have trouble comprehending medication information.[87] A similar study by Dellasega and associates documented that in the hospital, 60% of elders had trouble following the process for correct medication use.[88] For patients with chronic conditions, adherence with ongoing medication regimens is often a problem.

Medication nonadherence can take many forms, such as failure to fill the original prescription, failure to refill a prescription, failure to take the dose as prescribed, failure to take the dose at the appropriate time, failure to follow directions for taking the medication, and failure to follow warnings. The barriers causing medication nonadherence vary widely and are especially relevant for older adults. They fall in the realms of prescription issues, patient–provider communication issues, and disability issues. Some of the barriers to correct medication use reported in the literature for older adults are regimen complexity, miscommunication (gaps in the patient education process), unresolved patient concerns (inability of patient to express concerns),[83] hearing impairments (interfere with the patient counseling process),[89] vision impairments (may make medication labels difficult to read; lack of color discrimination may lead to administration errors),[90,91] functional impairments (difficulty opening containers or administering the medication as prescribed, e.g., bronchodilators),[92] and cognitive impairments (memory problems).[93] Table 17-2 summarizes the various factors contributing to nonadherence in the older patient.[94]

TABLE 17-2   Factors Influencing the Ability to Comply with a Medication Regimen
Three or more chronic conditions
More than five prescription medications
Twelve or more medication dosages per day
Medication regimen changed four or more times during past 12 months
Three or more prescribers involved
Significant cognitive or physical impairments (e.g., memory, hearing, vision, arthritis)
Living alone in the community
Recently discharged from the hospital
Low literacy
Medication cost
Adapted from Bero LA, Lipton HL, Bird JA. Characterization of geriatric drug-related hospital readmissions. Med Care 1991;29:989-1003.

In general, drug-related admissions secondary to noncompliance have been reported to occur in 3% to 28% of elderly patients.[95-97] Noncompliance was the most common cause of avoidable hospitalizations (6%).[98] Col and coworkers[97] found that 11% of admissions were related to noncompliance, with the mean cost per admission associated with medication noncompliance being $2,150. Even preventing half of the avoidable serious adverse events related to medication noncompliance would result in significant savings.

ADVERSE DRUG EVENTS

When used appropriately, drugs may be the single most important intervention in the care of an older patient, but when used inappropriately they no longer provide therapeutic benefit and may even endanger the health of the older patient by causing an adverse drug event (ADE). Because the use of medications increases with age, older patients are at greater risk for developing adverse events, which are often incorrectly attributed to the aging process or to a progression of the disease.[98] It is estimated that between 5% and 35% of older community-dwelling individuals experience an ADE.[99] Factors believed to be responsible for increased adverse events in elderly patients are polypharmacy (including prescription, OTC, and herbal medications), increased drug–drug interactions, pharmacokinetic factors, pharmacodynamic factors, the pathology of aging, and noncompliance.[100] ADEs can have serious consequences for the elderly. The mildest form of an ADE could be an unanticipated side effect of a medication, such as nausea. More ominous ADEs have been documented in many published reports.[94,101-105] Appropriate use of medications is such an important issue for older adults that it was targeted in the *Healthy People 2000* report.[106] The Joint Commission specifically recommends that institutions establish programs to monitor, track, and prevent adverse drug events and medication errors.[107]

Costs of Adverse Drug Events

It has long been established that drugs may cause or contribute to negative adverse events such as significant morbidity and increased costs of care in this population by increasing health care utilization.[102,108-111] It is estimated that drug-related morbidity and mortality costs $76.6 billion annually (1994 dollars) in the ambulatory setting in the United States. The largest component of this total cost is associated with drug-related hospitalizations,[109] with 28% of these ADEs being preventable.[102] Preventable costs account for an estimated 47% of the total annual costs.[112] Classen and colleagues found that patients with ADEs had a significantly prolonged length of stay, increased costs, and a twofold increased risk of death compared with matched controls.[113] A General Accounting Office study indicated that hospitalizations due to ADEs in the elderly account for $20 billion dollars each year.[114]

PHARMACEUTICAL CARE

Pharmacists are in a pivotal role to help improve communication as well as medication adherence among older adults. Pharmacists interact with patients, family members, healthcare professionals, and other pharmacists. Because of the presence of pharmacies in many community settings, pharmacists are viewed as the most accessible healthcare providers. The pharmacist's active role is critical in providing pharmaceutical care to older adults.

It is commonly known that older adults see multiple providers and use multiple medications. The fragmentation of health care leads to poorly coordinated care and is associated with an increased rate of hospitalization as well as other healthcare costs.[115] This is one of the reasons why the American Geriatrics Society published a position statement on the role of interdisciplinary care for older adults with complex needs.[116] This position statement supports the interdisciplinary care model because it can meet the complex needs of older individuals with multiple medical comorbidities, improve healthcare processes and outcomes for geriatric syndromes (e.g. falls), benefit the healthcare system as well as caregivers of older adults, and provide training and education of future healthcare providers to care for the needs of older adults.

SUMMARY

Healthcare professionals have obvious opportunities to improve the health care of older adults through health promotion strategies that target primary, secondary, and tertiary prevention. Ongoing initiatives to increase public awareness and to set objective measurements have been implemented through *Healthy People 2010*, a set of health objectives for the United States that builds on initiatives pursued over the past two decades.[117] The initiatives include the 1979 Surgeon General's Report, *Healthy People*, and *Healthy People 2000: National Health Promotion and Disease Prevention Objectives*. These national health objectives serve as the basis for the development of state and community plans and recently have been utilized to generate a report, *The State of Aging and Health in America 2007*.[118] This report has provided a national report card on how successful the various states have been in meeting 15 *Healthy People 2010* objectives related to health status, health behaviors, preventive care and screening, and injuries in adults older than 65. These guidelines and tools can be accessed on the website of the Agency for Healthcare Research and Quality (AHRQ).

Pharmaceutical care (or patient-directed pharmacist care) for the older adult requires the pharmacist to have an understanding of the differences in this population with respect to diversity, education level, health status, and the variety of medications available (prescription, OTC, herbal/supplements). The baby boomer generation will bring a new type of older patient who will be a more educated consumer of health-care services, will have different expectations of the healthcare system and its practitioners, and will have access to an unprecedented number of treatment options. There will be ongoing drug development for conditions of aging, providing new medications on the market along with prescription medications becoming increasingly available over the counter. In addition to billions of dollars spent annually on research and development of new medications, pharmaceutical companies spent $4.2 billion in 2005 on direct-to-consumer advertising.[119] It is not only the medications themselves that are important, but where they are purchased. Virtual pharmacies are a growing market on the Internet, with pharmaceuticals being the fourth largest product category advertised. Medications purchased through virtual pharmacies accounted for 45% of electronic healthcare transactions in 2004 (producing $349 million), and the percentage is expected to rise exponentially in the coming years. The prospect of cost savings and convenience associated with the Internet is appealing to older adults, but they could also be putting themselves at risk.

It is anticipated that healthcare reform will likely result in an increase in managed care environments, with an expected reduction in costly services such as inpatient care. As the delivery of health care continues to evolve, more emphasis will be directed toward lower-cost alternatives such as home care and assisted living arrangements. In this ever-changing climate, the challenges and opportunities for experts in geriatric pharmacotherapy will increase dramatically and will need to be met to serve the needs of the growing older adult population.

REFERENCES

1. Trends in aging—United States and worldwide. MMWR Morb Mortal Wkly Rep 2003;52(6): 101-4, 106.
2. Wan H, Sengupta M, Velkoff VA, DeBarrow KA, Bureau of the U.S. Census. 65+ in the United States: 2005. Washington, DC: U.S. Government Printing Office, 2005. (Current Population Reports.)
3. Mueller C, Schur C, O'Connell J. Prescription drug spending: the impact of age and chronic disease status. Am J Public Health 1997;87(10):1626-9.

4. Schraeder C, Dworak D, Stoll JF, Kucera C, Waldschmidt V, Dworak MP. Managing elders with comorbidities. J Ambul Care Manage. 2005;28(3):201-9.

5. Agency for Healthcare Research and Quality. Physical activity and older Americans: benefits and strategies. (Accessed at http://www.ahrq.gov/ppip/activity.htm.)

6. Social Security Administration. The origins of the retirement age in Social Security. (Accessed at http://www.ssa.gov/history/age65.html.)

7. Susman R, Riley MW. Introducing the oldest old. Millbank Memorial Fund Q 1985;63:177-86.

8. Avorn J. The elderly and drug policy: coming of age. Health Aff (Millwood) 1990;9(3):6-19.

9. Salom IL, Davis K. Prescribing for older patients: how to avoid toxic drug reactions. Geriatrics 1995;50(10):37-40, 43; discussion 44-5.

10. Kaufman DW, Kelly JP, Rosenberg L, Anderson TE, Mitchell AA. Recent patterns of medication use in the ambulatory adult population of the United States: the Slone survey. JAMA 2002;287(3):337-44.

11. Ruscin JM, Semla TP. Assessment of medication management skills in older outpatients. Ann Pharmacother 1996;30(10):1083-8.

12. Nikolaus T, Kruse W, Bach M, Specht-Leible N, Oster P, Schlierf G. Elderly patients' problems with medication. An in-hospital and follow-up study. Eur J Clin Pharmacol 1996;49(4):255-9.

13. Lewin Group. CMS review of current standards of practice for long-term care pharmacy services: long-term care pharmacy primer. (Accessed August 15, 2008, at http://www.cms.hhs.gov/Reports/downloads/LewinGroup.pdf.)

14. Roe CM, McNamara AM, Motheral BR. Gender- and age-related prescription drug use patterns. Ann Pharmacother 2002;36(1):30-9.

15. Aira M, Hartikainen S, Sulkava R. Community prevalence of alcohol use and concomitant use of medication—a source of possible risk in the elderly aged 75 and older? Int J Geriatr Psychiatry 2005;20(7):680-5.

16. Culberson JW. Alcohol use in the elderly: beyond the CAGE. Part 1 of 2: prevalence and patterns of problem drinking. Geriatrics 2006;61(10):23-7.

17. Pringle KE, Ahern FM, Heller DA, Gold CH, Brown TV. Potential for alcohol and prescription drug interactions in older people. J Am Geriatr Soc 2005;53(11):1930-6.

18. Forster LE, Pollow R, Stoller EP. Alcohol use and potential risk for alcohol-related adverse drug reactions among community-based elderly. J Community Health 1993;18(4):225-39.

19. Adams WL. Potential for adverse drug-alcohol interactions among retirement community residents. J Am Geriatr Soc 1995;43(9):1021-5.

20. Brown RL, Dimond AR, Hulisz D, et al. Pharmacoepidemiology of potential alcohol-prescription drug interactions among primary care patients with alcohol-use disorders. J Am Pharm Assoc 2007;47:135-9.

21. Lantz M. Prescription drug and alcohol abuse in an older woman. Clin Geriatr 2005;13(1):39-43.

22. Colliver JD, Compton WM, Gfroerer JC, Condon T. Projecting drug use among aging baby boomers in 2020. Ann Epidemiol 2006;16(4):257-65.

23. Astin JA, Pelletier KR, Marie A, Haskell WL. Complementary and alternative medicine use among elderly persons: one-year analysis of a Blue Shield Medicare supplement. J Gerontol A Biol Sci Med Sci. 2000;55(1):M4-9.

24. Foster DF, Phillips RS, Hamel MB, Eisenberg DM. Alternative medicine use in older Americans. J Am Geriatr Soc 2000;48(12):1560-5.

25. Bouchayer F. Alternative medicines. Compl Med Res 1990;4:4-8.

26. Astin JA. Why patients use alternative medicine: results of a national study. JAMA 1998; 279(19):1548-53.

27. Marinac JS, Buchinger CL, Godfrey LA, Wooten JM, Sun C, Willsie SK. Herbal products and dietary supplements: a survey of use, attitudes, and knowledge among older adults. J Am Osteopath Assoc 2007;107(1):13-20.

28. Huxtable RJ. The myth of beneficent nature: the risks of herbal preparations. Ann Intern Med 1992;117(2):165-6.

29. Hasegawa GR. Uncertain quality of dietary supplements: history repeated. Am J Health Syst Pharm 2000;57(10):951.

30. Miller LG. Herbal medicinals: selected clinical considerations focusing on known or potential drug-herb interactions. Arch Intern Med 1998;158(20):2200-11.

31. Fugh-Berman A. Herb-drug interactions. Lancet 2000;355(9198):134-8.

32. Arcury TA, Grzywacz JG, Bell RA, Neiberg RH, Lang W, Quandt SA. Herbal remedy use as health self-management among older adults. J Gerontol B Psychol Sci Soc Sci 2007;62(2):S142-9.

33. Kuo GM, Hawley ST, Weiss LT, Balkrishnan R, Volk RJ. Factors associated with herbal use among urban multiethnic primary care patients: a cross-sectional survey. BMC Complement Altern Med 2004;4:18.

34. Eisenberg DM, Davis RB, Ettner SL, et al. Trends in alternative medicine use in the United States, 1990–1997: results of a follow-up national survey. JAMA 1998;280(18):1569-75.

35. Sawhney R, Sehl M, Naeim A. Physiologic aspects of aging: impact on cancer management and decision making, part I. Cancer J 2005;11(6):449-60.

36. Watson GR. Low vision in the geriatric population: rehabilitation and management. J Am Geriatr Soc 2001;49(3):317-30.

37. Sass SM, Legge GE, Lee HW. Low-vision reading speed: influences of linguistic inference and aging. Optom Vis Sci 2006;83(3):166-77.

38. Helzner EP, Cauley JA, Pratt SR, et al. Race and sex differences in age-related hearing loss: the Health, Aging and Body Composition Study. J Am Geriatr Soc 2005;53(12):2119-27.

39. Anstey KJ, Luszcz MA, Sanchez L. Two-year decline in vision but not hearing is associated with memory decline in very old adults in a population-based sample. Gerontology 2001; 47(5):289-93.

40. Lieto JM, Schmidt KS. Reduced ability to self-administer medication is associated with assisted living placement in a continuing care retirement community. J Am Med Dir Assoc 2005; 6(4):246-9.

41. Kramer AF, Boot WR, McCarley JS, Peterson MS, Colcombe A, Scialfa CT. Aging, memory and visual search. Acta Psychol (Amst) 2006;122(3):288-304.

42. Cooper C, Carpenter I, Katona C, et al. The AdHOC Study of older adults' adherence to medication in 11 countries. Am J Geriatr Psychiatry 2005;13(12):1067-76.

43. Hebert LE, Scherr PA, Bienias JL, Bennett DA, Evans DA. Alzheimer disease in the US population: prevalence estimates using the 2000 census. Arch Neurol 2003;60(8):1119-22.

44. Rosenberg PB, Johnston D, Lyketsos CG. A clinical approach to mild cognitive impairment. Am J Psychiatry 2006;163(11):1884-90.

45. Fillit H, Hill J. Economics of dementia and pharmacoeconomics of dementia therapy. Am J Geriatr Pharmacother 2005;3(1):39-49.

46. Kirchstein R. Disease specific estimates of direct and indirect costs of illness and NIH support. Fiscal year 2000 update. (Accessed April, 2007, at http://ospp.od.nih.gov/ecostudies/ COIreportweb.htm.)

47. Lewin Group. Saving lives, saving money: dividends for Americans investing in Alzheimer research. Washington, DC: Commissioned by the Alzheimer's Association, 2004.

48. Maioli F, Coveri M, Pagni P, et al. Conversion of mild cognitive impairment to dementia in elderly subjects: a preliminary study in a memory and cognitive disorder unit. Arch Gerontol Geriatr 2007;44(suppl 1):233-41.

49. Joyce GF, Keeler EB, Shang B, Goldman DP. The lifetime burden of chronic disease among the elderly. Health Aff (Millwood) 2005;24(suppl 2):W5R18-29.

50. MacLaughlin EJ, Raehl CL, Treadway AK, Sterling TL, Zoller DP, Bond CA. Assessing medication adherence in the elderly: which tools to use in clinical practice? Drugs Aging 2005; 22(3):231-55.

51. Wetzels R, van Eijken M, Grol R, Wensing M, van Weel C. Self-management is not related to lower demand for primary care in independent-living elderly. J Am Geriatr Soc 2005;53(5): 918-9.

52. Institute of Medicine. Unequal treatment: confronting racial and ethnic disparities in health care. Washington, DC: National Academies Press, 2002.

53. Dunlop DD, Manheim LM, Song J, Chang RW. Gender and ethnic/racial disparities in health care utilization among older adults. J Gerontol B Psychol Sci Soc Sci 2002;57(4):S221-33.

54. Lavizzo-Mourey R, Knickman JR. Racial disparities—the need for research and action. N Engl J Med 2003;349(14):1379-80.

55. Shi L, Green LH, Kazakova S. Primary care experience and racial disparities in self-reported health status. J Am Board Fam Pract 2004;17(6):443-52.

56. Bach PB, Pham HH, Schrag D, Tate RC, Hargraves JL. Primary care physicians who treat blacks and whites. N Engl J Med 2004;351(6):575-84.

57. Blustein J, Weiss LJ. Visits to specialists under Medicare: socioeconomic advantage and access to care. J Health Care Poor Underserved 1998;9(2):153-69.

58. Gornick ME, Eggers PW, Reilly TW, et al. Effects of race and income on mortality and use of services among Medicare beneficiaries. N Engl J Med 1996;335(11):791-9.

59. Michielutte R, Diseker RA, Stafford CL, Carr P. Knowledge of diabetes and glaucoma in a rural North Carolina community. J Community Health 1984;9(4):269-84.

60. Ontiveros JA, Black SA, Jakobi PL, Goodwin JS. Ethnic variation in attitudes toward hypertension in adults ages 75 and older. Prev Med 1999;29(6 pt 1):443-9.

61. Goodwin JS, Black SA, Satish S. Aging versus disease: the opinions of older black, Hispanic, and non-Hispanic white Americans about the causes and treatment of common medical conditions. J Am Geriatr Soc 1999;47(8):973-9.

62. Crystal S, Sambamoorthi U, Walkup JT, Akincigil A. Diagnosis and treatment of depression in the elderly medicare population: predictors, disparities, and trends. J Am Geriatr Soc 2003; 51(12):1718-28.

63. Gesler W, Arcury TA, Koenig HG. An introduction to three studies of rural elderly people: effects of religion and culture on health. J Cross Cult Gerontol 2000;15:1-12.

64. Gallo JJ, Bogner HR, Morales KH, Ford DE. Patient ethnicity and the identification and active management of depression in late life. Arch Intern Med 2005;165(17):1962-8.

65. Institute of Medicine, Committee on Health Literacy. Health literacy: a prescription to end confusion. Washington, DC: National Academies Press, 2004.

66. Paasche-Orlow MK, Parker RM, Gazmararian JA, Nielsen-Bohlman LT, Rudd RR. The prevalence of limited health literacy. J Gen Intern Med 2005;20(2):175-84.

67. Wolf MS, Gazmararian JA, Baker DW. Health literacy and functional health status among older adults. Arch Intern Med 2005;165(17):1946-52.

68. Baudouin A, Vanneste S, Pouthas V, Isingrini M. Age-related changes in duration reproduction: involvement of working memory processes. Brain Cogn 2006;62(1):17-23.

69. Iezzoni LI, O'Day BL, Killeen M, Harker H. Communicating about health care: observations from persons who are deaf or hard of hearing. Ann Intern Med 2004;140(5):356-62.

70. Jacobson J. Counseling the deaf and hearing-impaired. Am J Health Syst Pharm 1999; 56(7): 610-1.

71. Chewning B, Wiederholt JB. Concordance in cancer medication management. Patient Educ Couns 2003;50(1):75-8.

72. Peterson MA, Dragon CJ. Improving medication adherence in patients receiving home health. Home Healthc Consult 1998;5(9):25-7.

73. Mittelman MS, Ferris SH, Shulman E, Steinberg G, Levin B. A family intervention to delay nursing home placement of patients with Alzheimer disease. A randomized controlled trial. JAMA 1996;276(21):1725-31.

74. Centers for Medicare and Medicaid Services. Dual eligibility. December 14, 2005. (Accessed April 14, 2007, at http://www.cms.hhs.gov/DualEligible/.)

75. Centers for Medicare and Medicaid Services. Summary of H.R.1: Medicare Prescription Drug, Improvement and Modernization Act of 2003; Public Law 108-173. (Accessed Aug 14, 2008, at http://www.cms.hhs.gov/MMAUpdate/downloads/PL108-173summary.pdf.)

76. Lamy PP. Institutionalization and drug use in older adults in the U.S. Drugs Aging 1993;3(3): 232-7.

77. Medicare. Long-term care. January 22, 2007. (Accessed April 14, 2007, at http://www.medicare.gov/LongTermCare/Static/Home.asp?dest=NAV%7CHome%7CWhatIsLTC#TabTop.)

78. Schneider EL, Guralnik JM. The aging of America. Impact on health care costs. JAMA 1990; 263(17):2335-40.

79. Perlman R. Introduction to part I. In: Perlman R, ed. Family home care: critical issues for services and policies. New York: Hawthorne Press, 1983:1-12.

80. Mihalich LK. The role of long-term care hospitals. Dennis Barry's Reimbursement Advisor 2007;22(7):6-9.

81. Tumlinson A, Woods S. Long-term care in America: an introduction. Washington, DC: Avalere Health, 2007.

82. American Society of Consultant Pharmacists. Guidelines for medication therapy management services in long-term care facilities. Alexandria, VA: American Society of Consultant Pharmacists, 2007.

83. Berg JS, Dischler J, Wagner DJ, Raia JJ, Palmer-Shevlin N. Medication compliance: a healthcare problem. Ann Pharmacother 1993;27(9 suppl):S1-24.

84. van Eijken M, Tsang S, Wensing M, de Smet PA, Grol RP. Interventions to improve medication compliance in older patients living in the community: a systematic review of the literature. Drugs Aging 2003;20(3):229-40.

85. Greenberg RN. Overview of patient compliance with medication dosing: a literature review. Clin Ther 1984;6(5):592-9.

86. Garrard J, Harms S, Hanlon J. Medication management of community based elderly people in managed care organizations. Paper presented at How Managed Care Can Help Older Persons Live Well with Chronic Conditions; October 27-28, 1998; Washington, DC.

87. Royall DR, Cordes J, Polk M. Executive control and the comprehension of medical information by elderly retirees. Exp Aging Res 1997;23(4):301-13.

88. Dellasega C, Orwig DL, Heller DA. OBRA guidelines: How do community prescribers compare? Pharmacoepidemiology and Drug Safety. 1999; 8:S131.

89. Uhlmann RF, Larson EB, Rees TS, Koepsell TD, Duckert LG. Relationship of hearing impairment to dementia and cognitive dysfunction in older adults. JAMA 1989;261(13):1916-9.

90. Luscombe DK, Jinks MJ, Duncan S. A survey of prescription label preferences among community pharmacy patrons. J Clin Pharm Ther 1992;17(4):241-4.

91. Jinks MJ, Evenson LM, Campbell RK, Kreager MC. Prescription labels for aging eyes. Am Pharm 1989;NS29(5):31-3.

92. Meyer ME, Schuna AA. Assessment of geriatric patients' functional ability to take medication. DICP 1989;23(2):171-4.

93. Maddigan SL, Farris KB, Keating N, Wiens CA, Johnson JA. Predictors of older adults' capacity for medication management in a self-medication program: a retrospective chart review. J Aging Health 2003;15(2):332-52.

94. Bero LA, Lipton HL, Bird JA. Characterization of geriatric drug-related hospital readmissions. Med Care 1991;29(10):989-1003.

95. Dartnell JG, Anderson RP, Chohan V, et al. Hospitalisation for adverse events related to drug therapy: incidence, avoidability and costs. Med J Aust 1996;164(11):659-62.

96. Tafreshi MJ, Melby MJ, Kaback KR, Nord TC. Medication-related visits to the emergency department: a prospective study. Ann Pharmacother 1999;33(12):1252-7.

97. Col N, Fanale JE, Kronholm P. The role of medication noncompliance and adverse drug reactions in hospitalizations of the elderly. Arch Intern Med 1990;150(4):841-5.

98. Courtman BJ, Stallings SB. Characterization of drug-related problems in elderly patients on admission to a medical ward. Can J Hosp Pharm 1995;48(3):161-6.

99. Hajjar ER, Hanlon JT, Artz MB, et al. Adverse drug reaction risk factors in older outpatients. Am J Geriatr Pharmacother 2003;1:82-9.

100. Beyth RJ, Shorr RI. Epidemiology of adverse drug reactions in the elderly by drug class. Drugs Aging 1999;14(3):231-9.

101. Lindley CM, Tully MP, Paramsothy V, Tallis RC. Inappropriate medication is a major cause of adverse drug reactions in elderly patients. Age Ageing 1992;21(4):294-300.

102. Bates DW, Cullen DJ, Laird N, et al. Incidence of adverse drug events and potential adverse drug events. Implications for prevention. ADE Prevention Study Group. JAMA 1995;274(1): 29-34.

103. Lazarou J, Pomeranz BH, Corey PN. Incidence of adverse drug reactions in hospitalized patients: a meta-analysis of prospective studies. JAMA 1998;279(15):1200-5.

104. Lesar TS, Lomaestro BM, Pohl H. Medication-prescribing errors in a teaching hospital. A 9-year experience. Arch Intern Med 1997;157(14):1569-76.

105. Cullen DJ, Sweitzer BJ, Bates DW, Burdick E, Edmondson A, Leape LL. Preventable adverse drug events in hospitalized patients: a comparative study of intensive care and general care units. Crit Care Med 1997;25(8):1289-97.

106. U.S. Department of Health and Human Services. Healthy People 2000: national health promotion and disease prevention objectives. Washington, DC: Government Printing Office, 1991.

107. Joint Commission. Section I: treatment of patients. Medication use. Accreditation manual for hospitals. Oakbrook Terrace, IL: 2003:1-25.

108. Walker J, Wynne H. Review: the frequency and severity of adverse drug reactions in elderly people. Age Ageing 1994;23(3):255-9.

109. Johnson JG, Spitzer RL, Williams JB, et al. Psychiatric comorbidity, health status, and functional impairment associated with alcohol abuse and dependence in primary care patients: findings of the PRIME MD-1000 study. J Consult Clin Psychol 1995;63(1):133-40.

110. Atkin PA, Shenfield GM. Medication-related adverse reactions and the elderly: a literature review. Adverse Drug React Toxicol Rev 1995;14(3):175-91.

111. Hanlon JT, Schmader KE, Koronkowski MJ, et al. Adverse drug events in high risk older outpatients. J Am Geriatr Soc 1997;45(8):945-8.

112. Bootman JL, Harrison DL, Cox E. The health care cost of drug-related morbidity and mortality in nursing facilities. Arch Intern Med 1997;157(18):2089-96.

113. Classen DC, Pestotnik SL, Evans RS, Lloyd JF, Burke JP. Adverse drug events in hospitalized patients. Excess length of stay, extra costs, and attributable mortality. JAMA 1997;277(4):301-6.

114. General Accounting Office. Prescription drugs and the elderly: many still receive potentially harmful drugs despite recent improvements. Washington, DC: U.S. General Accounting Office, 1995.

115. Wolff JL, Starfield B, Anderson G. Prevalence, expenditures, and complications of multiple chronic conditions in the elderly. Arch Intern Med 2002;162(20):2269-76.

116. Mion L, Odegard PS, Resnick B, Segal-Galan F. Interdisciplinary care for older adults with complex needs: American Geriatrics Society position statement. J Am Geriatr Soc 2006;54(5): 849-52.

117. U.S. Department of Health and Human Services. Healthy People 2010: understanding and improving health. 2nd ed. Washington, DC: U.S. Government Printing Office, November 2000.

118. Centers for Disease Control and Prevention and the Merck Company Foundation. The state of aging and health in America 2007. Whitehouse Station, NJ: Merck Company Foundation, 2007.

119. General Accounting Office. Prescription drugs: improvements needed in FDA's oversight of direct-to-consumer advertising. Washington, DC: U.S. General Accounting Office, December 14, 2006. (GAO-07-54.)

CHAPTER 18

Death and Dying

Albert I. Wertheimer, PhD, MBA

HISTORICAL DEVELOPMENT OF THE FIELD

In the 19th century it was quite common to learn that an individual had died from "natural causes." When a person aged 50 years or older died and there was no obvious violence, criminal activity, or observable pathology, it was reported that the patient had died of natural causes. Today, of course, we would not be satisfied with this cause of death because we are able to learn a great deal more about the pathology involved. Similarly, death in the 19th century was handled as a family activity. The deceased was displayed for a few days in the parlor of the house of a relative, and a burial took place shortly afterward. That quaint phenomenon no longer exists; a number of developments in both clinical medical practice as well as in the commercial world have replaced this tradition. In the 21st century no one would think of having a funeral and visitation take place without the involvement of a funeral parlor or mortuary. Funeral directors have taken over and arrange everything regarding the disposition of the newly departed.

However, there are a number of matters that cannot be solved or dealt with by the funeral director. Because diagnosis has become more precise, it is often possible to learn well in advance of the actual time of death of that impending event—even two or three years in advance. Naturally, the patient has an opportunity to react to this news, which is exactly what happens. Thanks to the work of Dr. Elizabeth Kübler-Ross, who began receiving widespread recognition in 1969, we know a great deal about the phases and activities involved in the dying process.[1]

The practicing pharmacist is often able to determine that a patient is in a terminal situation when the prescriptions for narcotic analgesics call for ever-increasing dosages and the patient appears to be in deteriorating health. What does the pharmacist say to the patient or to family members picking up the medications? Fortunately, through the work of Kübler-Ross, Moody,[2] Woodson,[3] and other pioneers in this discipline, we have some information that enables us to assist the dying patient and his or her family.

Kalish tells us that the dying process is like any other stage in human development: it is influenced by numerous decisions and other variables.[4] Well, what do we know? Actually, there is quite a robust literature on this topic. Numerous articles prior to the work of Kübler-Ross dealt with death and dying, but it was considered to be a morbid topic or a taboo area. In fact, some studies indicated that terminal patients were stigmatized and that nurses and other healthcare workers attempted to avoid them.[5] A 1963 study indicated that nurses took longer to respond to call lights or messages from terminal patients than nonterminal patients.[6] Some individuals have perceived the lives of younger people to be worth more in time and expense than the lives of the elderly, since the former are thought to have more social value. Glaser and Strauss reported that treatment of children and adolescents elicits more sympathy and attracts more workers than does treatment of the aged.[7]

Numerous reports in the literature indicate differential treatment of persons of different races and ethnic groups in all age groups. Even gender plays a role, in that society expects women to seek medical care when there is a need, whereas men are expected to be stoic. Some feel that men may die sooner partially as a result of their adherence to the male role model of "toughing it out" and not seeking care from a physician promptly. One's financial situation can influence whether one will seek care immediately or postpone it, as can whether one does or does not have adequate health insurance.

WHAT IS DEATH?

Death always has been and always will be with us. It is an integral part of human existence and has always been a subject of deep concern to all of us. Since the dawn of humankind, the human mind has pondered death, searching for the answer to its mysteries. The key to the question of death unlocks the door of life. Now, when humankind is surrounded by death and destruction as never before, it becomes essential that we study the problems of death and try to understand its true meaning.

Religious Perspective

Long before we had information or inferences from scientists and clinicians about death, what we knew or thought about death and dying came from religious teachings and from the writings of ancient philosophers. Full acceptance of the fact of death is seen as required in both Buddhism and Hinduism. It is felt that a person robs himself or herself of a purposeful live if the individual attempts to ignore death or deludes himself or herself into believing that he or she will endure forever. Only he who accepts death as an integral part of life, calmly and courageously, gains a purposeful life.

Buddhist teaching sees death as the cutting-off of the life force of a physical body, which is then transformed or displaced to continue functioning in another form. In this way, every birth is really a rebirth.[8]

The Hindu belief is that there are differences in the quality of deaths, depending on the degree of disciplined versus undisciplined living. Hindus pray for mercy at the hands of Yama, the God of Death, but recognize that after death, all persons are born again in the next world in a situation related to their deeds in this world. It is believed that an individual aspires toward the Supreme Person. When the individual finds the "self" and understands it truly, and thereby all worlds and desires, he or she gains immortality, which is understood to be freedom from the continuous chain of rebirth. For most Hindus, death is seen as a necessity and as a blessing. It is necessary because the world would run out of space and resources if no one died, and it is a blessing because it is an opportunity to move to a higher level of incarnation.[9]

Judaism teaches facing death in a straightforward manner and encourages the family to be present to support the dying person. Moreover, the deathbed confessional is considered important in the transition to the world to come. The dying person is expected, if possible, to seek repentance, to go through confession, to put his or her material matters in order, and to provide ethical instruction and blessing of the family. This enables the patient to express fears, find comfort and inner strength, and communicate meaningfully with those close to him or her. Orthodox Jews discuss an afterlife, but this is not a central tenet of the religion.[10]

The Christian view of death is probably most well known to the readers of this book. The concept of leading a good life in order to be admitted to heaven and of seeking rewards for the good or pure life on earth is recognized widely. The Catholic Last Rites when death is imminent are meant to assist in the path to heaven. The concept of a hell where "bad" people end up is the subject of numerous stories, jokes, and myths.

Scientific Perspective

In 1969 Kübler-Ross published her book *On Death and Dying*, which became a catalyst for an enormous body of subsequent work on this topic. She provided a grid or structure regarding the phases in the attitudes and behavior of the patient upon learning of the diagnosis of a terminal illness. The five phases are as follows:

- Denial
- Anger
- Bargaining
- Depression
- Acceptance

Denial is often accompanied by shock. Maybe the lab tests were wrong, perhaps the medical charts got mixed up. It can't be me—last week I was completely healthy. There is quite often a sensation of loneliness, recognizing that no one else can help and that the dying person is in this dilemma alone. There is considerable internal conflict while the patient ponders his or her new reality and health status. Guilt enters the consciousness. Did I do something to deserve this? I should have treated my parents/neighbors/teachers better or with more respect. There may be some degree of meaninglessness, where a person wonders if any efforts might postpone the inevitable and whether it would make any difference in the world even if that were possible.

Eventually, these emotions turn into anger: I worked so hard and never had that dreamed-of vacation. I won't be able to spend that money I've been saving for a comfortable retirement. I will not be able to meet my grandchildren, see graduations or weddings. It was a mistake to spend so much time on my career (or business) at the expense of family activities.

Some feel that it is not fair, and become angry because he or she is a "good" person, but that crook down the block is perfectly healthy at age 89. Anger can be directed at a dying person's loved ones, caregivers, and business associates, or randomly at persons he encounters as he is reminded of the situation by their vitality and energy or when he hears others making plans for the future. Anger is a phase that eventually fades and dissipates when the dying person realizes that it is not productive in changing the inevitable future course or in enhancing relationships with those he deals with.

At some point, the anger recedes, while not totally disappearing, being taken over by the bargaining phase. The wise or sensitive person comes to realize that others will avoid her if she can only talk about her problems. This whining makes others uncomfortable and contributes nothing toward a solution to the basic problem. It is a natural human instinct to attempt to bargain in an effort toward self-preservation. The patient says to her God, If you spare me, I will go to church every Sunday for the rest of my life, or if you let me live, I will volunteer my skills to poor or homeless persons, or I will be better at doing this or that. Many of us have met people who no longer eat candy or who teach Sunday religious school as a volunteer because "their prayer was answered or fulfilled."

It goes beyond the focus of this chapter to discuss the effectiveness of such offered bargains. The religiously devout will probably endorse them and suggest that a prayer might not have been fulfilled because the supplicant's life until that point in time was not sufficiently worthy. For those who tend to trust science and facts for the most part, such bargaining may appear to be a waste of time, but an activity that causes no harm.

Assuming that the prognosis remains bleak, next comes a gradual but steady realization of the actual consequences ahead and the dying person's powerlessness to modify that eventuality. This leads to a phase of depression. The person's life is about to end shortly and the quality of life between now and then may be most undesirable and limited. Most terminal patients conquer this depression and move toward the final phase prior to death—that of acceptance. These persons redevelop an increased self-awareness, and entry to this stage is observable as contact with others increases or as broken contacts are reestablished.

During acceptance, there is increased self-reliance and proactive efforts toward benefiting from the limited time available. Financial matters are put into final order; instructions to family and colleagues are given and pending matters are closed. The patient may want to learn about his disease in greater detail; he may volunteer his time for worthy causes so that more people will remember him as a kind and generous person (not, as in the earlier bargaining phase, in return for a reprieve). Patients often want to assist others with the same condition or to help prevent it, for example, by speaking to young people's groups about the dangers of cigarette smoking. Acceptance may include comforting those in the dying individual's immediate family, telling them to move on with their lives, and informing them that the patient is prepared for this finality.

Clearly, this model, as is the case with all models, is not accurate for all terminal persons or at all times. It is possible that someone might remain in the anger phase until the end, or until the final day. Also, many factors modify the application of this five-stage model. Those with ultrastrong religious views may act and feel differently from a nonreligious individual or from a devout believer in science.

The United States is composed of a large number of diverse ethnic and racial groups from all over the world. As one might expect, most of these numerous ethnic and racial groups have culturally learned practices and beliefs about death and dying. These practices and beliefs are too numerous to permit us to go into detail about any one of them, but the major differences lie in whether death is seen as a transition to another existence or as an end, and whether death is a type of punishment or whether it is a recognition that the individual might be ready for the next, possibly higher, life. Between these extremes, many different practices and beliefs coexist. To us as objective scientists and practitioners employing evidence-based treatments, it is frustrating, because we will not be able to know what is best, if anything is best.

Lynn Payer described a difference between British and American care for the terminally ill that should have great significance for us: "The lesser belief in medicine's ability to prolong life and the greater belief in medicine's role in making life nicer are undoubtedly the reason that hospices for the dying grew up first in Britain, not America. To accept the idea of hospice, one must accept the fact that people die. . . . American physicians seem to regard death as the ultimate failure of their skill. British doctors frequently regard death as physiological, sometimes even devoutly to be wished."[11]

Now in the 21st century, and with the benefit of religious scholars, scientists, philosophers, psychologists, clinicians, and laypersons having near-death experiences, we still ask: What is death and how should we think about it? Should we fear it or welcome it? Is death the end or a transition? For all of these questions, there are no definitive answers. Toynbee has described how humans have sought to reconcile themselves to the fact of death.[12] One strategy is hedonism—to enjoy life as much as possible before death comes into the picture. Another mechanism is the use of pessimism—convincing oneself that life is so distasteful that death is a relief from the unfortunate state of living. Suicide is an operationalization of such pessimism. Some may attempt to circumvent death through physical countermeasures such as serious exercise, proper nutrition, stress reduction, and healthy lifestyles.

One area of special interest is the death of children and young people. Death is seen as a natural consequence of aging. Were one to observe the obituary notices in any city newspaper, it is most likely the case that most of the deceased would be in their late 60s, or in their 70s or 80s. However, when we read about the death of a 12-year-old child, we have additional feelings of loss and remorse that such a young and "unlived" life was lost so soon. It is said that the greatest source of pain and anguish to parents is the death and burial of their child.

In all of the pages of this chapter to this point, death has been understood to mean the loss of life to some disease or from the sequelae of an automobile accident or other unintentional event. Yet, we all know that not all deaths are passive events. There are numerous examples of suicide or euthanasia (assisted suicide), and, of course, there are vastly different cultural reactions to the taking of one's own life. There is also death from military hostile activities and capital punishment by the civil authorities, all of which cases are not directly addressed in this chapter.

Perhaps one of the most difficult situations for a pharmacist to understand is a patient's intentional lack of medication adherence when the proper use of the medication could keep a life-threatening disease or condition at bay indefinitely. When nonadherence will surely lead to early health status decline and death, we ask how someone might elect to destroy themselves in such a way. The most vivid example is the intentional lack of adherence with antiretroviral drugs for patients with HIV/AIDS. With the proper use of the drugs, patients today can live fairly normal lives for an extended period of time—perhaps for 10 or more years. Why would someone fail to take his or her medications knowing that such behavior is a certain death sentence? Complex, multiple-drug therapy may cause such a decline in the quality of life from drug reactions that the patient may decide that life with painful drug side effects is too uncomfortable and that there is little or no hope for the future. Guilt may play a role, for example, in cases where a person may have unknowingly infected other persons with a life-threatening condition; rather than living with the guilt, the patient may elect to end his or her possibly pitiful existence.

BIOETHICS AND NEW TECHNOLOGIES

It seems strange that there can be anything new about death. It has been present since the existence of the first living being. Yet, scientific developments have raised new issues that did not require attention in earlier days. First of all, there is debate about the definition of death. As is widely known, a person may still have a functioning heart while in a coma or vegetative state even though there is no evidence of brain function. Persons can be maintained by respirators nearly indefinitely. There have been cases where this has been done for nearly two decades. The question of the time or definition of death has particular meaning for the families of those who are or might be deceased, and to the medical community as well. This latter interest becomes important when the patient at or near death is an organ donor.

The matter of new technologies to maintain life must be considered. Today, the medical armamentarium includes agents that are expected to extend the lives of terminal cancer patients by two months, at enormous expense and with a very limited quality of life. Should that therapy be undertaken, and who should make that decision? In recent times, some of these decisions have been made by the payers—the health insurance company or managed care organization that decides whether to pay for the therapy or not. Society will have to come to grips with these issues and questions.

The mirror image of that question is the matter of euthanasia—for example, when the kind and empathetic physician decides to increase the morphine level of a terminal patient in excruciating pain. Most often the request comes from the patient himself or herself or from close family members. The legalization of euthanasia (mercy killing) has been the source of passionate battles in the states where it has been considered. The law must provide protection to the caregiver who follows such a request so that he or she is not prosecuted for murder under existing laws.

It appears that Europeans have made more strides in the euthanasia debate than Americans. In the Netherlands, for example, a patient who is determined to be sane and aware of his decision can try to persuade his physician and a panel of other physicians that the prognosis is totally hopeless and that he can no longer endure the pain and suffering and the financial drain of his continued custodial, palliative care on him and his surviving family. The panel then reaches a decision to find a respectful response to his request so that he may die with dignity.[13]

SUMMARY

After thousands of years of recorded history, we still know very little of what happens during death and what follows it, if anything. The social sciences have given the pharmacist important facts, findings, and techniques to assist the terminal patient and the family in dealing with the process of dying. Understanding the different cultural and religious perspectives on death, the psychological and physical phases of the death and dying continuum, and the philosophical challenges that patients and families experience during the dying process can assist pharmacists in optimizing their support and care to a dying patient and his or her caregivers at the end of life.

REFERENCES

1. Kübler-Ross E. On death and dying. New York: Macmillan, 1969.
2. Moody RA. Life after life. Harrisburg, PA: Stackpole Books, 1976.
3. Woodson R. Concept of hospice care in terminal disease. In: Veath JM, ed. Breast cancer. Basle, Switzerland: Karger, 1976:16-179.
4. Kalish RA. Death and dying in a social context. In: Binstock RH, Shanas E, eds. Handbook of aging and the social sciences. 2nd ed. New York: VanNostrand, 1985:149-170.
5. Feifel H, ed. The meaning of death. New York: McGraw-Hill, 1959.
6. Aldrich CK. The dying patient's grief. JAMA 1963;184:329.
7. Glaser B, Strauss A. Time for dying. Chicago: Aldine, 1968.
8. Kübler-Ross E. Death: the final stage of growth. Englewood Cliffs, NJ: Prentice Hall, 1975:66.
9. Ibid., 68.
10. Shneidman ES. Death: current perspectives. Palo Alto, CA: Mayfield, 1980:36.
11. Payer L. Medicine and culture. New York: Penguin, 1989:120.
12. Toynbee A. The relation between life and death, living and dying. In: Toynbee A, Mant AK, Smart N, et al. Man's concern with death. New York: McGraw-Hill, 1968.
13. van der Heide A, Onwuteaka-Philipsen B, Rurup M, et al. End-of-life practices in the Netherlands under the Euthanasia Act. New Engl J Med 2007;356(19):1957-65.

CHAPTER 19

Care for Individuals with Mental Illness

Nathaniel M. Rickles, PharmD, PhD, BCPP

Every day, in practically every pharmacy setting, a pharmacist will interact with an individual who has a mental illness. We may not know for certain that the individual has a mental illness, because physical and mental illnesses share the same properties of being associated with conditions that are both observable and not observable. Mental illness affects millions of Americans and has no demographic boundaries: it affects the young, the old, males, females, different ethnic groups, different educational levels, and different geographic areas. Certain mental illnesses may be more common in one group than another, such as depression, which is twice as prevalent in women than men.[1] The care of those with mental illness is the subject of a booming pharmaceutical industry and a wide range of psychological services aimed at controlling symptoms and reducing the societal costs associated with uncontrolled symptoms. At the outset, it is important to note that the reader be conscious of efforts being made throughout this chapter to avoid labeling individuals as "schizophrenic" or "mentally ill" and, rather, to refer to this population as "individuals with mental illness." The identity of individuals is much more than their illness; the illness should not define them but rather be a part of them. Individuals with mental illness are mothers, fathers, sisters, brothers, friends, employees, and so on. A discussion about labeling and its consequences and why this change in language is important appears later in this chapter.

To fully appreciate the current mental health system and pharmacy's role in it, it is important to spend the first part of this chapter understanding the historical development of the U.S. mental healthcare system. Such history will also bring forward the key psychosocial issues that affect all stakeholders in the mental health system, including pharmacists. This historical context forms the basis for the second part of the chapter, which focuses on current issues in mental health care, and the third part, which deals with the roles of pharmacy in mental health care.

HISTORY OF MENTAL HEALTH CARE IN AMERICA _____

Colonial America

Many of the attitudes and behaviors of the early colonists toward individuals with mental illness stemmed from European attitudes that developed over centuries. Documents written in 15th-century Europe, such as the *Malleus Maleficarum* (Witches' hammer), stated that demons representing the devil could invade the souls of individuals and result in deviant acts.[2] European society identified individuals with mental illness as deviant, persecuted these individuals, and burned them at the stake for being "Satan's representatives."[2] Given such origins, it is not surprising that the colonists believed mental illnesses flowed from natural and supernatural sources such as the devil.[3] The colonists would eventually come to believe that individuals with mental illness were not passive recipients of these spirits but rather that they had individual control over these impulses.

In general, individuals who were "distracted" and "lunatick" were perceived as an individual rather than a societal problem. There were no social policies to deal with individuals with mental illness.[3] Subsequently, individuals with mental illness who were unable to support themselves were viewed as the primary responsibility of their family. Based on British principles of collective responsibility, both the poor and individuals with mental illness who threatened public safety and were not cared for by their families were helped by local communities.[3] This latter civic philosophy of the colonists led to the development of institutional care for individuals with mental illness. Institutional care for individuals with mental illness came largely in four forms during the mid- and late 1700s: general hospitals, private institutions, public hospitals (the first public hospital for individuals with mental illness was founded in Virginia in 1769), and prisons.[3] Because of the low population density in the colonial and early American period, the number of individuals identified with mental illness was low.

Nineteenth-Century America

As the population of the new America grew and the industrial revolution led to shifts from farms to factories, individuals became more geographically mobile and less likely to remain home. Such transformations led to the need for more institutions to care for people with mental illnesses. The 1800s brought about a surge in the number of public and private institutions (asylums) caring for individuals with mental illness.

This increase in asylums was also supported by two other factors: (1) the thinking that therapeutic approaches for mental illnesses required a well-ordered institution and (2) beliefs from the arrival of the religious Second Great Awakening suggesting that individuals are capable of overcoming their weaknesses and being cured.[3]

Because the government saw itself as having an obligation to care for all its citizens, more and more individuals were admitted into the local asylums. City asylums became overcrowded and were poorly staffed. These conditions and the efforts of consumer advocate Dorothea Dix led to the development of more state-funded asylums in the geographic centers of different states to ensure equal access for all citizens.[3] These early asylums were focused on "moral treatment," which consisted of religious exercises, recreation, and mechanical restraint. The institutionalization of individuals with mental illness was largely made by family members, with only a small role played by the legal system. The asylums were generally composed of diverse patient populations with multiple diagnoses and cultures; some asylums were segregated along racial and ethnic lines. In particular, the number of older adults committed to asylums grew because local authorities saw the benefit of redefining problems in the elderly as being psychiatric in nature and having the state pay for such care.

As the size and diversity of the asylums grew, the social organization and treatment philosophy of the asylums became more rigid and coercive. For example, overworked attendants would often respond to behavioral problems with force and heavily resort to straightjackets and seclusion rooms. In contrast, there were also some cases where close interpersonal relationships were formed between patients and staff.

The Rise of American Psychiatry

Many of the early physicians treating individuals with mental illness saw their roles as curing mental illnesses through two main mechanisms: guiding patients regarding appropriate behaviors and correcting imbalances in the physical-mental system through the use of chemicals or biological procedures. Among an organization of asylum directors (the Association of Medical Superintendents of American Institutions for the Insane, or AMSAII), there seemed to be a lack of national consensus about how asylums could optimally provide care to individuals with acute and chronic mental illnesses.[3] This conflict in treatment ideology, the lack of curative treatments, and the growing numbers in the asylums contributed to the characterization of asylums as depressing, hopeless "snake pits" where staff members were focused on maintaining the patients' daily routines.

The first approach to treating mental illnesses—guiding patients toward appropriate behaviors—developed from a growing scientific interest during the late 19th century in understanding the psychological and social roots of human behavior.

During this period numerous physicians were exploring different systematic approaches to talking with patients to work through their mental illnesses and help them return to better functioning. It is hard to identify precisely the birth of psychotherapy; however, contrary to popular thought, Sigmund Freud was not the founder of psychotherapy. Such confusion about the origins of psychotherapy are largely a result of how the media and textbooks have popularized Freud's early 20th century use of psychoanalysis and "lying on the couch" techniques to investigate the meanings of hidden or subconscious impulses and dreams. Today, there are over 400 known approaches to psychotherapy.[4] These psychotherapeutic approaches differ in the extent to which they apply behavioral, cognitive, and emotional modalities to helping improve patient functioning. Multimodal approaches that use a combination of psychotherapeutic techniques are common. For example, cognitive-behavioral therapies are one of the more widely used and effective psychotherapeutic modalities employed in the care of consumers with various mental health concerns (e.g., life adjustments, role conflicts, stress management) and psychiatric illnesses.

During the late 1800s, the second mechanism of treating mental illnesses—chemical or biological treatments—became more widely used as physicians began exploring the possibility that there were biological causes of mental illness. Such interests were promulgated by the extensive debate as to whether President Garfield's assassin, Charles Guiteau, had mental illness or not at the time of the assassination.[5] During this time the field of neurology began to emerge and individuals such as Dr. Emil Kraepelin began to scientifically explore what later became known as schizophrenia.[2] This period was also marked by the identification of various areas and functions of the brain, as reflected in the works of Drs. Alois Alzheimer, Carl Wernicke, and Alfred Meyer. To reflect this shift toward a more biological basis for behavior, AMSAII became the American Medico-Psychological Association in 1892. The American Medico-Psychological Association was the precursor to the modern-day American Psychiatric Association, which was founded in 1921.[3] Psychiatry was seen as a dynamic continuum between normal and abnormal, and its scientific study took place more and more in research institutes and psychiatric hospitals.

Mental illnesses were beginning to be seen as hereditary and thus as occurring from one generation to the next.[3] Therefore, supporters of the eugenics movement called for laws regulating the marriage and involuntary sterilization of the mentally ill. Another aspect of this movement was its focus on prevention of mental illnesses, which gradually developed greater predominance in mental health services. In 1909, a National Committee for Mental Hygiene (NCMH) was formed with the goals of protecting individuals with mental illness, improving hospitals for the mentally ill, promoting research on treatment and prevention, and establishing state societies of mental health.[3]

Transition to Community-Based Mental Health Care

Several forces brought about change in the nature and extent of mental health services delivered to individuals with mental illness. The economic depression of the 1930s and World War II brought about reductions in hospital funding to carry out services, provide staffing, and add physical facilities. Such reductions and the growing numbers of patients led to poor treatment conditions such as lack of cleanliness and abusive staff. The author Mary Jane Ward depicted such poor conditions in her book *The Snake Pit*, which became a motion picture in 1948.[3] These conditions contributed to growing tensions between state governments and asylum psychiatrists regarding the proper amount of professional autonomy and accountability.

World War II also brought about changes in how psychiatrists viewed the treatment trajectory of many mental illnesses. Military psychiatrists came from the battlefields reporting brief treatment of such symptoms as irritability, anxiety, and nightmares and then sending soldiers back to the battlefields. Such reports helped the mental health treatment community begin to think that more treatment of individuals with mental illness could occur in the community and not necessarily require hospitalization. Psychiatrists were beginning to think that early treatment might even prevent hospitalization.

During the 1930s and 1940s new biological treatments also were being explored, such as insulin shock treatments, electric shock therapy, fever therapy, and frontal lobotomies. Although these approaches were found to have serious side effects and risks, they were important steps by psychiatry to explore how changes in body chemistry and structure lead to potential therapeutic changes in patient behavior. Psychiatrists were beginning to explore the use of existing medications to treat symptoms of mental illness. Chlorpromazine, an antihistamine, was typically used to relax surgical patients experiencing surgical trauma. Psychiatrists examined chlorpromazine's benefits in helping to sedate patients with schizophrenia. The success of chlorpromazine in schizophrenia made many physicians realize the potential for drugs that affect behavior to treat the symptoms of mental illnesses. As a result, many more drugs began to be developed to manage psychiatric symptoms, such as the tranquilizer reserpine and antidepressants such as iproniazid and imipramine.

In conjunction with the increase in biological treatments of mental illnesses, there was also a shift toward greater diagnostic classification of symptoms in mental disorders.

The American Psychiatric Association's first edition of the *Diagnostic and Statistical Manual of Mental Disorders* (DSM) was developed in 1952 and identified 128 diagnostic categories. In 1994, the DSM-IV had 357 categories/diagnoses of mental illnesses, organized according to five main axes:

Axis 1: Clinical disorders, other conditions that may be a focus of clinical attention
Axis 2: Personality disorders, mental retardation
Axis 3: General medical conditions
Axis 4: Psychosocial and environmental problems
Axis 5: Global assessment of functioning

Since the first DSM edition, there have been numerous changes in what and how illnesses are classified.[6]

The increase in biological treatments and the diagnostic classification of mental illnesses were both a part of a growing movement toward the "medicalization" of mental illness, in which doctors targeted patients' symptoms with treatments and failed to view the psychosocial aspects of the patient's experience.[7] The promise of psychopharmacology in managing psychiatric symptoms and the poor conditions in state hospitals were contributors to the realization that the country needed greater federal resources to ensure greater scientific research and training involving these new treatments as well as improvements in hospital care. The National Institute of Mental Health was founded in 1949 and pledged to train more mental health professionals through fellowships and grants and to support research relating to the cause, diagnosis, and treatment of mental illness.[3] In addition, President Kennedy's 1961 Joint Commission on Mental Illness and Health called for larger investments in basic research, more training programs and guidelines for treatments, and greater public education about mental illness.[3] Such federal initiatives led to rapid expansions in various mental health occupations, such as clinical psychology, psychiatric social work, and psychiatric nursing.

There was also a growing focus on community health care, stimulated in part by the Hill-Burton Act of 1946, which brought about a general increase in community hospitals and their development of psychiatric units.[3] These inpatient units admitted patients with severe and persistent mental illnesses. The 1960s brought greater development of community psychiatry through the construction of community mental health centers (CMHCs). These CMHCs largely provided care to those with substance abuse and life issues such as marital problems and other personal stressors. The increase in community-based sites for mental health care helped improve access to early intervention services and avoid long-term psychiatric hospitalizations. At the same time that community-based psychiatry was taking shape, the Social Security Act of 1965 encouraged the states to reduce costs by shifting the care of older adults with mental illnesses from state-operated psychiatric hospitals to federally funded nursing homes. This combination of changes led to four major points of access to mental health services and, thus, the types of patients served by the setting: CMHCs for individuals with less severe illnesses, inpatient community-based hospitals for individuals with more severe illness but requiring limited treatment, state-based psychiatric facilities for young and middle-aged individuals with mental illness requiring more extensive treatment, and nursing homes for older adults with mental illnesses.

Transition to Greater Consumerism in Mental Health Care

During the 1960s and 1970s, there were significant challenges to the medicalization of mental illnesses. Erving Goffman's 1961 book *Asylums* highlighted how prolonged psychiatric hospitalizations led to individuals losing their self-identity and esteem and contributed to acts of deviance.[8] Goffman described how individuals living for months and years in psychiatric hospitals became "institutionalized" and lost critical skills and abilities needed to function outside the hospital. Others during this time, such as psychiatrists R. D. Laing and Thomas Szasz and philosopher Michel Focault, questioned the diagnosis and treatment of mental illnesses. They saw such medical diagnoses and treatments as a way for society to label and control people who may think and behave differently from those in the mainstream culture. One example supporting such arguments is the American Psychiatric Association's decision to include homosexuality as a psychiatric illness in the DSM until 1980, when it was removed from the third edition of the DSM.

Additional challenges to psychiatry were seen in the courts and on television. The court case of *Rouse vs. Cameron* (1966) supported the expectation that individuals with mental illness who were committed to psychiatric hospitals had a right to adequate treatments.[3] Ken Kesey's book *One Flew Over the Cuckoo's Nest* and the subsequent 1975 movie based on it powerfully presented the unjust and involuntary treatment of individuals with mental illness.

Because of these challenges to the mental healthcare system, the National Alliance on Mental Illness (NAMI) was formed in 1979 and became the largest national grassroots mental health organization dedicated to "improving the lives of persons living with serious mental illness and their families."[9] This organization widely publishes brochures, books, and other materials to promote awareness about mental illnesses and their consequences. The Mental Health Systems Act of 1980 provided protection of patient rights and support services for vulnerable groups.[3] In particular, mental health advocates were concerned that commitment procedures were often vague and arbitrary, that individuals should have a right to refuse treatment, and that care should be provided in a confidential manner.

Modern Psychiatric Care

In the late 1970s concerns mounted about the quality of institutional care and consumer rights. Concurrently, several effective medications were being brought to market that targeted the symptoms of various mental illnesses. These factors led to the government perceiving the need and value of releasing long-term institutionalized persons from state facilities and having them enter the community. This "deinstitutionalization" process resulted in many state psychiatric hospitals closing and individuals with mental illness being released into the streets without follow-up care, shelter, and other resources necessary for their successful integration into communities. Many of these individuals would return to the hospital quickly because of poor follow-up and inadequate management of symptoms. These individuals would go in and out of the psychiatric hospitals multiple times (known as the "revolving door" phenomenon) and often leave clinicians and hospital staff frustrated.[10]

In response to these concerns, the National Institute of Mental Health initiated a federal/state partnership to develop programs for those with severe and persistent mental illnesses related to housing, financial assistance, treatment, and support services. The State Comprehensive Mental Health Services Plan Act of 1984 and its 1989 modification were designed to test the effectiveness of the different approaches.[3] One program that served as a model for several outpatient mental health programs was the Program for Assertive Community Treatment (PACT) founded in Madison, Wisconsin, in 1980.[11] PACT was designed to prevent hospitalizations by teaching individuals with mental illness skills and providing support services to enable these individuals to live in the community. Some of these services included ongoing monitoring, crisis intervention, and family involvement in care. Results showed that PACT enabled individuals with mental illness to have better personal relationships, greater satisfaction with care, and lower rates of hospitalizations. Today, there are several community-based programs that attempt to better target exacerbation of symptoms and reduce hospitalizations.

The current mental health system involves a mix of state psychiatric facilities, private psychiatric facilities, inpatient psychiatric units in community hospitals, community mental health centers, and a variety of clinics and short-term stay facilities. Since the 1950s revolution in psychiatric medicines, hundreds of psychiatric medicines have come to the market to treat a variety of mental illnesses. Newer psychotropic medicines have fewer side effects and fewer drug interactions and are useful in targeting specific symptoms of illnesses. Much of the literature recommends that ideal treatments for a variety of psychiatric illnesses should involve both cognitive and behavioral therapies along with medications. Also, numerous public health efforts have improved the screening and detection of mental illnesses.

The historical context of the first part of this chapter lays the foundation for appreciating the development of the modern mental healthcare system in the United States. Such context also shapes some of the key contemporary trends and issues in mental health, such as the focus on labeling and reducing stigma, searching for etiologies of mental disorders, facilitating patient recovery, establishing parity in mental health insurance, and determining the best psychotropic prescribing practices.

CONTEMPORARY ISSUES IN MENTAL HEALTH CARE

Labeling and Reducing the Stigma of Mental Illness

Labels identify or define who we are. How do we define mental illness? What does a person with mental illness look like and how is he or she different from a physically ill person? People typically respond to such questions by saying that individuals with mental illness look odd and unkempt, talk to themselves, and act strangely. They will also respond that physically ill individuals have something visibly wrong, such as a broken leg, look pale, and appear weak. Although these generalizations (stereotypes) of individuals with mental and physical illness hold true in many cases, there are many situations in which it becomes difficult to distinguish who has mental or physical illness. For example, in both cases of high blood pressure and depression or anxiety, the symptoms may not be evident; thus, it is difficult to discern that the individual has either or both illnesses. Individuals also confuse the distinctions between developmental disorders, such as Down syndrome or autism, and mental disorders.

Definitions of mental illness also change depending on both clinical and sociocultural perspectives. For example, the American Psychiatric Association defines mental illness in clinical terms as:

> A clinically significant behavioral or psychological syndrome or pattern that occurs in an individual and that is associated with present distress (e.g., a painful symptom) or disability (i.e., impairment in one or more important areas of functioning) or with a significantly increased risk of suffering death, pain, disability, or an important loss of freedom.[6]

Conversely, Eaton uses a sociocultural perspective and defines mental illness as including two components: "(1) a collection of emotions or behaviors that meet all three conditions: rare, culturally deviant, inexplicable and (2) leads to one or more of following consequences: loss of control over environment, detachment from social networks, and interference with the individual's sense of biography/self."[2]

Regardless of which definition and perspective we wish to accept and the extent to which we include various illnesses as a part of the spectrum of mental illness, we are faced with the question of what it means to label someone as having mental illness. The signs and symptoms of most mental illnesses are often viewed as "deviant" because they fall outside the typical boundaries of expected human cognition and behavior. For example, most people would not report that their thoughts are being broadcast on television (a symptom of schizophrenia) and would consider this symptom as deviant thinking. Any form of deviance is dependent on culture because norms are defined by the culture. Some cultures may view individuals with mental illness as possessing special powers. In other words, an individual acting bizarrely is only considered deviant if the culture that surrounds that individual believes the behavior is deviant. Why does society develop such labels for acts considered deviant? Society determines what is deviant in large part so it can ensure structure, order, and context to daily living and expectations.

Stigma is a negative consequence of labeling and is associated with three components: it (1) sets a person apart from others, (2) links the marked person to undesirable characteristics, and (3) rejects and avoids the labeled individual.[12] A person may have consciously or unconsciously stigmatized an individual with mental illness when he or she sees a poorly dressed man talking angrily to himself and thinks that the man is acting strange and is potentially dangerous, and therefore avoids going near him. Stigma is a matter of degree because it often depends on how much the individual being marked is linked with the undesirable characteristics. An individual may feel less prejudice toward a person who acts a little strange but quietly sits on a bench than toward a person who talks angrily to himself because the former may be perceived as less dangerous.

Scales measuring stigma have been developed and validated.[13] One hears and sees stigma communicated on a daily basis throughout our culture through words such as *nut*, *crazy*, *cuckoo*, *psycho*, and *sicko*. One key source of stigma is the portrayals of individuals with mental illness in television, movies, and novels. Hollywood has often presented individuals with mental illness as deranged, dangerous, impulsive, and uncontrollable.[14] Examples of such movies are *Friday the 13th: A New Beginning* (1985), *Psycho III* (1986), *Misery* (1990), and *Silence of the Lambs* (1991). There have been some more positive movie images of individuals with mental illness, such as *A Beautiful Mind* (2001). Novels such as William Heffernan's *Ritual* (1988) and Jeff Raines's *Unbalanced Acts* (1990) both describe murderers with significant psychopathology.

Although clinicians are thought to be unconditional and not affected by such negative attitudes, the literature provides evidence that clinicians express similar discomfort with those with mental illness as the general public.[15] There has been some research exploring the attitudes of those in pharmacy toward individuals with mental illness. Several studies show that pharmacists and pharmacy students have generally positive views toward those with mental illness.[16-20] However, Phokeo and colleagues found that

Canadian community pharmacists were significantly more uncomfortable discussing symptoms and medications with consumers with mental illness than with those who had cardiovascular concerns.[18] As a result, it appeared that individuals with mental illness received fewer pharmacy services than those with cardiovascular illnesses.

In recent years, there have been numerous local, state, and national campaigns by consumer advocacy organizations to increase screening for mental illness and reduce its stigma. There have been numerous direct-to-consumer advertisements regarding mental illnesses and treatments for mental illnesses. Further, the National Institute of Mental Health continues to encourage research regarding the study and reduction of the stigma of mental illnesses. These combined efforts may be associated with the significant increases in the number of consumers receiving various psychotropic medications such as antidepressants and antianxiety agents.[21] All these changes would presumably reduce the stigma associated with mental illnesses. In particular, because most individuals know one or more individuals taking antidepressants, it would be expected that the stigma associated with depression would be much less prevalent than in previous years. However, Bell and associates found that pharmacy students and pharmacists did not distinguish between individuals with severe depression and schizophrenia.[20] The lack of a difference in stigma in this study may be because schizophrenia was compared with severe depression and not more common types of depression. It is likely that the level of symptom severity and/or the uncontrollable nature of behaviors can affect the degree of stigma associated with a mental illness. Future research will also need to explore how stigma affects pharmacists' willingness to provide services to individuals with mental illness.

Searching for Etiologies of Mental Illness

Although there has been much progress in mental health care over the last century, we are still unclear about the role of many structures in the brain, and about how various mental illnesses develop and respond to treatments. The mechanisms of action of most psychotropics also remain unknown. To answer these and other questions about the etiology and treatment of mental illnesses, neuroscientists have been actively engaged in considerable research exploring the use of brain imaging technologies and radioactive lab techniques to help link brain structures and functions with behavior and patient outcomes. Another important area of research in the etiology of mental illness has explored the concept of stress and how stress contributes to mental illness.

This latter research area has yielded both biological and social definitions of stress. Hans Selye, in *The Stress of Life*, described stress biologically as a disruption in the normal homeostasis of organisms and described three phases of the stress response, also known as the general adaptation syndrome (GAS): a general and widespread alarm stage, a specific response stage involving defense of tissues, and exhaustion if the stressor is not removed.[22] In related work, Seligman reported that individuals who are ineffective in terminating a stressor will eventually give up and accept the stressor (he called this learned helplessness).[23] Selye also found that many different stressors or mental representations of stressors led to the same GAS, that the entire organism was affected, and that GAS could lead to exhaustion in the absence of the stressor.[22] It is believed that these consequences of GAS explain in large part some of the symptoms of depression and anxiety.

In addition to these biological conceptualizations of stress, most social scientists have defined stress as it relates to feelings of being overwhelmed by circumstances. For example, Mechanic defines stress as "a discrepancy between the demands impinging on an individual, and his/her potential responses to those demands."[24] Wheaton defines stress as "conditions of threat, demands, or structural constraints that, by the very fact of their occurrence or existence, call into question the operating integrity of the organism."[25] Although there is general agreement on what defines stress socially or biologically, individuals vary considerably on how they interpret various stressors, with some events being more or less stressful. There has been considerable research in mental health care on identifying how different life events in isolation and cumulatively contribute to the risk for mental illnesses. The diathesis stress model is a well-known model that has added considerably to how researchers and clinicians think stressors result in mental illnesses.

In this context, *diathesis* refers to genetic or inherited vulnerability to respond to stress in maladaptive ways.[2] The model demonstrates that the manifestation of mental illness is a combined result of stress, a genetic risk for mental illnesses (such as schizophrenia, bipolar illness, depression, anxiety, etc.), how severely those disorders get manifested based on stress, and the protectiveness of one's environment. At high levels of stress (such as prolonged combat or a new transition) or in those having a significant genetic predisposition to mental illness, many individuals may meet the criteria for having a mental disorder. Individuals exposed to a high level of stress and possessing a strong genetic predisposition to mental illness may be more likely to experience the more severe forms of a mental illness. Only those individuals who have little genetic predisposition to an illness or are exposed to low environmental stress may avoid symptoms of mental illness. It is possible that individuals who have high genetic predisposition to a mental illness may avoid meeting criteria for the disorder if they live in a protective environment that provides adequate support.

Although the diathesis stress model is a useful way to conceptualize the interaction of genetics and stress in predicting the likelihood of mental illness, Kendler and Eaves note that the model is built on the questionable assumption that genes and the environment act additively and independently of each other.[26] This assumption is problematic because individuals often select their own environments, and such environments then act differently with their genetic predispositions; therefore, it becomes unclear how much of the vulnerability to mental illness is associated with environmental stress and how much is due to genetic predisposition.

Facilitating Patient Recovery

The concept that individuals can recover from mental illnesses is not new; it has been around since the 1980s, when studies and first-person accounts highlighted that individuals with mental illness can come out of the system relatively intact and return to a sense of self and self-worth.[27,28] This concept of recovery is central to many of the current outreach and public education efforts of organizations advocating for individuals with mental illness and their families. Jacobson and Greenley's model of recovery suggests that *recovery* refers to both the internal and external conditions that enable a person to return to fuller functioning in society.[29]

The internal conditions of recovery include hope, healing, empowerment, and connection. *Hope* refers to the individual's belief that recovery is possible. Having such a belief often means that individuals have accepted that there is a problem and involves committing to change, focusing on the positives, and avoiding the negative aspects of their past experiences. Jacobson and Greenley indicate that *healing* means not necessarily a return to baseline functioning but rather overcoming internalized stigma toward oneself for having mental illness and regaining self-esteem, self-respect, control over symptoms, and/or managing the social and psychological effects of stress.[29] These authors refer to *empowerment* as an internal capacity to take greater control and responsibility for oneself. *Connection* is that part of recovery in which the individual reconnects with the social world by filling various roles in society, including employment, family, religion, and community participation.

External conditions of recovery are those conditions outside the individual that help the individual achieve recovery. These conditions include human rights, a supportive culture, and the availability of recovery-oriented services. *Human rights* include those efforts to (1) reduce and eliminate stigma and discrimination against persons with psychiatric disabilities, (2) promote and protect the rights of those in the mental health system, (3) provide equal opportunities for individuals in education, employment, and housing, and (4) ensure access to needed resources such as food, shelter, and services that facilitate recovery (job training, subsidized housing, health services, etc.). A *supportive culture* highlights the need to incorporate individual rights into all decisions and incorporate informed consent as a part of daily practice. The need for informed consent has been especially important given past media reports that individuals with mental illness were not adequately informed of being put on placebos in clinical trials evaluating drug efficacy and toxicity. Another aspect of a supportive culture is the development of collaborative relationships regarding all aspects of care among individuals with mental illness, their families, and the health-care team. This approach views the individual with mental illness as capable of active participation in decision making.

The provision of *recovery-oriented services* is typically directed at symptom relief, crisis intervention, case management, rehabilitation, protection of rights, and support. Models of psychiatric rehabilitation integrate services provided by professionals, consumers, and collaboratively between providers and consumers.[29] Professionals often provide services related to medication management, therapy, and case management. Consumer-run services are developed and implemented by consumers for consumers and include peer support programs, hospitalization alternatives, hotlines, online support groups, and other programs involving role modeling and mentoring. Collaborative services are provided by and for consumers, professionals, family members, friends, and other members of the community. These latter services include recovery education and training, crisis planning, development of recovery and treatment plans, consumer rights, and so on.

The internal and external conditions of recovery are interdependent. A movement toward facilitating an external condition can help bring about positive change in an internal condition of recovery; likewise, a change in internal conditions can lead to a change in the external conditions of recovery. Two examples illustrate this interdependence. First, a local community's effort to reduce stigma can help individuals with mental illness heal and gain a better sense of self. Second, as more individuals enter recovery, they will provide more models for policy-related efforts to facilitate recovery services and a larger supportive culture for healing.

Establishing Parity in Mental Health Insurance

Since the birth of the managed healthcare movement in the 1970s and 1980s, health insurance companies have explored multiple ways to increase their profit margins by controlling the rising costs of health care. Such cost-containment approaches include setting up restricted lists of medications that are less expensive (formularies), restricting the number of office visits and procedures, and sharing costs with consumers through copayments and deductibles. Although these approaches have been applied to both physical and mental health care, there is evidence that the health insurance industry has not applied these and other approaches equally across physical and mental illnesses. Some of these inequities may be due in part to the fact that physical and mental health care have been handled separately by many health insurance plans. That is, many health insurance plans, including government-based plans, have contracted out ("carved out") the management of mental health services to behavioral healthcare organizations in an effort to identify more cost-efficient systems to specifically manage growing mental health costs. These contracted service providers or managed behavioral healthcare organizations are under significant pressures to contain mental healthcare costs to maximize profits.

These pressures and the stigma regarding mental illnesses are thought to be some of the key reasons for the insurance industry's greater health coverage for physical illnesses than mental illnesses. Such actions have left individuals with mental illness with restricted access to mental health care—for example, limited numbers of psychotherapy visits, medication management visits, and days of psychiatric hospitalization. Research has shown that limits in mental health insurance have caused individuals to limit their use of medications and other treatments, which puts them and the health system at risk for negative outcomes, including worsening symptoms and higher health costs.[30] Consumers and their families have advanced numerous successful efforts at local, state, and federal levels to enact legislation requiring greater parity in health insurance between physical and mental illnesses. Until more national health reforms are made, this debate over parity of coverage will likely remain a significant concern for consumers and providers throughout the mental health system.

Psychotropic Prescribing Practices

Psychiatrists, medical doctors specializing in mental health, traditionally were the main prescribers of psychotropic medications. In the last two decades, however, there have been significant changes in psychotropic prescribing. First, psychiatrists are not the only medical doctors prescribing medications for individuals with mental illness. There have been significant increases in the prescribing of antidepressants and anxiety medications by primary care physicians.[21] It is not entirely clear whether this increase is a result of an increase in public recognition of depression and anxiety disorders (via direct-to-consumer advertising), of primary care physicians having a better understanding of depression and greater comfort with antidepressants and their relatively safer medication profiles than in years past, or of the insurance industry's effort to limit patient access to specialists such as psychiatrists, or a combination of these reasons. In addition, physicians of all practice types are using psychotropic medications for medical conditions such as pain management and sleep disorders. There is growing concern that psychotropic medications are being prescribed without clear and documented indication that the individual patient needs the medication.

Nurse practitioners and physician assistants are two professions within the allied health professions that have prescribing privileges throughout the United States and thus contribute to a significant amount of psychotropic prescribing. Pharmacists in several states have collaborative practice agreements with physicians that allow them to prescribe under limited situations. Pharmacists have prescribing privileges in Veteran Affairs Medical Centers and in specialized settings such as state facilities for individuals with developmental disabilities. Psychologists have lobbied in several states to have prescribing privileges for psychotropic medications. These individuals are typically required to take courses and pass certification requirements to be allowed to prescribe these medications.

The American Psychiatric Association and the American Medical Association have initiated successful lobbying efforts to thwart many of these legislative initiatives for other practitioners to have prescribing privileges. Physicians may feel threatened that other professionals are encroaching on their roles as prescribers and affecting their ability to generate income from prescribing. They also argue that these other health professionals lack the education and training to prescribe safely. Pharmacists interested in prescribing privileges have argued persuasively through a growing number of demonstration projects and published interventions that pharmacist management of medication therapy can have a significant impact on many patient outcomes, including lower costs, improved clinical outcomes, and improved adherence.[31-35]

PHARMACY ROLES IN MENTAL HEALTH CARE

Pharmacists in mental health care have been involved in numerous collaborative services with physicians, including (1) monitoring and reducing side effects, (2) assessing drug serum concentrations, (3) identifying drug interactions, (4) assisting in the development of treatment plans, and (5) identifying ways to improve medication adherence. Over the past three decades, clinical pharmacists performing these kinds of collaborative services to individuals with mental illness have been shown to have a significant and positive impact on several patient and health system outcomes.[36-40] These studies have specifically demonstrated that psychotropic monitoring by clinical pharmacists was significantly associated with reductions in the number and doses of medications, hospitalizations, and side effects and in improved medication adherence and clinical symptoms. Community pharmacists have also been shown to have a significant and positive impact on psychotropic education and monitoring.[41-43] These latter studies have shown that community pharmacists can significantly improve patient knowledge, beliefs, and sense of treatment progress. More multicenter cost-effectiveness trials are needed to further demonstrate the role of pharmacists in mental health care.[40]

Since the late 1970s and early 1980s, there have been increased postgraduate opportunities in pharmacy practice, such as psychiatric pharmacy residencies and fellowships throughout the country to increase the number of trained pharmacists in mental health care. These psychiatric residencies and fellowships provide pharmacists an opportunity to train specifically in the area of mental health care. In the late 1990s, pharmacists who had extensive experiences in mental health care and/or had completed specialty residencies in psychiatric pharmacy became eligible to demonstrate their competencies in national certification exams on psychiatric pharmacy. A successful completion of these certification exams allows individuals to become board certified in psychiatric pharmacy (BCPP) for a 7-year period until they are required to meet requirements for recertification. The number of psychiatric pharmacists has grown considerably since the late 1990s and was the impetus for the development of an association in 1998, the College of Psychiatric and Neurologic Pharmacists (CPNP), dedicated to the following mission: "to promote excellence in pharmacy practice, education and research to optimize treatment outcomes of individuals affected by psychiatric and neurologic disorders."[44]

SUMMARY

This chapter has, it is hoped, enlightened the reader concerning the rich and complex history of care provided to individuals with mental illness in the United States. Much of this history shows a field struggling with definitions of what it is to have mental illness and how we as a culture should respond to these definitions in terms of diagnosis, treatment, and prevention. The mental health system is still considered by many to be quite fragmented, leaving individuals with mental illness with critical gaps in care. Current and future pharmacists should view themselves as a part of an interdisciplinary solution that resolves these gaps by helping to provide continuity in medication-related services and maximizing pharmacotherapy outcomes that facilitate the recovery of individuals with mental illness.

REFERENCES

1. Depression Guideline Panel. Depression in primary care: volume 1. Detection and diagnosis. Clinical practice guideline, number 5. Rockville, MD: U.S. Department of Health and Human Services, Public Health Services, Agency for Healthcare Policy and Research, 1993. (AHCPR publication no. 93-0551.)
2. Eaton WW. The sociology of mental disorders. 3rd ed. Westport, CT: Praeger Publishers, 2001.
3. Grob GN. The mad among us: a history of the care of America's mentally ill. New York: Free Press, 1994.
4. Corsini RJ. Introduction. In: Corsini RJ, Weddig D, eds. Current psychotherapies. 5th ed. Itasca, IL: F.E. Peacock Publishers, 1995.
5. Waldinger RJ. Sleep of reasons: John P. Gray and the challenge of moral insanity. J Hist Med Allied Sci 1979;34:163-79.
6. American Psychiatric Association. Diagnostic and statistical manual of mental disorders. 4th rev. ed. Washington, DC: American Psychiatric Association, 1994.
7. Conrad P, Schneider JW. Looking at levels of medicalization: a comment on Strong's critique of the thesis of medical imperialism. Soc Sci Med 1980;14A:75-9.
8. Goffman E. Asylums: essays on the social situation of mental patients and other inmates. New York: Random House, 1961.
9. National Alliance for the Mentally Ill. About NAMI. (Accessed January 24, 2008, at http://www.nami.org/Content/NavigationMenu/Inform_Yourself/About_NAMI/About_NAMI.htm.)
10. Glazer WM, Ereshefsky L. A pharmacoeconomic model of outpatient antipsychotic therapy in "revolving door" schizophrenic patients. J Clin Psychiatry 1996;57:337-45.
11. Stein LI, Test MA. Alternative to mental hospital treatment. I. Conceptual model, treatment program, and clinical evaluation. Arch Gen Psych 1980;37:392-7.
12. Jones E, Farina A, Hastorf AH, Markus H, Miller DT, Scott RA. Social stigma: the psychology of marked relationships. New York: Freeman, 1984.
13. Link BG, Cullen FT, Struening E, Shrout P, Dohrenwend BP. A modified labeling theory approach in the area of the mental disorders: an empirical assessment. Am Soc Rev 1989;54; 400-23.
14. Wahl OF. Media madness: public images of mental illness. New Brunswick, NJ: Rutgers University Press, 1995.
15. Chin SH, Balon R. Attitudes and perceptions toward depression and schizophrenia among residents in different medical specialties. Acad Psych 2006;30:262-3.
16. Bryant SG, Guernsey BG, Pearce EL, Hokanson JA. Pharmacists' perceptions of mental healthcare, psychiatrists, and mentally ill patients. Am J Hosp Pharm 1985;42:1366-9.
17. Crismon ML, Jermain DM, Torian SJ. Attitudes of pharmacy students toward mental illness. Am J Hosp Pharm 1990;47:1369-73.
18. Phokeo V, Sproule B, Raman-Wilms L. Community pharmacists' attitudes toward and professional interactions with users of psychiatric medication. Psychiatr Serv 2004;55:1434-6.
19. Cates ME, Burton AR, Woolley TW. Attitudes of pharmacists toward mental illness and providing pharmaceutical care to the mentally ill. Ann Pharmacother 2005;39:1450-5.
20. Bell JS, Johns R, Chen TF. Pharmacy students' and graduates' attitudes toward people with schizophrenia and severe depression. Am J Pharm Educ 2006;70(4):1-6.

21. Pincus HA, Tanielian TL, Marcus SC, et al. Prescribing trends in psychotropic medications: primary care, psychiatry, and other medical specialties. JAMA 1998;279(7):526-31.

22. Selye H. The stress of life. New York: McGraw-Hill, 1956.

23. Seligman MEP. Helplessness: on depression, development, and death. San Francisco: W.H. Freeman, 1975.

24. Mechanic D. Medical sociology. 2nd ed. New York: Free Press, 1978.

25. Wheaton B. The domains and boundaries of stress concepts. In: Kaplan HB, ed. Psychosocial stress: perspectives on structure, theory, life course, and methods. New York: Academic Press, 1996.

26. Kendler K, Eaves LJ. Models for the joint effect of genotype and environment on liability to psychiatric illness. Am J Psychiatry 1986;143(3):279-89.

27. Harding CM, Brooks GW, Ashikaga T, Strauss JS, Breier A. The Vermont longitudinal study of persons with severe mental illness, II. Long-term outcome of subjects who retrospectively met DSM-III criteria for schizophrenia. Am J Psychiatry 1987;144:727-35.

28. Deegan PE. Recovery: the lived experience of rehabilitation. Psychosocial Rehab J 1988;11(4):11-9.

29. Jacobson N, Greenley D. What is recovery? A conceptual model and explication. Psychiatr Serv 2001;52:482-5.

30. Soumerai SB, McLaughlin TJ, Ross-Degnan D, Casteris CS, Bollini P. Effects of limiting Medicaid drug-reimbursement benefits on the use of psychotropic agents and acute mental health services by patients with schizophrenia. New Engl J Med 1994;331:650-5.

31. McKenney JM, Slining JM, Henderson HR, Devins D, Barr M. The effect of clinical pharmacy services on patients with essential hypertension. Circulation 1973;48:1104-11.

32. Berringer R, Shibley MCH, Pugh CB, Rafi JA. Outcomes of a community pharmacy-based diabetes monitoring program. J Am Pharm Assoc 1999;39:791-7.

33. Narhi U, Airaksinen M, Tanskanen P, Erlund H. Therapeutic outcomes monitoring by community pharmacists for improving clinical outcomes in asthma. J Clin Pharm Ther 2000;25:177-83.

34. Nola KM, Gourley DR, Portner TS, Gourley GK, Regel B. Clinical and humanistic outcomes of a lipid management program in the community pharmacy setting. J Am Pharm Assoc 2000;40:166-73.

35. Bluml BM, McKenney JM, Cziraky MJ. Pharmaceutical care services and results in Project ImPACT: hyperlipidemia. 2000;40(2):157-65.

36. Bond CA, Salinger RJ. Fluphenazine outpatient clinics: a pharmacist's role. J Clin Psych 1979;40:501-3.

37. Saklad SR, Ereshefsky L, Jann MW, Crismon ML. Clinical pharmacists' impact on prescribing in an acute adult psychiatric facility. Drug Intell Clin Pharm 1984;18:632-4.

38. Lobeck F, Traxler WT, Bobiner DD. The cost-effectiveness of a clinical pharmacy service in an outpatient mental health clinic. Hosp Community Pharm 1989;40(6):643-5.

39. Finley PR, Rens HR, Pont JT, et al. Impact of a collaborative pharmacy practice model on the treatment of depression in primary care. Am J Health Syst Pharm 2002;59:1518-26.

40. Finley PR, Crismon ML, Rush AJ. Evaluating the impact of pharmacists in mental health: a systematic review. Pharmacotherapy 2003;23(12):1634-44.

41. Bultman DC, Svarstad BL. Effects of pharmacist monitoring on patient satisfaction with antidepressant medication therapy. J Am Pharm Assoc 2002;42:36-43.

42. Rickles NM, Svarstad BL, Statz-Paynter J, Taylor LV, Kobak K. Pharmacists' telemonitoring of antidepressant use: effects on patient feedback and other outcomes. J Am Pharm Assoc 2005; 45(3):344-53.

43. Rickles NM, Svarstad BL, Statz-Paynter J, Taylor LV, Kobak K. Improving patient feedback regarding antidepressant treatment: an experiment in eight community pharmacies. J Am Pharm Assoc 2006;46(1):25-32.

44. College of Neurologic and Psychiatric Pharmacists. CPNP mission and objectives. (Accessed January 24, 2008, at http://cpnp.org/about/mission.htm.)

CHAPTER 20

Medication Use Among Culturally Diverse Patients

Ilene Abramson, PhD

In recent years, pharmacists in both community and ambulatory settings have expanded their roles as participants in disease management programs and in various public health initiatives.[1] The success of these activities, however, depends heavily on practitioners' ability to interact with all patient groups, including the ever-increasing multinational populations across North America. To help you formulate your own plans for such endeavors, this chapter starts with an introduction to the term *culture* and then discusses models geared toward improving cultural competency in pharmacy practice.

OVERVIEW OF CULTURAL COMPETENCY

An abstract term, *culture* escapes a precise definition acceptable to all clinical sociologists. For the pharmacist, we can best describe it as "the way of life, customs, and script of a group of people."[2] Inherent in this concept is *diversity*, or "the existence of different cultures or ethnicities within a group or organization."[3] Cultural competency requires the pharmacist to remain cognizant of "patients with diverse values, beliefs, and behaviors, including tailoring delivery to meet patients' social, cultural, and linguistic needs."[4]

Certainly, one's knowledge of specific cultural beliefs can assist in particular situations. For example, if a healthcare provider knows that the Cambodian healing practice of coining involves dipping coins in mentholated oil and vigorously rubbing them on the skin, causing bruising and other mild skin abrasions, he or she is less likely to view a child with these markings as a victim of physical abuse. All providers, however, must avoid the false sense of total competence inadvertently created by some workshops highlighting a given population. In the following example, Melanie Tervalon and Jane Murray-Garcia illustrate the results of overestimating one's knowledge of patient characteristics:

> An African-American nurse is caring for a middle-aged Latina woman several hours after the patient had undergone surgery. A Latino physician . . . commented to the nurse that the patient appeared to be in a great deal of postoperative pain. The nurse summarily dismissed his perception, informing him that she took a course in cross-cultural medicine and "knew" that Hispanic patients "over express the pain they are feeling." The physician had a difficult time influencing the perspective of this nurse, who focused on her self-proclaimed cultural expertise.[5]

What does this mean for you, the pharmacist? Imagine yourself as the supervisor of a pharmacy with many patients of Slavic origin. An elderly limited-English-speaking man from this community approaches the counter with a physician's prescription for an antibiotic. In a parental tone, one of your staff pharmacists reiterates the importance of using the medication, "no matter what," during the brief talk to the gentleman. With confidence bordering on smugness, your coworker later mentions a cross-cultural colloquium he attended on "difficult" patients. This seminar included Eastern Europeans' attitudes toward prescription medications and how *those* people oppose antibiotics. Not surprisingly, the patient sensed your colleague's arrogance and took his business elsewhere from that point on.

This pharmacist possessed some facts, but sadly, little *cultural humility*: the abandonment of simplistic stereotyping for a continuous process of self-evaluation and analysis.[5] During his or her career, the pharmacist hoping to internalize this trait remains a lifetime learner. For a balanced comprehension of cultural competency as related to pharmacy practice, the material presented here refers to models. The following section introduces these models to enable you to improve your interaction with target populations.

Models of Cultural Competency

Cultural Brokering Model

A *cultural broker* is an activist, a go-between spanning the boundaries of two cultures—that of health care and that of the target community of which he or she is a member. He or she is a liaison guiding pharmacies and other clinical establishments as they interact with the broker's own ethnic or émigré population. The cultural broker understands the values of the broker's own group and of the healthcare system he or she has already navigated on behalf of himself or herself and his or her relatives.[6] This knowledge and abilities, like the acquisition of a second language, are never finite but are always in the process of growing toward higher levels of competence.[6] If implemented properly, cultural brokering programs increase understanding and compliance and set the foundation for rewarding patient experiences. These endeavors substantially help establish the pharmacist as a respected clinician sincerely attempting to reduce disparities in a given community.[6]

Cultural brokering is "the act of bridging, linking, or mediating between groups or persons of different cultural backgrounds for the purpose of reducing conflict or producing change."[7] In the case of pharmacies, this would involve the practitioner's increased use of cultural and clinical knowledge to negotiate an effective wellness plan with the patient and healthcare system.

The National Center for Cultural Competence (NCCC) envisions a particular model using a cultural broker who does the following:[6]

- Conducts a process for creating a shared vision for starting and maintaining a cultural brokering program
- Provides concrete data to show pharmacy administrators how a cultural brokering program benefits the establishment and the surrounding community
- Convenes a work group to define the parameters of a cultural broker program within the pharmacy setting and the community it serves
- Clarifies values and philosophy that support cultural brokering
- Creates, reviews, and amends policies that ensure the implementation of a cultural brokering program
- Launches an infrastructure to support cultural brokering that includes, but is not limited to, the following: staff recruitment and retention, professional development and staff training, location and scheduling of services, patient confidentiality and related state and federal statutes, and evaluation processes for continuous improvement of the practitioner–patient relationship
- Establishes objectives and timelines for implementing the program

Communication of Respect Model

During the time required to start a brokering program, you will greet ethnic patients whose backgrounds may radically differ from your own. According to folk wisdom, one never gets a second chance to make a first impression. The model offered by the Henry Ford Health System (Detroit, Michigan) helps ensure that the initial greeting between the patient and you sets a positive tone for the entire pharmacist–patient relationship. In their 1998 *Ethnic Resource Guide*, the Henry Ford Health System suggests the following steps:

- Assume people are U.S. citizens and speak English well unless you learn otherwise. The Detroit area has a large multi-generational Middle Eastern population which includes devout Muslim women born in Michigan or in another part of the U.S. They often choose to wear traditional religious clothing and, along with other citizens, can be deeply insulted if they are perceived as "foreigners" because of their appearance.
- Encounter each new patient with a "fresh" outlook. Do not pre-judge and do not let expectations from dealing with "similar" people lead you to act on stereotypes.
- Refer to a patient as a "man" or "young man," "woman" or "young woman." Avoid using "girl" or "boy" except for very young children. Never say "honey," "dear," or refer to an elderly person as "Mom," "Grandma," "Pops," or "Grandpa."
- Be cordial but not overly familiar. In many cultures, formality is a sign of respect, while informality is considered patronizing, as from a superior to an inferior.
- Most people in any culture need to feel that the clinician is sufficiently experienced in his or her field. The "first impression" should convey this; otherwise, there is a loss of faith in the skill level of the provider.[8]

Overcoming of Bias Model

This four-step model developed by Diggs and Berger[9] encourages pharmacists to improve cross-cultural interaction by first examining their own possible biases. The recommended measures are as follows.

Step 1: Realize that inequalities still exist for minority populations in the United States. The Institute of Medicine (IOM) states that ethnic minorities tend to have a poorer quality of care than Caucasians and that the most effective way to resolve these disparities is through better education of clinicians.[9]

Step 2: Try to grasp how a person's own roots might influence his or her judgment and interpretation of another culture.[9] Be aware of "ethnomyopia," the practice of looking at others through one's own cultural lenses. This approach often leads to *ethnocentrism*, a characteristic defined by Barger as "making false assumptions about others' ways based on our own limited experience."[10] The key word is *assumptions*, because we are not even aware that we are being ethnocentric.[10]

Step 3: Use a narrative communicative approach in addition to a biomedical approach to care. Encourage the patient to discuss personal beliefs regarding wellness and include these perceptions in the treatment plan.[9] The objectives of step 3 can readily be achieved by adopting the series of clinician–patient questions developed by Johnson, Hardt, and Kleinman:

1. What do you call the problem?
2. What causes the problem?
3. Why do you think it started when it did?
4. What do you think the sickness does? How does it work?
5. How severe is the sickness? Will it have a short or long course?
6. What kind of treatment do you think would be best for this problem?[11]

Keeping these questions in mind, envision a situation in which a patient with athlete's foot wants advice about an over-the-counter remedy. Some or all the questions may cause this person to feel awkward and to answer with an impatient statement such as "I don't know. You're the pharmacist!" Should this occur, you can emphasize the importance of both participants in the negotiation of a treatment plan. If your patient is still reluctant to speak, try asking about the opinion of a family member (e.g., "What does your eldest son think caused this problem?").[11]

Once the initial information is gathered, repeat these questions once more but now evaluate the patient's responses from a biomedical standpoint. In the end, call attention to incongruities and extract the best aspects of both the narrative and biomedical approaches.[11]

The following case study highlights the value of step 3 of the Diggs and Berger model, which advocates the use of the narrative communicative/explanatory model:

> Khaya Movshevna, an elderly émigré, had gone through open heart surgery and had been given a series of tests to verify her current condition. The physician's office later telephoned Khaya and informed her through the interpreter, a family member, that she would need to add warfarin to her long list of medicines. Khaya and her relative went to the community pharmacy, where the patient lamented having to ingest still another tablet. She feared a toxic reaction from this chemical overflow and asked the clinician to recommend some sort of juice or nectar to "neutralize everything." Upon hearing the patient's request via her bilingual companion, the pharmacist,

Bob, smiled pleasantly, told Khaya "don't worry," and handed the interpreter the medicine. Upon returning home, Khaya telephoned Regina, her friend and also an émigré, who agreed that "too much medicine is too much medicine." Regina promised to send a cleansing agent in the form of a liquid substance from "back home" that would prevent toxic reactions from the addition of warfarin to Khaya's other drugs. Evidently, the clinician either failed to follow the series of questions listed here in step 3 or did not even reach this point while interacting with Khaya. Until further discussion with her physician, Khaya remained noncompliant and the pharmacist lost a patient.

Step 4: Follow the Berlin and Fowkes *LEARN* model, the last point of the Diggs and Berger method:[12]

Listen to the patient.
Explain one's perceptions of the problem and one's advice for treatment.
Acknowledge the patient's concerns.
Recommend treatment while respecting the patient's individuality and
    cultural history.
Negotiate an agreement.

Sadly, Bob the pharmacist did not do so in the preceding scenario. If only he had:

- *Listened to the patient.* Bob's pleasant, noncondescending smile and automatic phrase were positive but failed to compensate for his not "listening" to Khaya's nonverbal signs of distress and mistrust. Moreover, his giving the medicine to her translator rather than to her displayed disrespect for the patient and set a negative tone, canceling any later constructive interaction that could have taken place during this or future encounters.

- *Explained his perceptions of the problem and advice for treatment.* The initial communication barrier between Bob and Khaya was the lack of a common language, both spoken and written. This situation is not unique. Nearly 30 million émigré and native-born adults in the United States can barely understand a simple pamphlet and thus may have difficulty comprehending certain medical terms.[13] Although one cannot evaluate literacy by looking, all clinicians need to be aware of this possibility and interact with patients accordingly. For more information, refer to "Alternate Wording for Medical Terms," developed by Barry Weiss for the American Medical Association.[14]

- *Acknowledged the patient's concerns.* The relationship between Khaya and Bob should have been collaborative rather than purely prescriptive.

- *Recommended treatment while respecting the woman's individuality and cultural history*. Bob failed to realize that Khaya would seek help elsewhere, most likely from a person in her own community. If he had set the mood for a constructive interchange and listened to her concerns, Bob could have formulated a plan suitable to both parties.
- *Negotiated an agreement*. One of Khaya's favorite phrases was "I understand my body best." Bob's initial inability to acknowledge her views and include her as a team player contributed to her nonadherence.[15] After the incident described in the case study, this elderly patient probably spoke negatively about her experience to other émigrés. Her words, in turn, may have created reluctance among other potential patients to deal with the pharmacy, thus costing the establishment a considerable amount of potential business. In addition to reduced revenue from the surrounding community and a tarnished reputation in the neighborhood, Bob missed the enjoyment he may have had from knowing Khaya for years to come.[15]

Few studies have been done to extract and emphasize the advantages of one model over another during clinician–patient interaction. But the benefits of continuously striving to improve cultural competency remain indisputable for pharmacists, the third largest health profession in the United States.[16]

Before leaving the topic of cultural competency models, we must call attention to one critical area—the physical layout of many pharmacies. Unlike a hospital or physician's office, many pharmacies, especially in popular retail settings, offer little patient privacy. Signs may direct patients to stand a few feet away from one another, but such distances cannot ensure confidentiality. You have probably witnessed the hard-of-hearing senior citizen shouting details of a health condition, therefore inadvertently sharing private issues with all bystanders. If you are interested in changing the layout of your pharmacy to avoid similar situations and extend privacy to patients, consult the State of Minnesota Board of Pharmacy's Mn Rule 6800.0700, Pharmacy Space and Security.[17] Their recommendations and accompanying blueprint could serve as a prototype for your own establishment.

DISPARITIES IN U.S. HEALTH CARE

Disparities are "differences between two or more population groups in health care access, coverage, and quality of care not due to different health needs" and "can include differences in preventative, diagnostic, and treatment services between population groups."[18] Dr. Martin Luther King Jr. once said, "Of all the forms of inequality, injustice [disparities] in health care is the most shocking and inhumane."[19] In 2006, the National Institutes of Health placed disparities "third among its top five organizational priorities."[20]

The IOM has reported that "ethnic minorities tend to receive a lower quality of health care than white Americans" regardless of insurance status, income, age, health condition, or symptom expressions."[9] David Satcher, the former U.S. surgeon general, reminds us that although "it's in our interests as a nation to make sure that all of our people are as healthy as they can be," many populations are far from this goal.[20] Among the reasons are historical discrimination against particular groups, bias that is still persistent today, and limited access to various sources of medical care and resources. As noted in this section, these inequities emerge in the frequencies of diseases, types of procedures performed, and the overall quality of care received by different groups.

Blacks, or African Americans, are individuals originating in any of the black racial groups from Africa. As of 2002, the U.S. Census Bureau reported the number of non-Hispanic blacks to be 36.6 million (about 12% of the entire population).[21] The overall mortality rates for blacks and whites has declined, but the racial gap is wider now than in 1950 for a number of diseases, including heart disease, cancer, diabetes, and cirrhosis of the liver.[22] Another inequality persists in the survival rates of newborns. In 2002, 14.1 black babies died per 1,000 live births, or 2.5 times the number of deaths among white infants. The incidence of sudden infant death syndrome (SIDS) was twice that reported among whites.[23] The following list highlights some of these health disparities.

- *High blood pressure and diabetes:* African Americans have the highest rate of high blood pressure of all groups studied by the Office of Minority Health and usually develop it earlier in life.[23] Diabetes is disproportionately found among African Americans.[23]
- *Cancer:* Cancer is the second leading cause of death for both African Americans and non-Hispanic whites, but the former suffer disproportionately from certain forms (colon/rectal, pancreatic, lung, prostate, breast, and cervical).[23] Looking at men alone, we find that African American men develop cancer 15% more frequently than white men.[24] However, the Minority Health Initiative reminds us that in numerous instances, all racial/ethnic minorities are less likely to undergo screening for cancer than non-Hispanic whites.[18]

- *HIV/AIDS:* HIV infection, the fifth leading cause of death for people in the United States between the ages of 25 and 44, is the primary cause of death for African American men aged 33 to 44. In 2003, black women were 18 times more likely to be diagnosed with AIDS than their non-Hispanic white counterparts.[23]

Focusing on disparities in clinical treatment, we find that African Americans received a lower quality of care than non-Hispanic whites for approximately 73% of quality measures.[25] For example, the former group was more likely *not* to be given pain medication when needed and was less frequently screened for prostate cancer. Most African Americans with asthma are never referred to an asthma specialist—even when they are insured. And despite their high morbidity and mortality from heart disease, blacks are seldom offered technologically advanced cardiac procedures.[18]

American Indian and Alaska natives (AI/ANs) are individuals with roots in one of the original populations of the Americas who maintain tribal or community affiliation.[26] In 2000, 4.1 million persons—1.5% of the U.S. population—reported their race as AI/AN in the U.S. census. The group encompasses over 550 federally recognized tribes that speak over 150 distinct languages.[27,28] In 2003, the U.S. Commission on Civil Rights exposed several inequalities among AI/AN populations.[29] Compared with non-Hispanic whites, AI/ANs are:

- 770% more prone to die from alcoholism
- 650% more likely to die from tuberculosis
- 420% more likely to die from diabetes
- 280% more likely to die in accidents
- 52% more likely to die of pneumonia or flu[29]

Additionally, the National Cancer Institute has disclosed that native Indian populations have the lowest cancer survival rates of any U.S. ethnic group.[24] One reason for these data is the federal government's allocation of funds for the Indian Health Services (IHS). In 2003, the federal government spent on average less for American Indians' and Alaska natives' medical care than for prisoners' health care ($1,914 for IHS patients versus $3,803 for inmates).[29]

Asian Americans are U.S. residents with origins in the Far East, Southeast Asia, or the Indian subcontinent (i.e., Cambodia, China, India, Japan, Korea, Malaysia, Pakistan, the Philippines, Thailand, and Vietnam). They represent 4.2% percent of the population, or 11.9 million inhabitants.[26] According to Samuel So of the Stanford

University School of Medicine, the disproportional occurrence of diseases such as chronic hepatitis B and associated liver cancer reflects the greatest health disparity between Asians and non-Hispanic whites.[30] Often endemic in the countries of origin but rarely discussed elsewhere, these conditions may begin receiving more attention as Asian ethnic populations expand in the United States. But even if the general public and clinical community significantly increased their awareness of these ailments, factors blocking effective treatment might still prevail: ignorance, lack of early symptoms, and issues regarding health access.[30] Other less pronounced but still significant disparities exist within this group, including the following:

- 61% of Asian women older than 40 received mammograms between 1999 and 2001, as compared with 67% of non-Hispanic white women.
- Vietnamese women suffer from cervical cancer nearly five times as often as white women.
- Second-generation Japanese men have diabetes at nearly four times the rate of men in Japan.
- Cambodians in California suffer strokes four times as often as the white population in the state.[31]

Historically, Asian Americans and native Hawaiian or other Pacific Islanders were placed together as a single population referred to as Asian Pacific Islanders (APIs).[32] The 2000 census showed this combined group to include 12.5 million U.S. residents, or 4.4% of the country's civilian, noninstitutionalized population.[33] Representing over 44 distinct ethnic groups, they are expected to become 10% of the entire populace by 2050.[34,35] Although sometimes overlooked as the "model minority" reflecting few disparities, API individuals do grapple with healthcare problems such as the following:

- Infant mortality rates exceeding the national average
- Disproportionately high rates of diabetes, cancer, tuberculosis, and hepatitis B
- Difficulty accessing clinical services because of language and cultural issues
- Lack of adequate health insurance (particularly among Koreans)[35]

Note that the country's 874,414 native Hawaiian and other Pacific Islanders (NHOPI), 3% of the larger, combined category just described, face their own distinct healthcare challenges.[32] The Hawaii State Department of Health reports twice the rate of tooth decay among Pacific Islander children aged 5 to 9 as compared with mainland children in the same group.[36] The highest tooth decay rate of all island residents occurs among native Hawaiian, other Pacific Islander, and Filipino boys and girls. Other conditions associated with poor oral health have been documented at higher rates among native Hawaiian, Samoan, and Filipino residents. These illnesses include, but are not limited to, diabetes, heart disease, kidney disease, obesity, tooth loss, and caries. We can assume that these inequalities stem from the population's high number of smokers, the lack of fluoridated drinking water in much of Hawaii, and the absence of a university-based dental school to address oral hygiene. The dearth of any solid research on this emerging population suggests a need for additional attention from clinicians.[36]

Hispanic, Latino, and *Spanish origin* are terms for individuals of Cuban, Mexican, Puerto Rican, and Central or South American descent, or from other Spanish-speaking cultures or origin. As of the 2000 census, they numbered 39 million in the United States and the Commonwealth of Puerto Rico.[26,37] The Institute for the Study of Migration at Georgetown University predicts that these communities will form 25% of the nation's population by 2050.[38]

Although some progress has been made in the area of health care, access to optimal treatment for this group remains deficient. The most salient problems, as compiled by the Centers for Disease Control and Prevention in 2004, are as follows.

- *HIV/AIDS:* In 1999, the morbidity for HIV was 32.7 per 100,000 for Puerto Ricans residing on the mainland. This was the highest incidence among *all* U.S. groups—six times the national average, and over 13 times the numbers for non-Hispanic whites.[37]
- *Diabetes:* In 2000, deaths from this disease were the highest among Puerto Ricans (172 per 100,000). The figures for Mexicans and Cubans were somewhat lower.[37]
- *Weight problems:* Latino girls are the second most overweight of all U.S. children. Mexican children are more overweight than white youngsters (23% versus 16%). Obese Mexican Americans, as well as African Americans and individuals with less than a high school education, are less likely to receive information about weight control than other overweight residents.[25,38]
- *Asthma:* Over half a million Latino children suffer from asthma. From 1993 to 1995, Hispanics in the northeastern United States showed an asthma death rate of 34 per million—over twice the rate for white Americans.[37,38]
- *Other issues:* In 2001, Latinos experienced more loss of life before age 75 than non-Hispanic whites due to a higher incidence of stroke, chronic liver disease and cirrhosis, diabetes, HIV, and homicide.[37]

Figures 20-1 and 20-2 summarize healthcare inequalities affecting the populations described in this section and within the nation's poorest communities.[25]

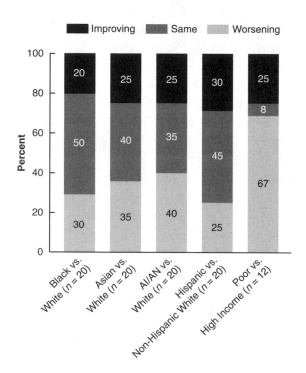

FIGURE 20-1   Change in Disparities in Core Quality Measures Over Time for Members of Selected Groups Compared with Reference Group

Source: Agency for Healthcare Research and Quality, 2006 National Healthcare Disparities Report. Rockville, MD: U.S. Department of Health and Human Services; Agency for Healthcare Research and Quality; December 2006. HRQ Pub. No. 07-0012;6–7.

Improving = Population-reference difference becoming smaller at rate greater than 1% per year
Same = Population-reference group difference not changing
Worsening = Population-reference group difference becoming larger at rate greater than 1% per year

Key: AI/AN = American Indian or Alaskan Native

Note: "Asian" includes "Asian or Pacific Islander" when information is not collected separately for each group. The most recent and oldest years of data available are compared.

n = number of core quality measures

REASONS FOR HEALTH DISPARITIES

Insurance

The Center for American Progress reports the absence of insurance covering clinical services and medications to be the primary access barrier.[19] As healthcare costs continue to rise, so has the number of uninsured individuals. In 2004, nearly 46 million people in

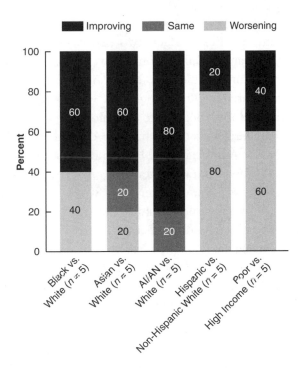

FIGURE 20-2   Change in Disparities in Core Access Measures Over Time for Members of Selected Groups Compared with Reference Group

Source: Agency for Healthcare Research and Quality, 2006 National Healthcare Disparities Report. Rockville, MD: U.S. Department of Health and Human Services; Agency for Healthcare Research and Quality; December 2006. HRQ Pub. No. 07-0012;6–7.

Improving = Population-reference difference becoming smaller at rate greater than 1% per year
Same = Population-reference group difference not changing
Worsening = Population-reference group difference becoming larger at rate greater than 1% per year

Key: AI/AN = American Indian or Alaskan Native

Note: "Asian" includes "Asian or Pacific Islander" when information is not collected separately for each group. The most recent and oldest years of data available are compared.

n = number of core quality measures

all age groups were unprotected—6 million more than in 2000.[39] Young men are more likely to lack coverage than any other age group, but women also face significant barriers when seeking insurance.[40,41] According to a Commonwealth Fund policy brief, women usually obtain coverage through their spouses' employer.[41] Even if insured by their workplace, however, women's coverage tends to be less comprehensive.

Inadequate insurance coverage is seen among the poorest populations and moderate to middle-income families. In fact, two of five working-age U.S. residents earning between $20,000 and $40,000 annually were uninsured for at least part of 2006.[42] Commonwealth Fund studies also discovered that nearly 16 million adults nationwide were underinsured in 2003. Among such adults, a staggering 59% did not fill prescriptions or reduced their dosages to save money.[42]

The lack of adequate health insurance has a specific and significant impact across populations such as Native Americans and Hispanics. Approximately 70% of Native Americans live off reservations and must travel to their home reservation for Indian Health Services. Because many Native Americans (80%) have no access at all to these centers and nearly one third lack health insurance for treatment at places other than the IHS, many individuals completely forgo necessary care.[26(p85)] The Pennsylvania State University School of Nursing has found that one third of all Hispanics have health insurance and that nearly 24% of the children are without coverage—the largest insurance-related disparity among youngsters in the country. This alone thwarts residents' attempts to maintain a usual source of care, a significant component in overall health status.[38,40]

Health Literacy

A report on the 2003 National Assessment of Adult Literacy exposes a third cause for disparities, namely health literacy. According to the IOM, "more than a measurement of reading skills, health literacy also includes writing, listening, speaking, arithmetic, and conceptual knowledge. Health literacy is defined as the degree to which individuals have the capacity to obtain, process, and understand basic information and services needed to make appropriate decisions regarding their health."[43]

It may be difficult to understand the emotional trauma of illiterate or semiliterate individuals. As the Russian proverb goes, "the well-fed person can never comprehend how the hungry person feels." To understand the embarrassment felt by those challenged by printed material, try to skim over the sentences in Figure 20-3, specifically developed by the American Medical Association Foundation for this purpose.[44] Then, imagine being forced to do this quickly in the presence of busy healthcare staff and a growing line of impatient strangers behind you at the pharmacy counter. How would you react if the provider asked, "do you understand everything?"

Keep in mind the following facts:

- As of 2003, nearly half of the population in the United States lacked the ability to follow specific medical treatments and advice promoting overall wellness.
- Most functionally and marginally literate adults are white, native-born U.S. residents.

> Your naicisyhp has dednemmocer that you have a ypocsonoloc. Ypocsonoloc is a test for noloc recnac. It sevlovni gnitresni a elbixelf gniweiv epocs into your mutcer. You must drink a laiceps diuqil the thgin erofeb the noitanimaxe to naelc out your noloc.

FIGURE 20-3 The text in the figure provides basic information about a colonoscopy but does so using words spelled backward. This should give an idea of what a person with limited literacy skills goes through when trying to read any healthcare information, including instructions on a medicine bottle.
From Weiss BD. Health literacy and patient safety: help patients understand. Manual for clinicians. 2nd ed. Chicago: American Medical Association and American Medical Association Foundation, 2007:23. Reprinted with permission from the American Medical Foundation Association.)

- Key risk populations affected by limited literacy are the elderly, low income, unemployed, high school dropouts, and minority groups (e.g., blacks, Hispanics, and limited English speakers).[14]
- Literacy is the best single predictor of overall wellness.[45]
- Those with low general literacy usually have low health literacy. The latter alone costs the U.S. healthcare system between $50 billion to $73 billion annually.[14]

Ironically, contemporary medical and technological advances can baffle even the most educated patient, compromise her understanding of medications, and thus place her in the category of those dealing with literacy-related health disparities.[14] Perhaps the most important fact to remember is that pharmacists, like all other clinicians, cannot tell by looking at people whether they are illiterate. Given this reality, the best response is to provide clear, understandable data to all patients.[46]

Language Assistance

As of 2006, an estimated 47 million U.S. residents did not use English at home.[47] Over 21 million struggle with verbal communication in all activities, including accessing health care. When they become patients, such individuals frequently express more frustration and overall dissatisfaction than those fluent in English. The lack of linguistically and culturally appropriate exchanges impairs interaction between limited English speakers and any clinician, including the pharmacist.

Insufficient verbal and nonverbal interaction readily leads to misunderstanding of medication use and to potentially fatal outcomes.[48] Glen Flores, national expert on language barriers in health care, cited an example of misunderstandings in a medical setting:

> In a case that cost a Florida hospital a $71 million malpractice settlement, Flores said an 18-year-old who said he was "intoxicado," which can mean nauseated, spent 36 hours in a hospital being treated for a drug overdose before doctors realized that he had a brain aneurysm.[48]

If this person had come to your pharmacy and spoken to someone unfamiliar with those Spanish words superficially resembling terms in English, your staff member might have accidentally offered an inappropriate over-the-counter remedy for a hangover. In the end, the family of this young man could have sued your pharmacy as well. To reduce the likelihood of such occurrences, resources are available such as the website for the Cross Cultural Health Care Program (CCHCP) in Seattle, Washington (www.xculture.org). Established in 1992, the CCHCP trains medical interpreters and assists multinational communities and their providers nationwide.

Despite the growing body of research addressing access issues, language ability, and patients' lifestyles, practitioners have yet to reach a complete understanding of health disparities among Latinos and other segments of the nation's population. In 2002, the IOM stressed that "racial/ethnic variations in medical care are infinitely more complex" than previously assumed by some clinicians and community members.[49]

DIVERSITY IN THE PHARMACY WORKFORCE

In 2003, a report from the American Society of Health-System Pharmacists (ASHP) stressed the need for more diversity in the pharmacy workforce: "healthcare organizations should implement strategies to recruit, retain, and promote at all levels of the organization a diverse staff and leadership that are representative of the demographic characteristics of the service area."[50] The IOM connects workforce diversity to "improved access to care for racial and ethnic minorities, greater patient choice and satisfaction, better patient-clinician communication, and improved educational experience for allied health students."[51]

Unfortunately, healthcare settings lag behind the general national workforce, which is already 50% staffed by minorities.[50] Table 20-1, from the Health Resources and Services Administration, notes a serious underrepresentation by the populations highlighted earlier in this chapter.[52] Consumers generally patronize an establishment whose culture and values resemble their own. In short, keeping a diverse pharmacy workforce is more than a response to the climate of the 21st century—it makes good clinical and business sense, too.

TABLE 20-1	**Race/Ethnicity of U.S. Health Professionals Compared to U.S. Population, 2000**				
	Non-Hispanic White (%)	Non-Hispanic Black (%)	Hispanic (%)	Asian/Pacific Islander (%)	American Indian/Alaska Native (%)
U.S. population (over age 18)	75.1	12.3	12.5	3.7	0.9
Chiropractors	91.9	1.2	2.9	2.7	0.6
Dentists	82.8	3.4	3.6	9.1	0.3
Medical and health services managers	78.5	10.8	5.9	3.1	1.0
Optometrists	86.5	1.7	2.7	8.1	0.4
Pharmacists	78.9	5.1	3.2	11.5	0.3
Physician assistants	76.2	8.6	8.1	4.8	0.6
Physicians and surgeons	73.6	4.5	5.1	15.3	0.3
Podiatrists	90.0	4.6	1.7	2.8	0.3
Registered nurses	80.4	9.0	3.3	6.0	0.8

Adapted from Association of American Medical Colleges. Minorities in medical education: facts and figures 2005. In: Health Resources and Services Administration. The rationale for diversity in the health professions: a review of the evidence. Washington, DC: U.S. Department of Health and Human Services, October 2006.

SUMMARY

This chapter reviewed the increasing diversity of U.S. residents and stressed the growing demand for care resonant with their needs. The three models offered herein outlined major approaches you can select and tailor to your clinical interviews. The focus of every model is twofold: cross-cultural perceptions of wellness and treatment plans respectfully designed for and consonant with patients' wishes.

Additionally, the chapter exposed significant disparities in the U.S. healthcare system and the urgency for reform. A pharmacist can be an active part of this change by learning about area residents and appropriately responding to their needs. Ongoing efforts to expand cultural awareness would inevitably help facilitate dialogue between pharmacists and other healthcare system professionals and between pharmacists and patients.

REFERENCES

1. McRee T. Pharmacy staffing: a silent but critical concern. San Francisco: UCSF Center for Health Professions, July 2002. (Accessed March 2007 at http://www.futurehealth.ucsf.edu/pdf_files/pharmacistIB.pdf.)
2. Hargie O, Dickson D. Skilled interpersonal communication: research, theory, and practice. New York: Routledge, 2003.
3. Yukl G. Leadership organizations. New Jersey: Pearson Prentice Hall, 2006:6. In: Rowe G, ed. Cases in leadership. Thousand Oaks, CA: Sage, 2007.
4. Bentacourt JR, Green AR, Carrillo JE. Cultural competence in health care: emerging frameworks and practical approaches. Commonwealth Fund, October 2002. Cited by: Diggs A, Berger B. Cultural competence: overcoming bias. Part 2: the pharmacist-patient relationship. US Pharmacist 2004;29(6):94-7.
5. Tervalon M, Garcia JM. Cultural humility versus cultural competence, a critical distinction in defining physician training outcomes in multicultural education. J Health Care Poor Underserved 1998;9(2):118.
6. Goode T, et al. Bridging the cultural divide in health care settings: the essential role of cultural broker programs. Washington, DC: National Center for Cultural Competence, Spring/Summer 2004.
7. Jezewski MA. Culture brokering in migrant farm worker health care. West J Nurs Res 1990;12(4):497-514. Cited by: Goode T, et al. Bridging the cultural divide in health care settings: the essential role of cultural broker programs. Washington, DC: National Center for Cultural Competence, Spring/Summer 2004.
8. Henry Ford Health System. General inter-cultural tips communicating respect. Ethnic resource guide. Detroit, MI: Henry Ford Health System, 1998.
9. Diggs A, Berger BA. Cultural competence: overcoming bias. Part 2: the pharmacist-patient relationship. US Pharmacist 2004;29(6):94-7.
10. Barger K. Ethnocentrism. What is it? Why are people ethnocentric? What is the problem? What can we do about it? December 20, 2004. (Accessed March 2007 at http://www.iupui.edu/~anthkb/ethnocen.htm.)

11. Johnson TM, Hardt E, Kleinman A. Cultural factors in the medical interview. In: Lipkin M, Putnam SM. Lazare A, eds. The medical interview: clinical care, education, and research. New York: Springer, 1995.

12. Berlin EA, Fowkes WC. Teaching framework for cross-cultural care: application in family practice. West J Med 1983;139:943-8. Cited by: Diggs A, Berger BA. Cultural competence: overcoming bias. Part 2: the pharmacist-patient relationship. US Pharmacist 2004;29(6):94-7.

13. Feller B. Study shows 11 million adults are illiterate. San Diego Union-Tribune, December 16, 2005. (Accessed August 2008 at http//www.signonsandiego.com/uniontrib/20051216/news_1n16literacy.html.)

14. Weiss BD. Alternate wording for medical terms. In: Health literacy: a manual for clinicians. Chicago: American Medical Association and American Medical Association Foundation, 2003:36.

15. Desmond J, Copeland LR. Communicating with today's patient: essentials to save time, decrease risk, and increase patient compliance. San Francisco: John Wiley & Sons, 2000.

16. Maryland Health Careers. Pharmacy careers. 2007. (Accessed May 2007 at http://www.marylandhealthcareers.org/html/student/pharmacy.main.html.)

17. Minnesota Board of Pharmacy. Checklist of legal requirements to be followed in opening a pharmacy. 2006. (Accessed January 2008 at http.//209.85.165.104/search?q=cache:SFYBPzNo0dwJ:www.phcybrd.state.mn.us/opening.pdf+Minnesota+Board+of+Pharmacy+Checklist+of+Legal+Requirements+to+be+Followed+in+Opening+a+Pharmacy&hl=en&ct=clnk&cd=1&gl=us&Ie=UTF-8.)

18. Families USA. Minority health initiatives. Quick facts: disparities in health care. January 2006. Available at http://www.familiesusa.org/assets/pdfs/minority-health-tool-kit/Quick-Facts-Care.pdf.

19. Center for American Progress. Community health interventions: prevention's role in reducing racial and ethnic disparities. Washington DC: 2007.

20. Institute of Medicine. Examining the health disparities research plan of the National Institutes of Health: unfinished business. March 2006. (Accessed March 2007 at http://www.iom.edu/CMS/3740/22356/33275.aspx?printfriendlly=true.)

21. U.S. Census Bureau. Guidance on the presentation and comparison of race and Hispanic origin data. 2003. (Accessed May 2007 at http://www.census.gov/population/www.socdemo/compraceho.html.)

22. Medscape Medical News. Black-white health gap as large as in 1950. 2000. (Accessed August 2008 at http://www.medscape.com/viewarticle/411748.)

23. Net Wellness Consumer Health Information. Health statistics on health disparities among African Americans. 2007. (Accessed April 2007 at http://www.netwellness.org/healthtopics/aahealth/currentstats.cfm.)

24. National Cancer Institute. NCI health information tip sheet for writers: cancer health disparities. 2005. (Accessed April 2007 at http://www.cancer.gov/newscenter/tip-sheet-cancer-health-disparities.)

25. Agency for Healthcare Research and Quality. Key themes and highlights from the *National Healthcare Disparities Report*. 2007. (Accessed February 2007 at http://www.ahrq.gov/qual/nhdr06/highlights/nhdr06high.htm.)

26. Institute of Medicine. Unequal treatment. Washington, DC: National Academy Press, 2002:34.

27. Ogunwole SU. The American Indian and Alaska native population: 2000. 2000. (ERIC ED469364 Census 2000 Brief.) (Accessed May 2007 at http://eric.ed.gov/ERICWebPortal/custom/portlets/recordDetails/detailmini.jsp?nfpb=true.)

28. Oropeza L. Clinician's guide: working with Native Americans living with HIV. Oakland, CA: National Native American AIDS Prevention Center, 2002.

29. Indianz.com. Report calls on U.S. to honor health care commitment; U.S. Commission on Civil Rights. 2004. (Accessed April 2007 at http://indianz.com/.)

30. Luo E. Healthcare outreach in ethnic communities. Next Gen 2007;3(5):1-5.

31. Daus GP. Issue brief: guidance for designing a national disparities report. Asian and Pacific Islander American Health Forum. April 2001. (Accessed April 2007 at http://www.apiahf.org/policy/healthaccess/200104brief_ahrq.htm.)

32. Ontai GP. Pacific American Research Center. 2001. (Accessed April 2007 at http://www.thepaf.org/Research/index1.htm.)

33. Reeves T, Bennett C. The Asian and Pacific Islander population in the United States: March 2002. Washington, DC: U.S. Department of Commerce, Economics and Statistics Administration, 2003. (Current Population Report P20-540.)

34. Wang E, Bormet M. Improving API health data in Minnesota. Minneapolis, MI: Department of Health and Family Support, 2006.

35. The White House Initiative on Asian Americans and Pacific Islanders. Asian American and Pacific Islander facts. U.S. Census Bureau, 2001. (Accessed April 2007 at http://www.aapi.gov/resources/aapifacts.htm.)

36. Harrigan RC, Eesa D, LeSaux C, et al. Oral health disparities and periodontal disease in Asian and Pacific Island populations. Ethn Dis 2005;15(4 suppl 5):39-46.

37. Centers for Disease Control and Prevention. Hispanic health disparities [fact sheet]. 2004. (Accessed April 2007 at http://www.cdc.gov/OD/OC/MEDIA/presskits/hhd/hhd=fs,htm.)

38. Institute for the Study of Migration, Georgetown University. Hispanic population. Cited by: Siantz ML. Understanding health disparities: the Hispanic experience. Presentation at the Woodrow Wilson Center, Washington, DC, April 4, 2006.

39. The Commonwealth Fund. Gaps in health insurance: an all-American problem. 2007. (Accessed March 2007 at http://www.cmwf.org/publications-show.htm?doc-id=367876&#doc367876.)

40. Henry J. Kaiser Family Foundation. Race, ethnicity, and health care: young African American men in the United States. July 2006. (Accessed March 2007 at http://www.kff.org.)

41. The Commonwealth Fund. Women and health coverage: the affordability gap. 2007. (Accessed April 2007 at http://www.cmwf.org/publications-show.htm?doc-id=478513&#doc478513.)

42. Davis K. Statement from Commonwealth Fund President Karen Davis on Census Bureau's revised estimates of uninsured. 2007. (Accessed March 2007 at http://www.cmwf.org/surveys/surveys_list.htm?attrib_id=15309.)

43. Nielsen-Bohlman L, Panzer AM, Kindig DA. Health literacy: a prescription to end confusion. Washington, DC: Institute of Medicine of the National Academies, 2004. (Accessed March 2007 at http://www.iom.edu/report.asp?id=19723.)

44. Weiss BD. Health literacy and patient safety: help patients understand. Manual for clinicians. 2nd ed. Chicago: American Medical Association and American Medical Association Foundation, 2007:23. (Accessed September 2008 at http://www.ama-assn.org/ama1/pub/upload/mm/367/healthlitclinicians.pdf.)

45. Schillinger D, Grumbach K, Piette J, et al. Association of health literacy with diabetes outcomes. JAMA 2002;288(4):475-82.

46. Agency for Healthcare Research and Quality. New AHRQ tools help pharmacies better serve patients with limited health literacy. Rockville, MD: U.S. Department of Health and Human Services, 2007. (Accessed September 2008 at http://www.ahrq.gov/news/press/pr2007/pharmtoolpr.htm.)

47. Flores G. Language barriers to health care in the United States. New Engl J Med 2006;355(3): 229-31. (Accessed August 2008 at http://content.nejm.org/cgi/content/full/355/3/229.)

48. Weise E. Language barriers plague hospitals. USA Today, July 20, 2006. (Accessed August 2008 at http://findarticles.com/p/articles/mi_kmusa/is_/ai_n16550847?tag=artBody;col1.)

49. Henry J. Kaiser Family Foundation, American College of Cardiology Foundation. Racial/ethnic differences in cardiac care: the weight of the evidence. Menlo Park, CA: Henry J. Kaiser Family Foundation, October 2002.

50. Vanderpool HK. Report of the ASHP ad hoc committee on ethnic diversity and cultural competence. Am J Health Syst Pharm 2005;62:1929.

51. Institute of Medicine. In the nation's compelling interest: ensuring diversity in the health care workforce. Washington DC: National Academy of Sciences, 2004. (Accessed August 2008 at http://www.nap.edu/openbook.php?isbn=030909125X.)

52. Association of American Medical Colleges. Minorities in medical education: facts and figures 2005. In: Health Resources and Services Administration. The rationale for diversity in the health professions: a review of the evidence. Washington, DC: U.S. Department of Health and Human Services, October 2006. (Accessed September 2008 at ftp://ftp.hrsa.gov/bhpr/workforce/diversity.pdf.)

PART IV

Public Policy Perspectives on Medical Practices

In each of the previous parts of the textbook, considerable attention has been paid to the larger public policy issues related to drug therapy and the pharmacy profession's efforts to respond to those issues. Part IV of this book continues to explore such large policy-related issues but with a specific focus on medication errors and various ethical issues facing public policy initiatives. Chapter 21 outlines key concepts and processes that result in and prevent medication errors. Chapter 22 examines several ethical issues facing pharmacy practice, such as dispensing emergency contraception pills and how to deal with the implications of pharmacogenetics on a patient's access to medications. Both chapters may introduce more questions than answers. It is hoped that this part of the textbook will be a starting point for more investigations on how public policy and pharmacy intersect. It should also create current and future challenges for various stakeholders trying to improve the safe and fair distribution of medications to those who need them.

PART IV

Public Policy Perspectives on Medical Practices

CHAPTER 21
A Psychosocial Approach to Medication Errors

CHAPTER 22
Ethical Issues Influencing Public Policy Initiatives

A Psychosocial Approach to Medication Errors

Elizabeth Flynn, PhD, Kraig L. Schell, PhD, and Jenny O. Rickles, MPH, CPHQ

B efore exploring the psychosocial issues related to medication errors, let us start with an understanding of what a medication error is and why it is important to patient care. The National Coordinating Council for Medication Error Reporting and Prevention defined a medication error as "any preventable event that may cause or lead to inappropriate medication use or patient harm while the medication is in the control of the healthcare professional, patient, or consumer. Such events may be related to professional practice, healthcare products, procedures, and systems, including prescribing; order communication; product labeling, packaging, and nomenclature; compounding; dispensing; distribution; administration; education; monitoring; and use."[1] It is important to recognize that medication error is just one type of medical error; other types of medical errors include wrong medical procedures, nonadherence to treatment guidelines, and so forth. Also, the reader should note that adverse drug events (ADEs) are injuries related to medication use and errors; not all medication errors result in an ADE.

Serious medication errors often gain national media attention. One example involved the death of three neonates after the administration of heparin overdoses in which the staff did not recognize that the heparin retrieved from an automated medication dispensing device was 1,000 times greater than the normally stocked concentration.[2] The death of *Boston Globe* health reporter Betsy Lehman at the Dana-Farber Cancer Institute as a result of an overadministration of cyclophosphamide (4,000 mg/m^2 instead of 1,000 mg/m^2) triggered widespread efforts to improve medication safety.[3]

Medication safety has received considerable attention and resources since the year 2000, when the Institute of Medicine (IOM) described the scope, severity, and impact of medical errors in its report *To Err Is Human*.[4] The impact of medication errors is astounding. Medication errors account for 20% of medical errors resulting in injury or death,[5] cause an estimated 7,000 deaths per year,[6] are associated with 3% to 7% of serious adverse events among those hospitalized,[7] and increase hospital costs in the United States by about $2 billion annually.[8] The IOM report *Preventing Medication Errors* contains a comprehensive summary of the frequency of a wide variety of types of medication errors and adverse drug events in hospitals, nursing homes, and pediatric, psychiatric, and community settings.[3]

This chapter presents errors from the individual, interpersonal, and system or organizational perspectives. As each perspective is described, we discuss errors as they relate to the drug delivery process, which includes medication prescribing, dispensing, and administration. We also describe types of errors, psychosocial causes of errors, and possible interventions and solutions. Table 21-1 provides the reader with definitions of error types and at what point in the drug delivery system a particular error can occur. It is important to understand that an error that occurs during administration could also have occurred at another stage in the drug delivery system (e.g., dispensing) but was not caught until the medication was administered. Throughout the chapter, we highlight the fact that the errors that occur can differ depending on the pharmacy setting (e.g., community, hospital, ambulatory care). The latter part of the chapter provides the reader information about detecting and reporting medication errors, as well as regulatory and policy implications.

Figure 21-1 illustrates the three domains (psychological, social, and organizational) with respect to their proximity to a hypothetical error event. It is adapted from a framework model proposed by Grasha and colleagues[9,10] and is based on the theories of error found in the literature.[11-13] The model suggests that some factors are proximal (near) to the error, whereas others are typically distal (far). The "distance" from the error should not be interpreted to mean that distal factors are less important to error capture and prevention. The reader should understand that this is a "direct-influence" proximity: the factors closer to the error are usually more directly predictive of it, whereas distal factors may only affect error by influencing the more proximal factors. Thus, our model should serve as an illustration of the typical relationship between the domains of influential factors as they relate to the individual, interpersonal, and system or organizational perspectives.

TABLE 21-1	Types and Definitions of Errors in the Drug Delivery System			
Error Type	**Definition**	**Prescribing**	**Dispensing**	**Administration**
Wrong drug	A medication that is different from that named by the prescriber is used to fill a prescription.[31]	✓	✓	✓
Wrong strength	A dosage unit containing a different amount of medication than the prescriber specified is used to fill a prescription (unless the pharmacist adjusts the instructions to accurately adjust for the difference).[74]	✓	✓	✓
Wrong dose	Any dose is given containing the wrong number of preferred dosage units (such as capsules) or an amount of medication that is different from what was ordered.[31]	✓	✓	✓
Wrong dosage form	A formulation of the medication dispensed deviates from the prescription.[31]	✓	✓	✓
Wrong quantity	The number or amount of medication ordered is different from what was dispensed to the patient when there is no other explanation for the difference (such as quantities that third-party payers will reimburse or patients request).[74]	✓	✓	✓
Wrong label instructions	Directions to the patient on the prescription label that deviate in one or more ways from what was prescribed, except for changes based on good pharmacy practice (e.g., adding the drug indication at the end of the instructions—"for pain").[32]		✓	

TABLE 21-1 Types and Definitions of Errors in the Drug Delivery System (cont.)				
Error Type	Definition	Prescribing	Dispensing	Administration
Wrong prescription label information (excluding instructions)	Detected by comparing the federal or state label requirements to the prescription.[32]		✓	
Deteriorated drug error	A medication has exceeded its expiration date, or a medication is stored in a location that is not in accordance with the manufacturer's recommendations (e.g., outside a refrigerator).[32]		✓	
Wrong patient	A medication is provided for a different patient than for whom it was ordered. May be viewed as an *unordered drug error* for the patient who received the dose, and a possible *omission error* for the patient for whom the dose was intended. [31]	✓	✓	✓
Extra dose	A dose is given in excess of the total number of times ordered by the physician, such as a dose given on the basis of an expired order, after a drug has been discontinued, or after a drug has been put on hold.[31]		✓	✓
Omission error	A patient fails to receive a dose of medication that was ordered by the time the next dose is due.[31]		✓	✓
Wrong route	A medication is administered to the patient using a different location or site than ordered.[31]	✓	✓	✓
Wrong time	Administration of a dose more than 60 minutes before or after the scheduled administration time, unless there is appropriate justification.[31]			✓
Wrong technique	An incorrect or omitted action by the nurse during the preparation or administration of a dose.[31]			✓

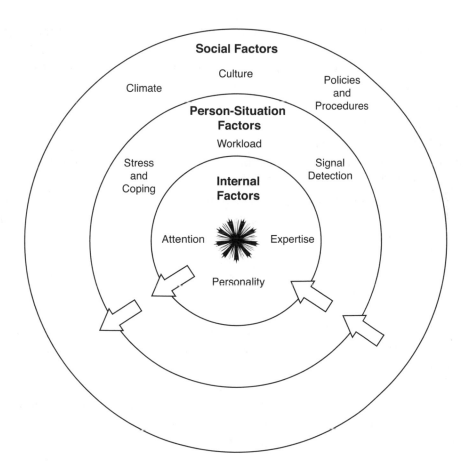

FIGURE 21-1 A Multilevel Framework of Influences on Error Occurrence in Organizational Systems

INDIVIDUAL PERSPECTIVES

Errors that can occur from the individual perspective can arise out of familiarity with procedures and materials. People have an innate tendency to perceive confirming evidence more readily than disconfirming evidence.[14] Confirmation bias can occur when an individual interprets information in a way that confirms his or her preconceptions or beliefs. This also occurs when individuals become familiar with procedures.[15] Individuals can have unconscious "slips," which are errors that occur as a result of distractions or failure to pay attention at critical moments. Conditions that make slips more likely are fatigue, substance abuse, illness, emotions, and environmental factors.

As illustrated in the model in Figure 21-1, three internally based factors can contribute to the occurrence of an error: attention, personality, and expertise. *Attention* refers to a person's focus on a particular stimulus; attention can be singly focused or focused across multiple tasks, and it can be sustained or varied across time.[16] With respect to medication error, individual differences in focused attention (i.e., resistance to attentional distraction) have been shown to be related to error rates in a stimulus checking task.[17] Attention is resource dependent,[16,18] requiring "cognitive fuel" to maintain itself for extended periods. Finally, attention can be captured by stimulus characteristics.[19,20]

Personality includes traits and predispositions that inform and influence a person's behavioral choices.[21] With respect to specific traits, there is evidence that an anxiety trait is related to error production in a simulated pharmacy task,[22] and that a self-regulation trait (the tendency to monitor and adjust behavior internally rather than relying on external information) is connected to increased false alarms, that is, identifying an error that does not really exist.[23]

Expertise is defined as the degree to which a skilled behavior has become routine and therefore requires fewer cognitive resources to effectively complete.[24] Researchers usually describe expertise as a shift from effortful processing to automatic processing of tasks.[25,26] Most pharmacy staff with even just 6 to 12 months of experience are likely to be in automatic mode as they work. Expertise is important because it facilitates multitasking without sacrificing accuracy,[27,28] and does so with no discernible strain on short-term memory. It also facilitates adaptive error management through enhanced knowledge structures,[29] making memory more efficient. Errors may decline naturally as a function of expertise, but it is too extreme to say that experts do not make mistakes. Although expertise is seen as a benefit, individuals who are considered to have expertise may feel a false sense of security, and the automatic mode in which they work could lead to errors.

Prescribing

From the individual perspective the root of an error may begin when a provider sees a patient and handwrites a prescription or when a provider calls a prescription into a community pharmacy. This type of error may occur because of medications with sound-alike or look-alike names. For example, a prescriber writes Taxol when he meant to prescribe Paxil. An error may also occur when prescribing medication doses that have zeros or decimal points. An example, a physician prescribes vincristine 2.0 mg, which later in the dispensing process is misread as vincristine 20 mg. In the case of the Betsy Lehman overdose mentioned previously, an ambiguous or incomplete order for cyclophosphamide caused the fatal error because the order was written 4 g/m^2 days 1–4. This led to ambiguity as to whether the medication was to be given for 4 days or whether the total amount was to have been divided by the 4 days. Errors can occur when mixing the metric and apothecary systems. For example, a pharmacist mistakes 2 of the 1/100 grain tablets (0.6 mg each or a total of 1.2 mg) as equivalent to one 1/200 grain (0.3 mg) tablet. Errors can also occur when using abbreviations. For example, U has been read as a 0, 4, or 6.[30]

Dispensing

Many different types of errors can occur during dispensing (see Table 21-1 for specific definitions). For example, an error can occur when a prescriber calls a medication into a community pharmacy and a wrong drug is dispensed as a result of the nature of the oral communication. Wrong dosage form errors can occur when giving a tablet when a suspension was ordered, or when administering plain aspirin instead of enteric-coated aspirin. Instances in which tablets are crushed are not considered wrong dosage form errors because of inadequate knowledge of the effect of crushing tablets.[31]

Dispensing errors can occur in different settings. In a community pharmacy setting there are many distractions and points in the dispensing of the medication where an error can occur. Many pharmacies experience high prescription volumes and thus have significant workload demands. Pharmacies have the additional burden of dealing with a multitude of insurance issues. These latter issues cause an enormous strain on the pharmacy staff and can lead to multitasking. Multitasking can then lead to errors because an individual's attention is dispersed and not focused on one step of the process at a time.

A national observational study of prescription dispensing accuracy in 50 community pharmacies found dispensing error rates ranging from 0% to 13%, with an overall error rate of 1.7% (77 errors on 4,481 prescriptions).[32] For example, a pharmacy dispensing 250 prescriptions per day would dispense 4 of them in error. Most deviations from the prescription were label errors, followed by wrong quantity,[33] wrong strength,[14] wrong drug,[34] omission,[35] and wrong dosage form.[4] Previous studies of error rates in prescription filling ranged from 1% to 24%.[36-39] Dispensing errors that could harm patients have been estimated to occur in 1.5% to 4% of erroneous prescriptions.[36,37,39]

Ashcroft and colleagues studied the possible causes of near misses and dispensing errors in community pharmacies in the United Kingdom.[40] The most common factors related to near misses and errors were misreading the prescription, similar drug names, selecting the wrong drug from the patient's profile, and similar drug packaging.

Dispensing errors can occur in an inpatient hospital setting for similar reasons as in community pharmacies: busy units, multitasking of staff, and the strain of discharging patients by a certain time because of insurance or Medicare constraints. Pharmacy error rates involving doses dispensed during the cart-filling process (picking errors) range from 0.04% to 2.9%.[41-46] In the most recent study, Cina and colleagues found a 3.6% pharmacy dispensing error rate (5,075 errors on 140,755 doses) on orders filled by pharmacy technicians.[47] Pharmacists inspecting these orders detected only 79% of the errors, for a final dispensing error rate of 0.75%. ADEs were judged to be possible on 23.5% of the undetected errors, with 28% of these deemed serious and 0.8% life threatening.

Some state boards of pharmacies have allowed technicians to check other technicians after filling patient medication drawers instead of requiring a pharmacist to perform this task.[48] A comparison of the unit-dose medication drawer checking accuracy of technicians and pharmacists found that the error rates detected by each group did not differ significantly: both found a 1.2% cart fill error rate.[49] Pharmacists overlooked errors more often than technicians: 107 errors on 49,718 doses (0.21% error rate) versus 50 errors overlooked by technicians on 55,470 doses (0.09% error rate). The authors noted that the percentage of missed errors that could have resulted in patient harm was not significantly different (25.2% for pharmacists versus 32.0% for technicians), but this means that 27 potentially serious errors were overlooked by pharmacists compared with 16 by technicians. Campbell and Facchinetti describe the use of process control charts for monitoring dispensing and checking errors in an inpatient pharmacy, including the introduction of artificial errors to evaluate accuracy.[50] The source of the medication profile information from which the cart is checked has also been studied. A study of missing dose rates measured a decrease from 0.93% to 0.33% when nursing and pharmacy personnel checked the cart against the patient's medication administration record.[51]

As illustrated in the model in Figure 21-1, there are three personal or situational factors that can affect the dispensing process: stress and coping behaviors, signal detection factors, and workload. *Stress and coping behaviors* refers to the interaction between stressful circumstances (stressors) and how an individual responds to them (coping).[52,53] The pharmacy literature includes a number of stress studies, most concluding that pharmacists must handle a considerable amount of stress at work.[54-56] However, one cannot assume that stress from work is the only relevant stress. Studies have shown consistently that stress from extra-work roles, such as family, can affect performance on the job.[57,58]

Signal detection factors refer to elements of the error detection environment that affect our ability to find errors among the "noise" of non-errors.[59] The theory suggests that we evaluate a stimulus on some criteria and then decide whether that stimulus is either a "target" or a "nontarget." In the case of pharmacy, the target would be an error, and the nontarget would be a correct prescription. Our threshold for making that decision varies depending on a number of factors, such that sometimes we will tend to be more conservative (hesitant to identify a possible error) and at other times we will tend to be more liberal (willing to identify a possible error).[60] From this theory and studies of simulated pharmacy performance, we know that error probability,[61] the costs and benefits of each decision possibility, as well as signal strength[62] can push a person toward either liberality (greater willingness to identify suspicious targets) or conservatism (lesser willingness to identify suspicious targets).

Workload can be composed of factors from a number of sources, including prescription volume, multiple tasks, interruptions and distractions, and poor environmental conditions for work. However, there is one pervasive assumption that persists about how workload affects errors in pharmacy. Workload is often thought by pharmacists to be a primary cause of error, but empirical investigations of this claim have shown that things are not quite that simple.[63] One study showed that the *lowest-volume* pharmacies produced the highest error rates, most likely through task disengagement and boredom.[64,65] Perceptions of workload are likely to be more important to errors in pharmacy because they are indicative of how stressful the workload is to the person.[66]

Administration

Medication administration errors are typically viewed as being related to drug administration in the hospital and are defined as any deviation from the prescriber's interpretable order.[33] Many different types of errors can occur during administration (see Table 21-1 for specific definitions). Administration errors can also occur at home when, for example, an older adult has multiple medications and confuses what should be taken or when to take her medication and takes too many, too few, at the wrong times, or forgets to take her medication altogether. Such errors can also occur when a patient is discharged from a hospital with multiple medications and the patient has medications at home and confuses doses.

In a hospital setting, a wrong technique error can occur. For example, if the wrong rate of infusion is used but the patient receives the correct dose, a wrong technique error has occurred. If the prescriber ordered that the patient's heart rate or blood pressure meet a specific criterion prior to drug administration and the action was omitted, a wrong technique error has occurred. If the heart rate is measured and the rate is too low for the dose to be given, but the nurse still administers the drug, an extra dose error has occurred.[31] One study defined intravenous drug errors as "any deviation in the preparation or administration of a drug from a doctor's prescription, the hospital's intravenous policy, or the manufacturer's instructions."[67] This study only considered a dose to be in error if it had the potential to adversely affect the patient.

Interventions and Solutions

From the individual perspective, there are many interventions or solutions that could help to reduce errors. During prescribing, a double-check system can be put into place in which a second person checks the written order. Read-backs are also an important intervention. For example, if a prescriber were to call a medication into a community pharmacy or hospital pharmacy, the pharmacist or pharmacy technician on the phone would write down the verbal order, then read back what he or she had written to receive confirmation of the correct prescription. This was incorporated into the Joint Commission's national patient safety goals in 2003. The goal was to implement a process for taking verbal or telephone orders and requires a verification read-back of the complete order by the person receiving the order.[30]

Another intervention or solution is a model of patient empowerment. In 2007, the Joint Commission added a patient safety goal that encourages patients' active involvement in their own care.[30] Initiatives can be put into place to encourage patients and families to speak up and become active participants in their care. For example, if a patient received a prescription and was not sure of the reason or dose, the patient would be encouraged to speak up and ask the prescriber or pharmacist.

A sense of accountability is equally important from the individual staff perspective. Staff should have a sense of accountability for their responsibilities and how their actions can affect others with whom they work and the patients who rely on them. A sense of accountability will help staff feel empowered. Staff empowerment includes feeling comfortable and safe to tell another staff member, even a supervisor, that one questions a particular dose or order that was written.

INTERPERSONAL PERSPECTIVES

Errors that can occur from the interpersonal perspective are complex. Interpersonal communications that occur between the pharmacist and patient, prescriber and patient, and prescriber and pharmacist all have their own particular challenges. For example, time and workloads limit the nature and extent of communication between different members of the healthcare team and between those members and the patient. Such communications are important for patient education, adequate provider assessment, and development of an optimal treatment plan. Inadequate patient education and patient assessment may lead to errors.

Communication and life stressors play a role in the interpersonal perspectives leading to errors. As described earlier, healthcare professionals continue to work in a fast-paced environment, with increasing volume and acuity of patients. This is compounded by the shortages of healthcare professionals in many disciplines. During these busy times, teamwork is essential. Communication among team members was added as a Joint Commission national patient safety goal in 2003 and then updated in 2006 to include the need to develop a standard approach for "hand-off" communication.[30] *Hand-off communication* includes communication between health professionals, caregivers, and others during transitions in care, which should allow enough time to ask questions and clarify issues. These and other interpersonal perspectives are discussed further in the next paragraphs.

Prescribing

The focus in prescribing is on interdisciplinary communication as well as communication with the patient. Let us take an example of a provider not counseling the patient on the medication she is prescribing, or giving confusing information. The patient may not understand why he is taking it and be unclear on the risks or benefits. The patient may think he is taking a particular medication and not realize that the medication he was prescribed was not the intended one. Errors can occur through lack of proper assessment of the patient's background, including medication history, adherence, illnesses, and barriers to taking medication.

Dispensing

Poor exchange of patient information across shifts (hand-off communication) can lead to errors.[30] In a hospital setting, errors can be made as a result of miscommunication among team members regarding what medications and doses are needed. In a community pharmacy setting, assumptions can be made about the medications being checked by someone else because of poor communication among staff members. An example of this is a prescriber assuming that a pharmacist has checked for drug interactions, whereas the pharmacist did not do so.

Administration

Errors can occur as a result of poor medication reconciliation between multiple healthcare providers. *Medication reconciliation* is a process in which each patient's list of medications is cross-checked by a healthcare provider during each interaction or transition. For example, a patient being admitted to a hospital is asked to list all his or her current medications, and then upon discharge the list is reconciled and decisions are made about what medications to continue, new medications to add, or other changes to make. A complete list of medications is communicated to the next provider of service when the patient is referred or transferred to another setting. Medication reconciliation was added by the Joint Commission as a national patient safety goal in 2006.[30]

Medication administration errors can occur when the pharmacist does not verify the patient's name upon pickup of medications. If the communication is poor between the patient and pharmacist and no counseling is performed during prescription pickup, errors can occur during medication consumption by the patient at home.

Interventions and Solutions

The situation-background-assessment-recommendation (SBAR) technique has long been used in the aviation industry and in recent years has gained attention from healthcare organizations. SBAR provides a framework for communication between healthcare team members.[15] An example of a situation in which one could use SBAR in a community pharmacy setting would be as follows: A pharmacist notices that the patient had recently refilled a prescription for a medication with similar mechanisms as the current prescription. The pharmacist may call the prescriber and say the following:

S (situation): "I am calling about Mr. Smith's prescription for fluoxetine."
B (background): "The patient is already on a similar drug, paroxetine, and refilled it 2 weeks ago."
A (assessment): "If we give this medication, then the patient may take both and have an interaction or excessive side effects."
R (recommendation): "I suggest eliminating one of the medications."

In a community pharmacy setting, some ways to reduce dispensing errors are reviewing one patient's medication(s) at a time, creating distraction-free and interruption-free zones whenever possible, verifying each patient's name at pickup, and thorough patient counseling. The performance of show-and-tell counseling includes verifying the patient's identity (e.g., by viewing a driver's license), comparing the filled prescription to the original order, showing the medication to the patient, reviewing the label information, and counseling on key points. This technique detected 89% of dispensing errors.[68]

SYSTEM OR ORGANIZATIONAL PERSPECTIVES

Errors that can occur from the system or organizational perspective are multifaceted and quite complex. Many organizations have systems in place that might have worked decades ago but are not feasible in today's environment. The healthcare environment has become more complex, and the regulations and policy implications (discussed later in the chapter) have increasingly become more prominent. For example, an assessment of the nuclear power plant incident at Three Mile Island in 1979 found that human errors are a result of major failures in design and organization long before the actual incident or error occurs. Faulty system designs contribute to errors and often make them difficult to detect; such faulty designs are referred to as *latent errors*.[15]

There are two main kinds of system failures: design failures and organizational or environmental failures. *Design failures* focus on process, task design, and environmental design. *Organizational or environmental failures* focus on psychological precursors, inadequate team building, and training. Many obstacles exist, such as the complexities of systems and the lack of ownership or accountability. Systems that are too complex may be open to failures because individuals do not find such complex systems intuitive and their processes easy to remember. Lack of ownership can lead to system failures because individuals do not feel a sense of responsibility for a system they may not have had any input in developing. Individuals may also feel that they are not accountable for failures if the system was faulty to begin with and open to such failures.

Tolerance of faulty practices is also possible. For example, a new staff member might begin working in your pharmacy and ask "Why do we take down the order in this particular area of the pharmacy but then need to walk across the pharmacy to input the order?" A person who has been working at the pharmacy a long time may have adjusted well to this faulty practice and be surprised by the concern raised by the new staff member.

We also may become less attuned to potential error-causing situations because of the infrequent occurrence of events that lead to errors. There may be new technology in the systems put into place and we may think that an error just could not occur and therefore become too comfortable. Fear of punishment is also a growing concern from an organizational perspective. Many have adopted a blame-free and just culture environment. Everyone can learn from errors when the staff is comfortable analyzing and reporting errors.[15]

As illustrated in the model in Figure 21-1, organizational culture and climate sound quite similar, but they differ in that *culture* describes the often-embedded and unnoticed aspects of how employees are supposed to see the world and interpret it. *Climate*, by contrast, describes the general perceptions of the work environment by the workers with respect to their behavior. Climate can tap into culture, but it need not do so completely.[69] There are many studies available suggesting that these two factors can affect employees' safety behaviors, particularly with respect to behaviors that might put themselves at risk, including one directly relevant to medication error.[70-72] Almost every organization must work within the constraints outlined by the regulatory entities that govern them, and pharmacy is no exception. Professionally, pharmacists must behave according to guidance from a number of these entities, and on a smaller scale, the activities of a particular store in a chain pharmacy are determined in part by the decisions of the administration of the chain. This can affect perceptions of autonomy and self-determination, the lack of which many pharmacists consider to be a source of dissatisfaction with pharmacy practice.[73]

Prescribing

Errors that can occur during prescribing from a system or organizational perspective are multifaceted. Errors can occur if a prescriber does not have access to the most current information or if the chart is not available, not updated, or incomplete. A prescriber may feel rushed as a result of the nature of clinical practice; this type of environment does not allow for proper assessments. Allergies not properly incorporated into the chart can lead to errors because this information would be missing during drug selection. Awareness of national guidelines for prescribing of medications is crucial. Many prescribers may not be aware and prescribe a medication that is not the preferred therapy for a particular illness. Similarly, a prescriber may choose a drug that is on the hospital formulary or based on the patient's insurance coverage and it may not be the drug of choice.

Dispensing

Errors can occur during dispensing at the system or organizational level when hospital floors use multiple-dose vials as floor stocks. Errors may also occur when dispensing is based on computer-generated labels rather than original prescriptions. Organizations may also be vulnerable to dispensing errors for similar reasons as mentioned earlier in discussing prescribing errors. Busy hospital units or busy community pharmacies can create an environment prone to errors. Many community pharmacies rely on double checks of the pharmacist after a pharmacy technician has filled the prescription order. Safeguards may exist in some settings to avoid dispensing errors, such as bar coding and automated dispensing systems.

Bar code–based inspection systems have been studied in inpatient pharmacies to determine the effects on dispensing accuracy. Poon and colleagues evaluated pharmacy dispensing errors before and after implementation of a bar code verification system.[74] Dispensing error rates for four filling processes assessed were 0.25% to 0.71% before implementation, and 0.018% to 0.026% after. A key recommendation of the study was to require bar code scanning of every dose dispensed, not just a single representative dose used to fill an order.[74]

Flynn and Barker conducted an observational study to assess the effect of an automated dispensing system (ADS) on dispensing error rates for all errors and for target errors (those the ADS was designed to prevent) in one independent pharmacy and one chain community pharmacy.[75] The ADS had robotic controls for the top 200 most commonly dispensed tablets and capsules, as well as a bar code–based control system for all other medications dispensed. At the independent pharmacy, the authors noted a significant decrease ($p<0.10$) in the dispensing error rate, from 2.9% before ADS (99 errors on 3,427 prescriptions) to 2.1% after ADS (68 errors on 3,241 prescriptions). At the chain pharmacy, there was no significant difference between the error rate before and after ADS: 1.9% before ADS (64 errors on 3,424 prescriptions) and 2.4% after ADS (74 errors on 3,028 prescriptions). Target error rates decreased significantly at both pharmacies ($p = 0.002$ and $p = 0.07$, respectively). The most frequent source of errors that occurred after the intervention involved the deliberate overriding of system controls by pharmacy staff. Most errors originated in the computer order entry process, which the ADS could not control.[75]

Teagarden and colleagues conducted an internal observational study of a high-volume, highly automated mail order pharmacy operation.[76] Using the same definitions and methods as the national accuracy study by Flynn and Barker, the authors found 16 errors on 21,252 prescriptions, yielding an error rate of 0.075%. The errors found were believed to have originated during the initial tasks performed by the staff, such as order entry. No errors were associated with the automated parts of the prescription filling system.[3,32]

Administration

Medication administration errors that may occur from the system or organizational perspective are briefly examined here. Storing similar-looking medications next to each other may lead to errors. In a pharmacy, medications for different patients placed simultaneously on the counter may lead to errors if they are not separated from each other (e.g., with bins). In hospitals or nursing homes, errors may occur when discontinued medications are not removed from patients' medication boxes.

Errors can occur because of manufacturer and instrumentation problems such as near-identical packaging (e.g., Warfarin, Merck products, antibiotic bags). Errors can also occur due to misprogramming of rates and concentrations into infusion pumps and patient-controlled analgesia systems.

Medication administration errors have been shown to be common, occurring at a rate of 2 per patient-day, based on the results of an observational study in 36 hospitals and skilled nursing facilities. The medication administration errors occurred at a rate of 19% overall (605 errors detected on 3,216 doses) or of 10% excluding wrong-time errors. The most frequent types of errors were wrong time (43%), omission (30%), and wrong dose (17%). Seven percent of the errors were judged to have the potential for resulting in ADEs, or more than 40 per day in a 300-bed hospital.[77]

Medication administration error rates in hospitals (excluding wrong-time errors) range from 0% to 18%, measured by observational studies conducted since 1980 in several countries. Error rates as low as two to three per patient per week have been achieved by installing unit-dose systems. Comparison of error rates between studies should be made cautiously, considering differences in error category definitions and methodologies.[31]

In addition to hospital and skilled nursing facility studies, medication administration errors have been studied in specific areas. Croskerry and colleagues described 15 adult and pediatric medication error cases in an emergency department, including discussions about how the errors can be prevented.[78]

Interventions and Solutions

There are several objectives in developing systems designed for safe medication practices. These objectives include making errors difficult to occur, creating redundancy (double checks) in the system, and creating systems to automatically correct (buffer) errors. For example, computerized physician order entry (CPOE) systems have been gaining increased importance in hospital settings. CPOE is a valuable resource in providing patient medication history and other pertinent data. CPOE systems also provide clinical information such as drug interactions, adverse drug reactions, guidelines, and formulary/generic drug information. CPOE can reduce dispensing errors that occur as a result of prescribers' poor handwriting. CPOE can also reduce errors by taking into account patient information and alerting the prescriber to potential errors. For example, if a prescriber ordered a medication dose based on the patient's weight and ordered an excessive dose, the system would prompt the prescriber to check the dosing. Some other key areas for systems or organizations to focus on to reduce medication errors are to create systems in which process steps are simplified, to standardize and simplify communication, and to create redundancies (such as double checks).[15]

In keeping with the framework displayed in Figure 21-1, interventions can be targeted at all three levels of analysis, but they will be most successful when they are supported by changes in the nontargeted levels simultaneously. At the most proximal level, error training has been used in other organizations to great effect.[79,80] The main idea of error training is to expose people to common errors in their tasks and allow for practice in handling those errors under controlled conditions. Keith and colleagues have reported not only better performance but deeper learning and development of expertise of error-trained individuals compared with control subjects.[80]

A second intervention approach, this one at the interactive level, is stress inoculation, which is similar to error training in that it allows staff to practice responses in controlled conditions.[53] However, the intent of stress inoculation is to prepare the staff to cope with work-related stressors of all kinds, not just errors. Research in other domains has supported this approach as useful and beneficial.[81] At the organizational level, a stress audit can be useful to pinpoint areas of the work environment that may contribute to perceived stress by employees. The stress audit can take a number of forms, but should include at least the following: an assessment of the stress capacity of the employees (including stress tolerance and coping abilities), a detailed assessment of the work environment, and a historical survey of possible stress-related outcomes (errors, work injuries, absences, turnover, etc.). Finally, culture and climate change can be instituted to support new approaches to error management.[82-84]

One concrete solution that can be installed to facilitate these changes is error management meetings. The purpose of the meetings is to encourage organizational learning and reduce the stigma associated with errors; by doing this, the organization can develop expertise as a unit and should be better able to detect and intercept harmful errors before they reach the consumer.[85] However, use of these meetings should be relatively frequent (i.e., once a week), include actual errors and "near errors" (captured before they exited the facility), and accompanied by clear changes in management priorities so as to emphasize their importance. Otherwise, they run the risk of being seen merely as superficial quality control devices. For example, in a hospital pharmacy setting, it is important to consistently meet to discuss and evaluate sources of errors, develop interventions to reduce errors, assess the impact of interventions on errors, and measure and track medication errors.

DETECTING AND REPORTING MEDICATION ERRORS

Detecting and reporting medication errors can be accomplished by many different methods. This section of the chapter focuses on the most common error detection and reporting mechanisms.

Anonymous Self-Reports

Methods such as questionnaires can be used to enable the person who made or witnessed the error to report it without being associated with it. Some advantages of this method are the low cost and the avoidance of fear of disciplinary action. A disadvantage is that the person witnessing the error can report it only if he or she is aware that an error was made.[15]

Incident Reports

Incident reports are the most commonly used method for documenting medication errors. An incident report is the official written legal report of a medication error as documented by hospital staff. When an error is detected by staff, a standard form required by the hospital is completed to report the incident. Incident reports may or may not be anonymous. Voluntary reporting of medication errors in a culture of safety without fear of disciplinary action is promoted by the Joint Commission, the Food and Drug Administration (FDA), the United States Pharmacopeia (USP), and the Institute for Safe Medication Practices. Medication-use system processes that may have led to the error are analyzed in an attempt to prevent similar errors.[86]

The primary limitation of the incident report method is the underdetection of errors. The number of incident reports filed is not an accurate representation of the actual frequency of errors, and should not be used in research to evaluate the effects of interventions on errors. Flynn and colleagues compared observation methods to incident reports, and found 1 error detected by incident reports in an examination of 2,557 doses in a total of 36 hospitals and skilled-nursing facilities. Observation detected 456 errors among these doses.[87] Comparable results have been reported in other studies.[88-90] Cullen and colleagues studied the frequency of reporting ADEs and found underreporting of ADEs as well.[91]

Several reasons may explain why only a small percentage of medication errors are reported. For example, in a hospital setting, nurses cannot report an error unless they are aware that an error has occurred. There is heavy reliance upon the nurse's motivation to report the error. Evidence suggests that the nurse is not likely to report the error if a physician advises against reporting the error, if the nurse believes that the drug involved will not lead to patient harm, or if the error involved is an omission or wrong-time error.[92] An ethnomethodologic study by Baker found some additional reasons that nurses do not report some errors, based on their own definition of what is and is not an error.[93] A survey of 1,105 staff nurses at 25 hospitals found three factors related to the frequency of error reporting: administrative response to reports, personal fears, and unit quality management.[94]

Incident reports have been used as a source of data in studies of the clinical significance and possible causes of medication errors. Descriptions of the use of incident reports are available in a number of settings, including anesthesia,[95,96] pediatrics,[97-99] tertiary care hospitals,[100] and community pharmacies.[101,102] An analysis of mortalities associated with medication errors from 1993 to 1998 in the FDA's Adverse Event Reporting System found that improper doses represented 41% of the fatal errors.[103] The USP publishes data and focused analyses from their national voluntary medication error reporting database and MEDMARX program on a regular basis.[104,105]

Chart Review

Chart review has been used to detect medication errors and adverse drug events. The chart review is focused on areas that are related to medication use, such as medication orders, laboratory test results, physician progress notes, nurse notes, and the medication administration record (MAR). Trained nurses or pharmacists review information looking for clues that an error might have occurred. Clues include sudden acute changes in a patient's condition, clarification of an order, and lab results that exceed normal values to a degree that it was likely that an error occurred (e.g., a blood glucose level above 400 could indicate an omitted insulin dose).[106] Orders for red-flag or trigger drugs such as naloxone and flumazenil may indicate that a medication error has occurred.[107] Chart review detected 24 medication administration errors, compared with 456 detected using direct observation of the same 2,557 doses in one study.[87] Chart review is best used when patient harm resulting from medication errors is the focus of the research. Grasso and colleagues found that retrospective chart review identified 2,194 errors over 1,448 patient-days, compared with 9 errors that were self-reported in a state psychiatric hospital.[108]

Observation

The observation technique was developed for the detection of medication administration errors by Barker and McConnell.[92] A nurse or pharmacist trained in the observation technique accompanies the person administering medications and witnesses the preparation and administration of each dose. The observer writes down exactly what the subject does, including all details of the medication, and notes consumption of the medication by the patient.[33] The observer's notes are then compared with the original prescriber orders to identify discrepancies. An error is counted if there are any differences between what was ordered and what was administered. The accuracy rate is calculated as the percentage of doses administered correctly.[109,110]

The observation method overcomes many of the limitations of the incident report method because it does not require the nurse to be aware of the error, be willing to report it, and to retain a memory of the error. As noted earlier, observation detects many more errors and types per unit time than other methods—it can detect 24 times more errors than chart review, and 456 times more than incident reports.[87] The potential disadvantages of the observation method include the following:[109]

- *Fatigue:* Observation is a physically and mentally demanding activity if performed for more than a few hours each day.
- *Staff:* A trained nurse or pharmacist is required, which may be difficult to arrange during staff shortages.
- *Influence of observer:* The effects of close observation upon subjects can be minimized by striving to remain unobtrusive and nonjudgmental.
- *Observer inference:* Careful training of observers and proper category definitions can minimize this problem.

Dean and Barber confirmed that if the observer is unobtrusive and nonjudgmental, the subject will resume normal work patterns within a brief period.[111,112]

How accurately do pharmacists fill prescriptions? Methods for answering this question include having a pharmacist double-check the filled orders,[32] self-report by pharmacists,[113] and analyzing patient reports of errors on prescriptions. Observation has also been used to identify system problems and technology workarounds that may contribute to medication errors.[114]

Computerized Error Monitoring

Computerized error monitoring detects medication errors and ADEs by screening for trigger drug orders and evaluating lab test results for outliers that may have resulted from an error. Hospital personnel are alerted that follow-up is needed to confirm the error and treat the patient if necessary.[115,116] Jha and colleagues compared computerized monitoring of ADEs to chart review and voluntary reporting.[117] Chart review identified the most ADEs (398), followed by computerized monitoring (275) and voluntary reporting, for a total of 21,964 patient-days.[47] Chart review and computerized monitoring identified 67 of the same ADEs, and 2 ADEs were detected by both voluntary reporting and computerized monitoring.[117] Retrospective computerized analysis of outpatient medication records for ADEs found a rate of 5.5 per 100 patients.[118]

Systems Approach to Error Detection and Reduction

Root cause analysis (RCA) can be used to identify critical underlying reasons for the occurrence of the adverse event or near miss. The major steps of an RCA are convening a team, documenting and researching the incident, and identifying its possible root causes. The RCA is an analytical approach used in organizations to find out what happened, why it happened, and what will prevent it from happening again. Key learning can occur from a RCA, and a system or organization can use the findings to improve its processes. The RCA should include all the key staff associated with the incident. The RCA also provides managers an opportunity to implement more reliable and cost-effective processes. For an RCA to be effective, an organization needs to be open to realizing that system flaws may be discovered by performing this analysis.[15]

The purpose of failure mode effects analysis (FMEA) is to discover potential risks in a product or system by identifying ways in which a failure could occur. FMEA is a risk assessment method that identifies where a potential error could occur at each step in a process. In an FMEA, one may ask what would happen if a prescriber were to mistake one medication for another because of similar packaging, administer a dose by the wrong route, or give a drug at the wrong time. Once these potential failures are identified, potential interventions can be put into place to assist in preventing an error.[15]

There are several promising interventions that could lead to reductions in medication error through enhancements in detecting and learning from the errors that occur. It is important to clarify that a successful intervention need not reduce the overall number of self-reporting errors; in fact, it may increase them. Thus, the most appropriate outcome measure is the ratio of errors that reach the patient to overall prescriptions produced; this is a batting average of sorts and considers the probability of error in its correct form. Data regarding the number of recurrences of the same error over time are also useful to chart the learning ability of the organization.

PUBLIC POLICY IMPLICATIONS

In recent years there has been an increase of publicly available data, in part as a result of Centers for Medicare and Medicaid Services (CMS) regulations. The move to publicly report data is a move toward transparency in hospital outcomes. In August 2008, CMS began displaying hospital mortality rates from certain disease groups and procedures. Many hospitals will now also receive a reduced payment from CMS for what are seen as preventable injuries (e.g., injuries from falls/fractures, hospital-acquired infections). Could publicly reporting medication errors and adverse events be next?[119]

A continuous quality improvement (CQI) program is a system of standards and procedures to identify and evaluate quality-related events (QRE). An example of a QRE is an incorrect dispensing of a prescribed medication that is received by a patient. In Massachusetts, CQI requirements were implemented for each pharmacy in the state as of December 2005. The implementation required each pharmacy to identify an individual or individuals to monitor CQI program compliance, identify and document QREs, minimize the impact of QREs on patients, and analyze QRE data to determine causes and identify interventions to prevent QREs, as well as an annual CQI education for pharmacy staff.[120]

SUMMARY

Why is it important for pharmacists to understand the importance and implications of medication errors? Could we have an error-free environment? Errors can occur at any time and to anyone. If we can understand why they occur, when they can occur, and how to detect and report an error, we can learn how these errors could potentially be prevented. In a fast-paced community pharmacy or hospital unit, we can all become familiar with processes and make critical judgments that can affect patients. The judgments would be based on the best available resources and information. One of the reasons why we all need to understand the importance of this chapter is that each of us is vulnerable to error. We are all going to be in situations where we rely on others to work together to provide the safest care possible in any number of the care settings mentioned. Medication errors are a vast topic that has received much attention over recent years. It is hoped that this chapter will guide the reader to learn more about the individual, interpersonal, and organizational perspectives of medication errors that occur throughout the drug delivery system and to discover innovative ways to reduce medication errors.

Portions of this chapter were adapted by permission from Cohen, MR. *Medication Errors*, 2nd edition. Washington, DC: American Pharmacists Association; 2007:20.

REFERENCES

1. National Coordinating Council for Medication Error Reporting and Prevention. What is a medication error? (c)1998-2008. (Accessed August 2008 at http://www.nccmerp.org.)
2. Davies T. Deaths of 3 babies in Indiana spotlight medication mix-ups. 2006. (Accessed May 23, 2007, at http://www.boston.com/news/nation/articles/2006/09/23/deaths_of_3_babies_in_indiana_spotlight_medication_mix_ups/.)
3. Aspden P, Wolcott J, Bootman JL, Cronenwett LR, eds. Preventing medication errors. Washington, DC: National Academies Press, 2007.

4. Kohn LT, Corrigan JM, Donaldson MS, eds. To err is human: building a safer health system. Washington, DC: National Academies Press, 2000.

5. Leape LL, Brennon TA, Laird N, et al. The nature of adverse events in hospitalized patients. Results of the Harvard Medical Practice Study II. N Engl J Med 1991;324:370-6.

6. Agency for Healthcare Research and Quality. Medical errors: the scope of the problem. 2000. (Accessed October 15, 2005, at http://www.ahrq.gov/qual/errback/htm.)

7. Bond CA, Raehl CL, Franke T. Clinical pharmacy services, hospital pharmacy staffing, and medication errors in United States hospitals. Pharmacotherapy 2002;22(2):134-47.

8. Quality Interagency Coordination Task Force. Report of the Quality Interagency Coordination Task Force (QuIC) to the President. February 2000. (Accessed October 15, 2005, at http://www.quic.gov/report/errors6.pdf.)

9. Grasha AF, O'Neill M. Cognitive processes in medication errors. US Pharmacist 1996;21:96-109.

10. Schell KL, Grasha AF, Reilley S, Tranum D. Improving accuracy in simulated product assembly tasks using workspace interventions to enhance the cognitive environment. Cincinnati, OH: Cognitive Systems Performance Laboratory, University of Cincinnati, 2001:1-13. (Technical report no. 06-1201.)

11. Reason J. Human error. New York: Cambridge University Press, 1990.

12. Reason J. Managing the risks of organizational accidents. Aldershot, England: Ashgate, 1997.

13. Moray N. Error reduction as a systems problem. In: Bogner MS, ed. Human error in medicine. Hillsdale, NJ: Erlbaum, 1994:67-92.

14. Bates DW, Cullen DJ, Laird N, et al. Incidence of adverse drug events and potential adverse drug events. Implications for prevention. ADE Prevention Study Group. JAMA 1995;274(1):29-34.

15. Cohen MR. Medication errors. 2nd ed. Washington, DC: American Pharmacists Association, 2007:112-639.

16. Johnson A, Proctor RW. Attention: theory and practice. Thousand Oaks, CA: Sage, 2004.

17. Schell KL, Kelley K, Hunsaker C. Focused attention and error detection in a prescription checking task. Poster presented to the annual conference of the Society for Industrial-Organizational Psychology, Los Angeles, CA, 2005.

18. Norman DA, Bobrow DB. On data-limited and resource-limited processes. Cogn Psychol 1975;7:44-64.

19. Franconeri SL, Hollingworth A, Simons DJ. Do new objects capture attention? Psychol Sci 2005;16:275-81.

20. Franconeri SL, Simons DJ. Moving and looming stimuli capture attention. Percept Psychophysics 2003;65:999-1010.

21. Ozer DJ, Benet-Martinez V. Personality and the prediction of consequential outcomes. Ann Rev Psychol 2006;57:401-21.

22. Schell KL, Grasha AF. State anxiety, performance accuracy and work pace in a simulated pharmacy dispensing task. Percept Motor Skills 2000;90:547-61.

23. Schell KL, Melton EC, Woodruff A, Corbin GB. Self-regulation, engagement, motivation and performance in a simulated quality control task. Psychol Rep 2004;94:944-54.

24. Ericsson KA, Charness N. Expert performance: its structure and acquisition. Am Psychol 1994;49:725-47.

25. Shiffrin RM, Schneider W. Controlled and automatic human information processing: II. Perceptual learning, automatic attending and a general theory. Psychol Rev 1977;84:127-90.

26. Logan GD. Attention and preattention in theories of automaticity. Am J Psychol 1992;105: 317-39.

27. Anderson JR. The architecture of cognition. Hillsdale, NJ: Lawrence Erlbaum, 1983.

28. Anderson JR. Rules of the mind. Hillsdale, NJ: Lawrence Erlbaum, 1993.

29. Shallice T. From neuropsychology to mental structure. Cambridge: Cambridge University Press, 1988.

30. The Joint Commission. National patient safety goals. 2008. (Accessed September 8, 2008, at http://www.jointcommission.org/AccreditationPrograms/Hospitals/NPSG/.)

31. Flynn EA, Barker KN. Medication error research. In: Cohen MR, ed. Medication errors. 2nd ed. Washington, DC: American Pharmaceutical Association, 2006.

32. Flynn EA, Barker KN, Carnahan BJ. National observational study of prescription dispensing accuracy and safety in 50 pharmacies. J Am Pharm Assoc 2003;43(2):191-200.

33. Barker KN, Flynn EA, Pepper GA. Observation method of detecting medication errors. Am J Health Syst Pharm 2002;59(23):2314-6.

34. Manasse HR. Medication use in an imperfect world: drug misadventuring as an issue of public policy. Part 2. Am J Hosp Pharm 1989;46:1141-52.

35. Nau DP, Erickson SR. Medication safety: patients' experiences, beliefs, and behaviors. J Am Pharm Assoc 2005;45(4):452-7.

36. Guernsey BG, Ingrim NB, Hokanson JA, et al. Pharmacists' dispensing accuracy in a high-volume outpatient pharmacy service: focus on risk management. Drug Intell Clin Pharm 1983;17(10):742-6.

37. Kistner UA, Keith MR, Sergeant KA, Hokanson JA. Accuracy of dispensing in a high-volume, hospital-based outpatient pharmacy. Am J Hosp Pharm 1994;51:2793-7.

38. Buchanan TL, Barker KN, Gibson JT, Jiang BC, Pearson RE. Illumination and errors in dispensing. Am J Hosp Pharm 1991;48(10):2137-45.

39. Allan EL, Barker KN, Malloy MJ, Heller WM. Dispensing errors and counseling in community practice. Am Pharm 1995;NS35:25-33.

40. Ashcroft DM, Quinlan P, Blenkinsopp A. Prospective study of the incidence, nature and causes of dispensing errors in community pharmacies. Pharmacoepidemiol Drug Safety 2005;14(5):327-32.

41. Woller TW, Stuart J, Vrabel R, Senst B. Checking of unit dose cassettes by pharmacy technicians at three Minnesota hospitals: pilot project. Am J Hosp Pharm 1991;48:1952-6.

42. Becker MD, Johnson MH, Longe RL. Errors remaining in unit-dose carts after checking by pharmacists versus pharmacy technicians. Am J Hosp Pharm 1978;35:432-4.

43. Mayo CE, Kitchens RG, Reese L, et al. Distribution accuracy of a decentralized unit-dose system. Am J Hosp Pharm 1975;32:1124-6.

44. Taylor J, Gaucher M. Medication selection errors made by pharmacy technicians in filling unit dose orders. Can J Hosp Pharm 1986;39:9-12.

45. Hassall TH, Daniels CE. Evaluation of three types of control chart methods in unit dose error monitoring. Am J Hosp Pharm 1983;40:970-5.

46. Hoffmann RP, Bartt KH, Berlin L, Frank BM. Multidisciplinary quality assessment of a unit dose drug distribution system. Hosp Pharm 1984;19:167-9, 173-4.

47. Cina JL, Gandhi TK, Churchill W, et al. How many hospital pharmacy medication dispensing errors go undetected? Jt Comm J Qual Patient Safety 2006;32(2):73-80.

48. Chi J. Tech-check-tech, as sanctioned practice, gaining in states. Hosp Pharm Rep 1994;8:14, 17.

49. Ness JE, Sullivan SD, Stergachis A. Accuracy of technicians and pharmacists in identifying dispensing errors. Am J Hosp Pharm 1994;51:354-7.

50. Campbell GM, Facchinetti NJ. Using process control charts to monitor dispensing and checking errors. Am J Health Syst Pharm 1998;55(9):946-52.

51. Pang F, Grant JA. Missing medications associated with centralized unit-dose dispensing. Am J Hosp Pharm 1975;32:1121-3.

52. Lazarus RS, Folkman S. Stress, appraisal and coping. New York: Springer, 1984.

53. Quick JC, Quick JD, Nelson DL, Hurrell JJ Jr. Preventive stress management in organizations. Washington, DC: American Psychological Association, 1997.

54. Wolfgang AP. Is pharmacist turnover a function of job stress? Am Pharm 1987;NS27:33-7.

55. Lapane KL, Hughes CM. Baseline job satisfaction and stress among pharmacists and pharmacy technicians participating in the Fleetwood Phase III study. Consult Pharm 2004;19:1029-37.

56. Lapane KL, Hughes CM. Job satisfaction and stress among pharmacists in the long-term care sector. Consult Pharm 2006;21:287-92.

57. Judge TA, Ilies R, Scott BA. Work-family conflict and emotions: effects at work and at home. Personnel Psychol 2006;59:779-814.

58. Somech A, Drach-Zahavy A. Strategies for coping with work-family conflict: the distinctive relationships of gender role ideology. J Occup Health Psychol 2007;12:1-19.

59. Davies DR, Parasuraman R. The psychology of vigilance. London: Academic Press, 1982.

60. Wickens CD, Hollands JG. Engineering psychology and human performance. 3rd ed. Upper Saddle River, NJ: Prentice Hall, 2000.

61. Bilsing-Palacio L, Schell KL. Signal probability effects on error detection performance in a quality control task. Psychol Rep 2003;93:343-52.

62. Schell KL, Hunsaker C, Kelley K. Extending effects of salience and payoffs on stimulus discrimination: an experimental simulation of prescription checking. Percept Motor Skills 2006; 103:375-86.

63. Marken RS. Errors in skilled performance: a control model of prescribing. Ergonomics 2003; 46:1200-14.

64. Prinzel LJ III, Freeman FG, Prinzel HD. Individual differences in complacency and monitoring for automation failures. Individual Diff Res 2005;3:27-49.

65. Young PT. Affective arousal: some implications. Am Psychol 1967;22:32-40.

66. Hart SG, Staveland LE. Development of NASA-TLX (Task Load Index): results of empirical and theoretical research. In: Hancock PA, Meshkati N, eds. Human mental workload. Amsterdam: North-Holland, 1988:139-83.

67. Taxis K, Barber N. Ethnographic study of incidence and severity of intravenous drug errors. BMJ 2003;326(7391):684-7.

68. Kuyper AR. Patient counseling detects prescription errors. Hosp Pharm 1993;28:1180-1, 1184-9.

69. Schneider B, Brief AP, Guzzo RA. Creating a climate and culture for sustainable organizational change. Organ Dynamics 1996;24:7-19.

70. Parker D, Lawrie M, Hudson P. A framework for understanding the development of organisational safety culture. Safety Sci 2006;44:551-62.

71. Wiegmann DA, Zhang H, von Thaden TL, Sharma G, Gibbons AM. Safety culture: an integrative review. Int J Aviation Psychol 2004;14:117-34.

72. Hofmann DA, Mark B. An investigation of the relationship between safety climate and medication errors as well as other nurse and patient outcomes. Personnel Psychol 2006;59:847-69.

73. Mott DA. Pharmacist job turnover, length of service, and reasons for leaving. Am J Health Syst Pharm 2000;57:975-84.

74. Poon EG, Cina JL, Churchill W, et al. Medication dispensing errors and potential adverse drug events before and after implementing bar code technology in the pharmacy. Ann Intern Med 2006;145(6):426-34.

75. Flynn EA, Barker KN. Effect of an automated dispensing system on errors in two pharmacies. J Am Pharm Assoc 2006;46(5):613-5.

76. Teagarden JR, Nagle B, Aubert RE, Wasdyke C, Courtney P, Epstein RS. Dispensing error rate in a highly automated mail-service pharmacy practice. Pharmacotherapy 2005;25(11):1629-35.

77. Barker KN, Flynn EA, Pepper GA, Bates DW, Mikeal RL. Medication errors observed in 36 healthcare facilities. Arch Intern Med 2002;162(16):1897-1903.

78. Croskerry PSM, Campbell S, LeBlanc C, et al. Profiles in patient safety: medication errors in the emergency department. Acad Emerg Med 2004;11:289-99.

79. Heimbeck D, Frese M, Sonnentag S, Keith N. Integrating errors into the training process: the function of error management instructions and the role of goal orientation. Personnel Psychol 2003;56:333-61.

80. Keith N, Frese M. Self-regulation in error management training: emotion control and metacognition as mediators of performance effects. J Appl Psychol 2005;90:677-91.

81. Southwick SM, Vythilingham M, Charney DS. The psychobiology of depression and resilience to stress: implications for prevention and treatment. Ann Rev Clin Psychol 2006;1:255-91.

82. Kaissi A. An organizational approach to understanding patient safety and medical errors. Healthcare Manager 2006;25:292-305.

83. Milligan FJ. Establishing a culture for patient safety—the role of education. Nurse Educ Today 2007;27(2):95-102

84. Vogus TJ, Sutcliffe KM. The Safety Organizing Scale: development and validation of a behavioral measure of safety culture in hospital nursing units. Med Care 2007;45:46-54.

85. Argyris C, Schon DA. Organizational learning II: theory, method and practice. Reading, MA: Addison-Wesley, 1996.

86. Phillips MA. Voluntary reporting of medication errors. Am J Health Syst Pharm 2002;59(23):2326-8.

87. Flynn EA, Barker KN, Pepper GA, Bates DW, Mikeal RL. Comparison of methods for detecting medication errors in 36 hospitals and skilled-nursing facilities. Am J Health Syst Pharm 2002;59(5):436-46.

88. Barker KN, Kimbrough WW, Heller WM. A study of medication errors in a hospital. Fayetteville, AR: University of Arkansas, 1966.

89. Barker KN, Harris JA, Webster DB, et al. Consultant evaluation of a hospital medication system: analysis of the existing system. Am J Hosp Pharm 1984;41:2009-16.

90. Borel JM, Rascati KL. Effect of an automated, nursing unit-based drug-dispensing device on medication errors. Am J Health Syst Pharm 1995;52(17):1875-9.

91. Cullen DJ, Bates DW, Small SD, Cooper JB, Nemeskal AR, Leape LL. The incident reporting system does not detect adverse drug events: a problem for quality improvement. Jt Comm J Qual Improve 1995;21(10):541-8.

92. Barker KN, McConnell WE. The problems of detecting medication errors in hospitals. Am J Hosp Pharm 1962;19:360-9.

93. Baker HM. Rules outside the rules for administration of medication: a study in New South Wales, Australia. Image J Nurs Scholarship 1997;29(2):155-8.

94. Blegen MA, Vaughn T, Pepper G, et al. Patient and staff safety: voluntary reporting. Am J Med Qual 2004;19(2):67-74.

95. Chopra V, Bovill JG, Spierdijk J, Koornneef F. Reported significant observations during anaesthesia: a prospective analysis over an 18-month period. Br J Anaesth 1992;68(1):13-7.

96. Currie M, Mackay P, Morgan C, et al. The Australian Incident Monitoring Study. The "wrong drug" problem in anaesthesia: an analysis of 2000 incident reports. Anaesth Intens Care 1993;21(5):596-601.

97. Wong IC, Ghaleb MA, Franklin BD, Barber N. Incidence and nature of dosing errors in paediatric medications: a systematic review. Drug Safety 2004;27(9):661-70.

98. Ross LM, Wallace J, Paton JY. Medication errors in a paediatric teaching hospital in the UK: five years operational experience. Arch Dis Child 2000;83(6):492-7.

99. Wilson DG, McArtney RG, Newcombe RG, et al. Medication errors in paediatric practice: insights from a continuous quality improvement approach. Eur J Pediatrics 1998;157(9):769-74.

100. Winterstein AG, Johns TE, Rosenberg EI, et al. Nature and causes of clinically significant medication errors in a tertiary care hospital. Am J Health Syst Pharm 2004;61(18):1908-16.

101. Kennedy AG, Littenberg B. Medication error reporting by community pharmacists in Vermont. J Am Pharm Assoc 2004;44(4):434-8.

102. Quinlan P, Ashcroft DM, Blenkinsopp A. Medication errors: a baseline survey of dispensing errors reported in community pharmacy. Int J Pharm Pract 2002;10(suppl):R68.

103. Phillips J, Beam S, Brinker A, et al. Retrospective analysis of mortalities associated with medication errors. Am J Health Syst Pharm 2001;58:1835-41.

104. Santell JP, Protzel MM, Cousins D. Medication errors in oncology practice. US Pharmacist 2004;29(4):NIL_0001-5.

105. Hicks RW, Cousins DD, Williams RL. Selected medication-error data from USP's MEDMARX program for 2002. Am J Health Syst Pharm 2004;61(10):993-1000.

106. Kaushal R. Using chart review to screen for medication errors and adverse drug events. Am J Health Syst Pharm 2002;59(23):2323-5.

107. Dalton-Bunnow MF, Halvachs FJ. Computer-assisted use of tracer antidote drugs to increase detection of adverse drug reactions: retrospective and concurrent trial. Hosp Pharm 1993;28:746-9, 752-5.

108. Grasso BC, Genest R, Jordan CW, Bates DW. Use of chart and record reviews to detect medication errors in a state psychiatric hospital. Psychiatr Serv 2003;54(5):677-81.

109. Barker KN. Data collection techniques: observation. Am J Hosp Pharm 1980;37:1235-43.

110. Mays N, Pope C. Qualitative research: observational methods in healthcare settings. BMJ 1995;311(6998):182-4.

111. Dean B, Barber N. Validity and reliability of observational methods for studying medication administration errors. Am J Health Syst Pharm 2001;58(1):54-9.

112. Kerlinger FN, Lee HB. Observations of behavior and sociometry. In: Foundations of behavioral research. 4th ed. Fort Worth, TX: Harcourt College Publishers, 2000:727-52.

113. Chua SS, Wong IC, Edmondson H, et al. A feasibility study for recording of dispensing errors and 'near misses' in four UK primary care pharmacies. Drug Safety 2003;26(11):803-13.

114. Patterson ES, Rogers ML, Chapman RJ, Render ML. Compliance with intended use of bar code medication administration in acute and long-term care: an observational study. Hum Factors 2006;48(1):15-22.

115. Classen DC, Pestotnik SL, Evans RS, Burke JP. Computerized surveillance of adverse drug events in hospital patients. JAMA 1991;266:2847-51.

116. Bates DW. Using information technology to screen for adverse drug events. Am J Health Syst Pharm 2002;59(23):2317-9.

117. Jha AK, Kuperman GJ, Teich JM, et al. Identifying adverse drug events: development of a computer-based monitor and comparison with chart review and stimulated voluntary report. J Am Med Inform Assoc 1998;5(3):305-14.

118. Honigman B, Lee J, Rothschild J, et al. Using computerized data to identify adverse drug events in outpatients. J Am Med Inform Assoc 2001;8(3):254-66.

119. Centers for Medicare and Medicaid Services. FY 2008 inpatient prospective payment system proposed rule improving the quality of hospital care. (Accessed September 8, 2008, at http://www.cms.hhs.gov/apps/media/press/factsheet.asp?Counter=2119.)

120. 247 CMR 15: Board of Registration in Pharmacy. Continuous quality improvement program. (Accessed September 8, 2008, at http://www.mass.gov/Eeohhs2/docs/dph/regs/247cmr011.pdf.)

CHAPTER 22

Ethical Issues Influencing Public Policy Initiatives

Robert I. Garis, PhD, MBA, Jeremy Popek, PharmD, and Richard L. O'Brien, MD, FACP

We are often faced with decisions of what is right and wrong in the practice of pharmacy. This is brought home to most of us in issues that we face in daily practice and in the public policy arena. Public policy issues affecting pharmacy include conscientious objection to contraception and abortion, patient privacy issues, and the practices of pharmacy benefit managers. To facilitate our discussion of the public policy issues, it will be useful to address some commonly used terms in the ethics vocabulary, examine ethical theories, introduce a decision-making process, and explore why good people disagree on moral issues. Finally, we introduce some of the current public policy issues that we, as pharmacists, face.

ETHICS: A PRIMER

Whether we are performing duties as a pharmacist, parent, or a concerned friend, we make decisions about what is right and wrong. We use personal *values* to guide our actions. Our values depend on our upbringing, our beliefs, the rules of our society, our religion, and our life experiences.

An assessment of whether a course of action is right or wrong is *ethics*, a systematic analysis that arose from the disciplines of theology and philosophy. The second edition of *Webster's New Universal Unabridged Dictionary* defines ethics as "the study of standards of conduct and moral judgment; moral philosophy."[1] Figure 22-1 provides a useful description of the relationship of morality, values, and ethics, as formulated by Purtilo.[2]

Understanding how people live together the best (morality) is influenced by our parents, the beliefs and organization of our society, and our religious and philosophical

Morality Interested in how persons can live successfully together
Values Customs, laws, beliefs, societal rules, etc. These differ depending on one's culture and religion.
Ethics A framework in which one can assess a moral situation and reach a conclusion that will facilitate the coexistence of persons.

FIGURE 22-1 The Relationship of Morality, Values, and Ethics
Source: Purtilo RB, Ethical dimensions in the health professions. 3rd ed. Philadelphia (PA): W.B. Saunders 1999. 81-9.

influences (values). As we arrive at decisions concerning what is "best," we use the tools of ethics. That is, ethics could be referred to as a framework in which we assess a moral situation and reach a conclusion intended to facilitate the coexistence of people.

ETHICAL THEORIES

We make decisions based on our value systems. We likely use tools from ethical theory whether we know it or not. This section provides short descriptions of five commonly used ethical theories and looks at how these theories help us arrive at rational decisions on morality.

Ethical theories are like theories in any other discipline: they attempt to provide a framework with which to observe and judge the world. We focus on normative theories, that is, theories that attempt to describe what is good and bad. A classic example of a normative principle is the Golden Rule, "we should treat others the way we would like to be treated."[3] Put another way, normative ethics answer the question "what kinds of things are good?"[4] This discussion focuses on five theories in common use: principlism, deontology, utilitarianism, contractarianism, and libertarianism.

Principlism

In some cases, persons subscribing to different ethical theories can arrive at different conclusions. Principlism is a theory that Beauchamp and Childress introduced seeking a common ground between theories discussed later in this chapter, deontology and utilitarianism.[5] Principlism attempts to use concepts that ethicists can generally agree upon.[4] These concepts are ethical principles considered to be behavioral norms that offer a common, basic language concerning a moral life.[2] Ethical principles are moral conditions that have gained acceptance in many societies. The four principles constituting the theory are autonomy, nonmaleficence, beneficence, and justice. The four principles attempt to describe the minimum moral conditions of the healthcare provider.[6]

Autonomy is freedom of self-direction, or moral independence. This independence is applicable when people are able to make decisions for themselves.[7] Healthcare professionals have an obligation to confirm that patients have the information they need to arrive at a decision. The fact that modern medicine can perform heroic acts and prolong life has made autonomy particularly important. Often drastic measures to keep the patient alive can result in increased suffering for the patient and a burden on family members and society. Pharmacists can face conflicts concerning patient autonomy. Conflicts occur when a patient wants to do something that a pharmacist knows is not in the patient's best interest. For example, a patient with a painful infection may want the pain medication filled in order to get immediate relief and not want to fill the expensive antibiotic that goes with the regimen.

Beneficence describes an action done to contribute to a person's welfare or to provide optimal care.[5,8] This principle requires the clinician to take an active role in patient care, to promote good, and prevent harm of the patient when it is occurring.[2] Autonomy and beneficence are in conflict in the situation in which the patient only wants the pain medication and not the antibiotic prescription. We have the obligation to respect the patient's wishes and also the obligation to advocate for the patient's well-being.

Above all (or first) "do no harm" (*nonmaleficence*) is a principle frequently cited as the first principle of health care.[5] This declaration of nonmaleficence is often attributed to the author of the Hippocratic Oath.[2] We distinguish nonmaleficence from beneficence: the latter requires the provider to actively promote good, whereas nonmaleficence requires that we do no harm. We do not dispense benzodiazepines to someone obviously under the influence of alcohol (do no harm). We actively advocate to the patient with the painful infection that the antibiotic is a necessity if he or she intends to get well (beneficence).

Justice is that which is rightfully due to a person. It is generally considered that there are two types of justice: distributive and compensatory. *Distributive justice* is concerned with the fair allocation of benefits and burdens in society. Tensions concerning distributive justice arise in situations of scarce resources and competition for those resources. In public policy this may occur when we address the funding of health promotion and healthcare initiatives. We are challenged with deciding what projects to fund among many worthy proposals, such as AIDS awareness education, immunization programs, upgrading substandard housing projects, and health screening for underserved populations. *Compensatory justice* is concerned with determining appropriate compensation for harm done.[7]

Principlism has been subject to criticism. Some writers have asked, what happens when the principles clash? Others argue that principlism does not give ethicists adequate guidance because it is not a systemized theory. Beauchamp and Childress answer the first criticism by saying that when principles clash, one needs to look for precedents. Responding to the second criticism, the authors defend their theory by saying that systemized theories cause too much disagreement; therefore, principlism is needed because it contains moral conditions upon which ethicists can agree.[5]

Deontology

Deontology is a framework for making moral decisions based on rules or duties to others (*deon* is Greek for "duty").[2,3] The rules that a person chooses as moral guides are assembled by the individual and are shaped by that person's value system. Persons who make decisions with this framework tend to be consistent in their decision making because they hold fast to the rules they value most in a particular situation. Each person has duties to himself or herself and to others, and therefore has rules for each situation. Pharmacists might hold to the rules of law as their professional guides. Still others might hold to the rules of their spiritual training or to the rules in their professional code of ethics. People who use this theory, either knowingly or unknowingly, may have problems selecting between competing rules they value. A basic premise of deontology is that a person should always be treated as an end and not the means to an end. The consequences of an act are less important than consistently following the rule one believes to be right.[4] Deontology is most closely associated with the 18th century German philosopher Immanuel Kant and 20th century American philosopher John Rawls.

Utilitarianism

The utilitarian theory is also known as a teleological or consequentialist approach to determining right and wrong; British philosophers Jeremy Bentham (1748–1832) and John Stuart Mill (1806–1873) were the principal proponents. This theory is based on the premise that an act is right if it brings about the best overall consequences. As opposed to deontology, in which one is concerned with making decisions congruent with one's duty, teleology is concerned with maximizing good consequences. An appeal of the utilitarian approach is that there are public and observable consequences of actions.[3] The utilitarian could be thought of as following three steps in arriving at a moral decision:

1. Identify the problem.
2. Determine the alternatives.
3. Identify the alternative that will yield the best consequences.

This theory presumes that the decision maker can identify all the possible courses of action and then accurately predict which action will maximize good. The inabilities of decision makers to predict the future and accurately measure the consequences of actions are weaknesses of this theory. Many times decision makers subscribing to either a deontological or utilitarian perspective will arrive at the same conclusion.[2]

Contractarianism

The *Stanford Encyclopedia of Philosophy* states that the basis for all contractarian theories is the following: "some scarcity or motive for competition . . . and there is some potential for gains from social interaction and cooperation."[9] Contractarians believe that consent in a society provides legitimacy regarding issues of right and wrong. This theory—or, more appropriately, family of theories—posits that the agreements or contracts established for the mutual benefit of citizens establish the rules for society. The contractarian views the provider–patient relationship as one of respectful communication between two rational individuals. Therefore, paternalistic treatment of the patient by a pharmacist—treating a patient as if he or she were ignorant or inferior to the pharmacist—is seen as a violation of the patient's autonomy. In line with respectful communication, the pharmacist and patient would, perhaps implicitly, enter into a contract. That contract requires the pharmacist to provide the technical and factual information. The patient, then, is responsible for his or her personal decision. In the previous example of the patient with a painful infection who only wanted the pain medication, it would be the pharmacist's role to educate the patient about the need to treat the cause of the pain with the antibiotic. The patient would have the ultimate choice.[9,10]

Contractarian theory has been criticized on several grounds. Patients and providers seldom start off on equal footing in an interaction because of asymmetry of information and weakness, fear, pain, and need on the part of the patient. Critics have also argued that the moral goals of beneficence and nonmaleficence are not given the weight they deserve in the contractarian view of health care. Thus, in the case of the patient with the painful infection, the pharmacist would have done his or her duty by simply informing the patient that only getting the pain medication would not effect a cure.[10]

Libertarianism

The libertarian believes that government should only promulgate rules that protect life, liberty, and the property of citizens in the society. The libertarian believes that competent persons should not be forced to do anything by the state except to prevent harm to other members of the society. Consistent with that philosophy, the libertarian does not believe the state should redistribute wealth, but rather that persons, of their own free will, should give to others out of a sense of compassion and justice. Libertarians see health care as a privilege and believe that healthcare insurance should be privately and voluntarily purchased—each person should pay his or her own way. Therefore, subscribers to this philosophy would oppose the statutory Medicare and Medicaid programs. Further, they believe that charity is a good and moral quality. However, "enforced beneficence" of citizens violates the principle of autonomy.[5] People having this perspective believe in an orderly and harmonious society with voluntary cooperation. Critics argue that this approach leads to inequalities and poverty—people not forced to share their resources will not do so.[11]

The five ethical theories discussed are a sampling of the theories developed to provide frameworks to assess wrong and right. There is considerable overlap among them, and using different ethical frameworks may lead one to different or to similar conclusions. The fact remains that we must make prudent decisions in a world that throws information at us in a seemingly haphazard fashion. Pharmacists can benefit from systematically organizing the facts and reflecting on ethical problems.

A SIX-STEP PROCESS FOR ETHICAL DECISION MAKING

The six-step process described here represents a way to identify the key issues of a problem more clearly—to focus on the important issues and stakeholders—and hence work toward ethical decisions. Ethical situations can be highly charged and arouse strong feelings; therefore, the tendency is to rely on gut instincts in the absence of a systematic evaluation. The process we describe relies on facts, one's values, and the framework of ethical theories to arrive at a decision.

Authors such as Jonsen, Siegler, and Winslade take a physician–patient perspective that stresses information gathering in four domains that affect the patient: medical indications, patient preferences, quality of life issues, and contextual features (e.g., family situation, finances, and religious influences).[12] Other authors have taken a general ethics approach.[13] Whether the problem-solving task deals specifically with patients or not, the processes used to arrive at moral decisions seem to have commonalities: the decision maker must get the facts of the situation and evaluate the moral options available.[2,14,15] Purtilo has outlined a six-step process that seems of particular value to pharmacists.[2] It uses the information-gathering steps articulated by Jonson and colleagues,[12] but with somewhat less emphasis on the aspects of diagnosis, prognosis, rehabilitation, and treatment. Table 22-1 summarizes the six-step process of arriving at moral decisions.

TABLE 22-1 Six-Step Process for Ethical Decision Making

Step	Activity	Questions to Facilitate the Activity
1	Get the facts.	What is the patient's health condition? What resources are available to the patient? Is the patient competent? What are the patient's wishes? Who are the stakeholders? Who are respected, insightful colleagues?
2	Identify the problem.	Is there really a problem? What is the ethical issue? Is there more than one correct action? Do I have the authority to act? Who are respected, insightful colleagues?
3	Apply ethics theories in analysis.	What ethics theories seem appropriate to this situation? Are the theories congruent with my value system? Who are respected, insightful colleagues?
4	Explore practical alternative solutions.	What are possible alternatives to resolve the situation? What does each stakeholder need? What will my job title allow me to do? Who are respected, insightful colleagues?
5	Take action.	Do I have the guts to live with my decision? What do respected colleagues think of my decision?
6	Evaluate the process and outcome.	Did the outcome go as expected? What could have been done better? How do the circumstances of this decision fit with other decisions I will make in professional life? Who are respected, insightful colleagues that have faced the same (or similar) circumstances?

As indicated in step 1 of Table 22-1, when one is faced with a moral decision, it is essential to gather as many facts as possible. Frequently, a pharmacist lacks the necessary information of the patient's medical record, family situation, care needs, and financial situation. To the extent possible, pharmacists should seek information from the patient, physician, and family members. Talk with colleagues who may be more familiar with a particular patient than you. Perhaps the elderly patient on seemingly heroic doses of anxiolytics has been carefully titrated upward and the current dose optimizes his or her functional capacity. Further, this seemingly extreme dose may be necessary to facilitate cooperation of the patient with home health nurses.

Step 2 in the process requires us to determine whether there is a problem. If there is a problem, pharmacists must decide whether action on their part is an option. In the case of a staff pharmacist, there may be organizational policies preventing action at this level of the organization, and the pharmacist may choose to discuss the problem with a supervisor. If action is within the pharmacist's purview, he or she needs to determine whether there is more than one resolution. For example, pharmacists must decide whether they should respect the patient's wishes to refuse the antibiotic for a painful infection (autonomy) or insist that the patient get the antibiotic (beneficence).

Step 3 in the decision-making process requires the pharmacist to use ethical theories to approach the problem. The approach depends greatly on a person's training. Some professionals lacking adequate orientation to ethics may revert to gut feelings or emotions to frame a decision. However, others who are not formally trained may rely on their value systems and exercise rational ethics logic without being aware that ethical theories exist. Pharmacists who have a basic knowledge of the theories are at a distinct advantage because the structure provided by theories may make them less likely to arrive at decisions based on emotion.

In step 4, the pharmacist is charged with developing alternatives to resolve the ethical problem. In pharmacy we are often torn between multiple constituencies: the patient, family members, immediate caregivers, the physician, our supervisors, and the policies of our employer. We may be limited in what we can do at times. Other times, we may be able to craft alternatives that are agreeable to most constituencies. Whether our impact on a situation is minor or quite significant, we must spend the necessary time consulting with stakeholders in such a situation (within the limits of confidentiality) as we formulate alternative approaches. The views of respected colleagues are valuable resources, as in other aspects of professional life.

Step 5 involves action. Ethical decisions are in many cases very difficult. Additionally, because the pharmacist is motivated enough to take action, he or she would likely have strong feelings (a sense of personal passion) about the "rightness" of his or her position. Therefore, criticisms of a pharmacist's decision could be particularly upsetting to the pharmacist. To take action in a very difficult situation requires considerable resolve.

The final step in this decision process is the "quality control" part of the exercise. In this step we critique what we did and determine how we might do it better in the future. Further, this step allows us to accumulate decision rules to apply in subsequent situations.

We have provided some basics upon which to consider public policy issues that affect pharmacy. We realize that ethics is, at best, a challenging topic; it takes years of study and practice to gain proficiency. However, we hope that this outline of decision making allows readers to more critically evaluate the issues presented in the following discussion of public policy. Given the various approaches to ethical decision making, it should be no surprise that people disagree about many issues.

WHY GOOD PEOPLE DISAGREE

However formal our theories of ethics and however structured our approaches to the analyses of specific ethical challenges, well-meaning, conscientious persons frequently arrive at profoundly conflicting moral conclusions. Because health care involves such deeply held values about freedom, well-being, and life itself, health professionals are often caught up in controversial ethical issues. Consider the roles of pharmacists in matters such as contraception, abortion, assisted suicide, euthanasia, and embryonic stem cell research.

Why is it that reasonable, well-intentioned people disagree and hold adversarial positions about these important issues? All persons are likely to hold desirable the avoidance of unwanted pregnancies and the suffering an unwanted child may experience; the prevention of psychological, social, or economic hardships that may result from bearing a child; the diminution of suffering at the end of life; and the development and application of effective cellular therapies to alleviate such debilitating conditions as diabetes or Parkinson disease. Ethical or moral disagreement is usually about the means rather than the end—that is, how to achieve desirable outcomes rather than the outcomes themselves.

Such controversies usually arise because people reason from different premises, hold different values, or weigh values differently. Contributing causes may be uncertainty about facts, different interpretations of available data, and differing ideological positions; the last may also be based on different values and the relative weights placed on values.

Uncertainty about facts and interpretation of data has led to considerable disagreement about the relative therapeutic potential of embryonic stem cells and adult stem cells. Some hold that only embryonic stem cells have the potential to be broadly applicable to replace diseased cells in all or most tissues.[16] Others believe that stem cells derived from cord blood or differentiated tissues possess therapeutic potential adequate to achieve the desired goals and thus obviate the need for deriving and using embryonic stem cells.[17] This kind of disagreement is, in principle, susceptible to resolution by gathering more scientific information. But even if adult stem cells are shown to be therapeutically effective, this will not resolve the moral disagreement about the use of stem cells derived from embryos that are destroyed in the process.

The mechanism of action of Plan B (levonorgestrel) emergency contraception is also subject to uncertainty and may thus lead to differing moral conclusions. Depending on when Plan B is used in a woman's ovulatory cycle, it may prevent ovulation, prevent fertilization of the ovum, or prevent implantation of a blastocyst.[18] Those opposed to contraception are likely to conclude that Plan B use is morally illicit under any circumstances. Some persons view contraception as morally acceptable but oppose destruction of a zygote or any subsequent stage of human development. Their moral objection to Plan B is likely to arise from the fact that it *may* block implantation and is considered tantamount to abortion.

The controversies over abortion, the use of abortifacients, and embryonic stem cell research usually derive from well-meaning persons reasoning from different premises about when a human being acquires moral status and human rights. Some contend that a zygote with the potential to develop into a unique human person has full human moral status. Others put the acquisition of moral status at other times or milestones along the continuum of development: implantation, formation of the neural tube, development of sensation or sensorium, extrauterine viability, birth. A few persons are even willing to accept or counsel infanticide "of severely disabled infants" or even an "older human being who has been profoundly intellectually disabled since birth."[19]

What, then, leads well-meaning persons to adopt such different premises about the acquisition of moral status? It may be religious teaching and belief, cultural tradition, or honest disagreement about how or when a human being becomes a human person with moral status.

Alternatively, differences may arise among people who accept the fact that a zygote, embryo, or fetus has moral status because they assign different values to different lives based on relative potential or realization of potential. Some may reason that a zygote or embryo constitutes a biologically distinct individual human being with potential for full development but conclude that, because there is a rather high rate of embryonal loss in nature (17% to 30%),[20-22] this limited potential is outweighed by the good another person may derive from aborting it or using an embryo formed extracorporeally as a source of stem cells that may help others. Or they may value the freedom to choose, the desires, and the social and economic well-being of a woman over the health and well-being of a fetus. The potential value of cellular replacement therapy to someone suffering from diabetes or Parkinson disease may be viewed more highly than the potential of an insensate early embryo to become fully human. These are essentially utilitarian arguments.

Differences in values and what weight to give them may also derive from different ethical or ideological approaches. There is disagreement in Western societies about whether humans have a right to health care. Libertarians value personal freedom; contractarians put a higher value on collective well-being and the common good. That is not to say that libertarians do not value the common good or that contractarians do not value personal freedom. Rather, they put different weights on competing values. In the case of a right to health care, disagreement stems from differences in weighing the benefit of a right of access to health care against the burden of supporting that right. Providing health care requires resources, and resources are not equally distributed. Providing health care to all means that some must provide more resources—that is, bear a greater (absolute) burden—than others of more modest means. Libertarians hold that the benefit is not worth the burden. Contractarians argue that the benefit *is* worth the burden. Others might argue that burdens are relative and that expecting contribution of greater resources from those of greater wealth is less of a burden than the burden imposed by limited access to health care.

Ideology may also give rise to disagreement because of different convictions about whether a desired outcome is more likely to ensue from a given course of action than another—for example, that a capitalist free market is more likely to generate and distribute wealth and societal resources effectively than a highly regulated social democratic economy. In such instances, finding mutually acceptable middle ground is exceedingly difficult. There is rarely willingness to rely on facts and experience to temper or moderate such positions or to reach compromise.

Ethical principles (e.g., autonomy) may also be interpreted as expressions of values as premises. Thus, the principle of autonomy poses the premise that each person has the right to make autonomous decisions even if there are effects (adverse, good, or neutral) on others, whether the others would want that decision made or not for their own reasons. For example, a person may decide that she does not want treatment for her leukemia because she believes the burden outweighs the potential benefit. Her husband and children, however, may prefer that she undergo treatment because it provides hope. The premise of autonomy is that the choice is hers and hers alone. Principles, like other premises, are not universally held. In some cultures, such decisions are expected to be made by the family or larger group of which an individual is a part.

Efforts are often made to resolve ethical conflicts, usually by attempting to find alternate and mutually agreeable means to reach an agreed-upon desirable end. For example, in the case of stem cell research, many scientists strive to find sources of stem cells that will not result in the destruction of an embryo with the potential for full human development.[23,24] This does not resolve the moral conflict about the legitimacy of using embryonic stem cells in research or treatment, however. It simply attempts to avoid or diminish conflict by finding an alternate means to the end.

There are some conflicts that are not resolvable because people start with different premises and values that derive from belief, personal conviction, or culture and are not subject to scientific or any sort of factual validation. In those instances individuals must reach the best conscientious conclusions that they can and act accordingly.

Pharmacists, like all health professionals, encounter moral conflicts in their practices. Conscientious objection to dispensing drugs that they believe are intended or will be used in ways they find morally objectionable is an example.

PUBLIC POLICY ISSUES

Pharmacists' Conscientious Objection

Pharmacists are frequently asked to dispense legally prescribed agents for purposes they find "morally, religiously, or ethically troubling."[25] These notably include routine or emergency contraception and drugs intended to be used in assisted suicide. They may also be asked to dispense drugs intended to produce superovulation for purposes of in vitro fertilization or to derive ova for embryonic stem cell research. In some nations, they may be asked to fill prescriptions intended for euthanasia.

Why is the filling of such prescriptions troubling? What grounds for conscientious objection can be made? If a pharmacist is morally, religiously, or ethically opposed to contraception, abortion, in vitro fertilization, the intentional termination of life, or the derivation of embryonic stem cells for research or treatment and is presented with prescriptions for drugs that are necessary agents in these practices, then to dispense them is to be complicit in an immoral act or to cooperate in an action that would not occur without his or her participation (known as material cooperation).

Many who are not opposed to such practices disagree with the concept of conscientious objection and insist that the professional prescription and dispensing of legal agents intended to be used for widely accepted legal purposes are morally licit and that access to such medications demands that such prescriptions be filled. Some argue that, as professionals formally sanctioned to serve society, pharmacists have a fiduciary duty to patients and must honor that duty above their own moral beliefs and principles.[26-28] Some suggest that pharmacists (and pharmacies) should be required by law to stock and dispense all legal agents for which they may be presented a prescription. Others go so far as to state that professionals who object to legal and widely accepted healthcare practices should leave the profession.[29,30]

More moderate voices suggest that conscientious decisions by pharmacists should be respected while simultaneously providing alternate means of acquiring the drugs that have been prescribed for those who hold different moral views. They argue that because each individual in our free and liberal society is empowered to make his or her own moral decisions and choices, conscientious objection should be legally approved and protected, that pharmacy owners have an obligation to honor conscientious objection by their employed pharmacists, and that any sort of retaliation against them should be prohibited. But to protect the right of others to choose legal drugs, pharmacists who object to dispensing particular drugs have an obligation to provide alternate means of honoring such prescriptions by referring patients to another pharmacist or pharmacy. If a pharmacy does not stock or dispense agents that its owner finds objectionable, it should post notice of such a policy in a publicly prominent place along with phone numbers and addresses of other pharmacies that do dispense such drugs.[31-35] This is the sort of conflict resolution noted earlier; however, it does not resolve the ethical conflict. Rather, it seeks alternate ways to achieve desired goals: honoring the conscience of all involved and allowing the free exercise of autonomous choices.

Unfortunately, this is not a satisfactory solution to many pharmacists with conscientious objections. To consciously and intentionally refer someone to another who will assist them to accomplish what the referring pharmacist believes is an immoral act is to some pharmacists the very essence of material cooperation.[36] A person who objects in good conscience to a given act cannot in good conscience provide the means to achieve it, even indirectly. If such an individual is employed in a pharmacy that stocks and dispense such drugs, he or she may simply explain to the patient why he or she cannot dispense the drug and suggest that another employed pharmacist who does not share that position may be able to help. That may seem like walking a fine line, and some pharmacists will not be comfortable with it.

Further, in some settings, referral to other pharmacists or pharmacies may not be feasible, particularly if a drug must be taken in a relatively short period of time to be effective. Such is the case with Plan B emergency contraception, which is most effective if taken 12 to 24 hours postcoitus and is at least partially effective up to 72 hours postcoitus. Those with limited means or living in geographic areas without easy access to other sources may find it impossible to travel to or obtain the drug within such time constraints. It has been proposed by some that, in those instances, pharmacists be required by their fiduciary obligation or law to dispense the drug.[34,37] Others argue that such coercion should not be used, that the threat to the health of the woman affected is not dire, that there is no certainty that she will become pregnant, and that if she does and still does not want to bear a child she has the option of abortion.[38] It may be argued in opposition that some women may oppose abortion but not contraception and that by denying them contraception, the pharmacist is forcing them to bear a child if they become pregnant or to face the agonizing choice of abortion.

Conscientious objection and the conflicting position that a person should have unfettered access to legal drugs is a particularly vexing policy problem. A number of states have passed "conscience laws" that allow pharmacists and other health professionals to opt out of providing services and products to which they have moral objection and protect them from retaliation. Some state laws provide alternative means to access the services or products prescribed. The fact that the Food and Drug Administration has approved Plan B for over-the-counter distribution to women aged 18 and older does not resolve the problem. It may relieve individual pharmacists of the burden, but pharmacies owned and operated by conscientiously objecting pharmacists may still refuse to stock, sell, or refer to another source. And it also does not address other uses of drugs to which some pharmacists conscientiously object. Some states have enacted laws that require pharmacists to stock and/or dispense all legal drugs. This creates a problem for conscientious objecting pharmacists and pharmacies in remote rural areas and in underserved urban areas. They are faced with the problem of violating their conscience or going out of the profession or business. This may leave underserved areas without access to any pharmacy professionals or products.

The vexing problem of honoring the consciences and needs of patients and the consciences of pharmacists is not subject to ready resolution. In our diverse society, it is important to respect all conscientiously reached moral decisions, even though we may disagree with them. Respecting differing moral viewpoints is not equivalent to cooperating with them. At the very least, conscientiously objecting pharmacists should treat those with whom they disagree with courtesy and respect, attempting to understand patients' needs and reasons for wanting the drugs they seek, explaining politely and noncoercively why he or she (the pharmacist) holds the position that he or she does, and taking no actions to obstruct access to agents that others find morally acceptable. Conversely, those who disagree with objecting pharmacists should treat them and their moral decisions with respect and without coercion.

Patient Confidentiality and Privacy: HIPAA

The importance of patient confidentiality was acknowledged in the Hippocratic Oath, in which the subscriber pledges to "hold as holy secrets" what the practitioner sees or hears. Confidentiality involves a relationship between the patient and healthcare provider that fosters trust that the provider will not divulge information about the patient unless that information is clinically necessary. That is, the provider will respect the privacy of the patient unless doing otherwise is necessary to keep the patient from harm (nonmaleficence) or to help the patient (beneficence).[2] This trust facilitates patient care, allowing patients to freely communicate with their providers.

Advances in computer technology over the last 20 years led to the development and use of electronic medical record keeping. The ease with which millions of electronic records can be misplaced or stolen has become apparent and raised security concerns. Media reports describing breaches of medical privacy, including a report of a computer purchaser discovering thousands of prescription records on a used computer, fueled consumer concern.[39]

In response to these concerns, Congress passed the Health Insurance Portability and Accountability Act of 1996 (HIPAA). HIPAA is a broad and complex set of rules and procedures for protecting the privacy of patient health information. Many healthcare entities and their employees, including any pharmacy or pharmacist, which transmits patient information electronically, must follow these privacy regulations. The finalized rules for the privacy regulations were released on August 9, 2002, and providers were required to comply with the regulations by April 14, 2003.[40]

The HIPAA regulations set a federal minimum on the protection of privacy. Thus, when other federal or state laws afford more protection for patients' privacy than HIPAA, the more protective federal and state laws will supersede.[41] Examples include federal laws protecting drug and alcohol treatment records, and state laws, such as special protections for mental health or genetic records.

Serious security breaches have occurred since the enactment of HIPAA. Two such occurrences involving Veterans Administration (VA) data were documented in 2006. In May 2006, a VA computer was stolen from an employee's home that contained 26.5 million records with patient names, birth dates, and Social Security numbers. In August 2006, a computer containing VA recipients' names, Social Security numbers, and health insurance data was lost from a VA computer vendor's facility.[42]

Pharmacists have a moral responsibility to protect the confidentiality of their patients. It seems clear from the previous discussion that legislated data transfer standards and security regulations can only do so much to protect patients. Practitioners must remember the basics of data security. They must be diligent in shredding sensitive information and shut down or lock computers when they are not in use. Pharmacists should be careful about making indiscreet comments, watching what they say and when they say it—an indiscreet comment can cause a patient distress and seriously harm the patient–pharmacist relationship. Pharmacists must be sensitive to negative perceptions that patients may develop when reports such as the loss of millions of patient records appear on the evening news. Pharmacists are positioned to play a greater role than ever in patient care, such as expanding pharmaceutical care activities. We must demonstrate to our patients that their trust is well founded and their right to privacy is taken seriously.

The Pharmacy Benefit Manager

The pharmacy benefit management industry has come under intense scrutiny in recent years. Particularly of interest are the cash flows the pharmacy benefit manager (PBM) takes in the process of administering "pharmacy card" programs for sponsors that include insurance companies, unions, private employers, and government. Although the cash flows taken by the PBM are allowed by nuances in their contracts, objections to these practices have been voiced by healthcare purchasers and academics.[43-45]

In the 1980s the public was outraged by excessive charges made by contractors to the Department of Defense (e.g., the $900 hammer). In the early part of the 21st century, U.S. corporate scandal robbed employees of their retirement funds. Currently there are serious allegations leveled at PBMs. These allegations, although perhaps not yet as well known as these other examples, could eventually lead to public outrage. PBMs are accused of retaining excessive cash flows. Inflated prescription costs could be particularly important in today's healthcare environment, a time when baby boomers are driving increased utilization of prescription drugs. There has been a significant drop in the number of employers offering health insurance coverage; particularly dramatic is the decline in coverage by smaller employers (3 to 199 employees) from 2000 to 2006.[46]

We first investigate three cash flows to the PBM (rebates, spread pricing, and sponsor data sales) that have captured the attention of the academic and popular press.[47,48] PBM cash flows raise the issue of distributive justice: Are the sponsors receiving a fair allocation of the benefits due them? Are the employees being forced to pay higher premiums because of these practices? One must also consider whether the cash flows to the PBM are proportional to the service the PBM provides the sponsors. It is up to the reader to determine whether the cash flows taken by the PBM are consistent with a fair allocation of resources in our healthcare system, but we will likely need more data to decide.

Rebates

The PBM develops a list of drugs, called a formulary, which represents the drugs that will be covered for all the PBM's clients. The PBM's clients represent thousands of plan sponsors (e.g., employers) that pay for the prescriptions of many millions of beneficiaries. The PBM negotiates with drug manufacturers to place the manufacturers' products on the formulary. In exchange for access to potential customers, the drug manufacturer pays the PBM rebates, of which only a part is paid to the sponsor by the PBM. The PBM has historically retained over 50% of the rebate and has only recently allowed the sponsor any information about rebates. Rebates paid to sponsors to lower the overall cost of drugs could represent a good value for the sponsor if the drugs chosen for the formulary were truly the best therapeutic and economic value. The problem is that the actual net cost of any given drug cannot be easily determined. PBMs will not release rebate information for specific drugs; the industry contends that releasing rebate information of that specificity would be a violation of the PBM's proprietary information.

Sponsors are beginning to question this practice of nondisclosure, and tension between sponsors and PBMs usually centers on the following two questions: Is the formulary drug selected on the basis of the best value for the sponsor or rebate maximization for the PBM? Is the sponsor getting a fair share of the drug manufacturer rebate? The "fair" share of drug rebate payments can only be determined after the PBM makes the payments known to the sponsor. The sponsor has every right to know the amount of the rebate. After all, it is the sponsor's money that purchases the drugs and generates the rebate in the first place.

Spread Pricing

Spread pricing is a practice in which the PBM charges the sponsor more than the pharmacy is paid for a prescription. For example, with a prescription for 100 enalapril 10 mg the sponsor could be billed $32 and the pharmacy paid $24. This would result in an $8 spread to the PBM for this one prescription; this cash flow to the PBM represents an $8 overcharge to the sponsor. Being able to track the prices of generic drugs is beyond the expertise of plan sponsors; therefore, this $8 is a cash flow "hidden" within thousands of prescriptions that the sponsor might generate. Because of the wide spread in pricing, the sponsor is unable to tell how much the PBM service is actually costing. Spread pricing occurs in addition to a per-prescription administration fee (e.g., $0.25 to $0.75) that is agreed to in the contract to compensate the PBM for executing the transaction. This administration fee is analogous to the fee charged by a credit card company to conduct a transaction. All the sponsor is aware of is the small prescription administration fee charged per prescription (e.g., $0.25 to $0.75). The sponsor is unable to make a rational choice in selecting a PBM. As far as the sponsor is concerned, the enalapril prescription cost 25 cents for the processing service; in fact, however, that prescription cost the sponsor $8.25 for the service ($8.00 in spread and 25 cents in administration fees).

The pharmacy benefit management industry would argue that this practice is fair and reasonable; all businesses make a profit. In most cases, the PBM never takes possession of the drugs and simply adjudicates an electronic prescription that is transmitted between the pharmacy and PBM. The retail pharmacies buy and take possession of the drugs, and the sponsor reimburses the PBM according to the bill from the PBM to the sponsor. How much value does the PBM provide? Is that value proportional to the charges?

Spread pricing appears to be an injustice suffered by both the sponsor and the pharmacy. In the spread pricing model, the PBM has the incentive to maximize what it charges the sponsors and minimize what it pays the pharmacies. In this environment, pharmacies have been forced to accept progressively lower reimbursement—a reduction in payment of 8.8% in the period from 1995 to 2003.[49]

Data Selling

PBMs routinely sell sponsor's de-identified prescription claims data. The data are quite valuable for both pharmacy chains and drug manufacturers. The claims data enable retail pharmacy chains to determine where to locate stores (e.g., close to areas of heavy prescribing). Drug manufacturers use these data to determine the prescription volume of their products in each Zip code (the physician's DEA number on the claim is linked to his or her office address). In other words, these data help drug manufacturers determine where intense sales efforts are needed. One should consider whether using pharmacy claims to target physicians in an attempt to influence their prescribing patterns is an appropriate use of industrial intelligence.

The sponsor has, historically, been unaware of the sales. Reasonable questions that arise in relation to data selling are as follows: Should sponsors be explicitly told about the sale of their data? Should sponsors be entitled to proceeds from the sale of their data?

Pharmacogenetics: Ethics and Policy

Pharmacogenetics holds exciting promise for tailoring drug therapy to individual patients. It should enable drug prescriptions based on genetic predictions of an individual patient's likelihood of a good therapeutic response or risk of adverse drug effects, making drug treatment both more effective and safer. It may also allow the use of drugs that have been removed from the market because of adverse reactions by identifying individuals who may benefit from the therapy and who are genetically determined not to be at risk of adverse responses.

Pharmacogenetics may also enable better and more efficient drug development. To the extent that knowledge of the mechanisms of drug action can be learned by studying the relationships of genotypes and drug responses, new drugs may be designed and developed for use in persons of specific genotypes. If specific genotypes are known to be better responders or to predispose individuals to adverse reactions to certain classes of drugs, drug developers may utilize genotype as an inclusion or exclusion criterion for participation in clinical trials, thus making trials safer and diminishing the numbers of enrollees and the time required to reach valid conclusions. The use of postmarketing surveillance may also benefit from pharmacogenetics by identifying genotypes in the larger population or alleles that affect drug response or risks.

The promise of pharmacogenetics is not absolute, however. The field is subject to a number of factors that may compromise or impede the effective realization of its promise. Further, it raises a number of ethical and policy issues. There have been two major comprehensive efforts to delineate ethical and policy issues, one by the Consortium on Pharmacogenetics[50] and another by the Nuffield Council on Bioethics.[51]

The scientific potential of pharmacogenetics may be mitigated by three important factors: (1) there is a wide range of genotypic variability and great variation in individuals' responses to drugs; (2) therapeutic and adverse responses may depend on the interactions of several genes, combinations of which are likely to vary from person to person; and (3) other environmental factors may affect the expression of genes so that their effects on drug responses may be significantly modified. Even with these mitigating factors, it is likely that pharmacogenetics will have practical value—in at least some instances, it already has.[52]

Pharmacogenetics also raises several ethical and policy issues. These include issues of confidentiality and privacy, access to insurance and care, adequately informed consent, potential constraints on autonomy, and quality of care. These are intimately intertwined.

Laws and regulations relating to confidentiality and privacy apply to genetic information just as they do to any other private health care information. However, in respect to genetic information, there is the opportunity for abuse by insurers and self-insured employers. The former have access to individuals' health information. If a drug response genotype is linked to one or another disease risk genotype, insurers may refuse to insure people who have those genotypes. Self-insured employers are required by HIPAA to erect firewalls between employees who have access to health records and other employees. However, many critics have serious concerns about the effectiveness of these barriers to information flow. The fear is that if they fail, employers may discriminate against employees with "bad" or "expensive" genotypes. The passage of laws protecting against genetic discrimination by insurers or employers is a possible solution to this concern. Confidentiality and privacy must also be part of the consideration of whether, and by whom, relatives should be informed of genetic results that may be of importance to them.

Knowledge that a given genotype predicts a modest response to a drug or a somewhat higher risk of side effects may induce insurers to require genetic testing and deny coverage to persons who are not "high" or "safe" responders, even though the prediction of response or risk may be relative, not absolute. This infringes on patient and professional autonomy and denies patients the right to consent. Alternatively, access to genetic testing may be affected if insurers decide not to cover it, reasoning that, at least for some conditions, the selection of drugs by trial and error is more cost efficient. Insurers and PBMs may constrain access by choosing not to include in their formularies drugs that are most appropriate for individuals with certain genotypes.

Access to care may also be affected by drug makers' decisions not to develop new drugs effective for certain genotypes if the frequency of the genotype is so rare that the market for it is too small to support the cost of drug development and testing. There may be "orphan" genotypes, as we currently have orphan diseases, which are so rare they do not justify the cost of drug development. Another concern is that certain genotypes may occur disproportionately in populations with poor resources to pay for new drugs, either in developed nations or developing nations. These concerns could be addressed by extending existing orphan drug laws to orphan genotypes and making drug development for such genotypes a priority for public funding.

Ensuring adequate informed consent will require substantial effort by physicians and other health professionals to ensure that patients are aware of the following issues: the specific genes that may be evaluated and the fact that this may subject them to the risks of disclosure to insurers and employers, and the psychological risk of learning that they have a low likelihood of responding to a given drug, an increased risk of side effects, or may be susceptible to disease associated with specific genotypes. Will patients have access to appropriate counseling? If they are participating in research, they should be informed whether their genetic information will become a part of their medical record. Some believe that specific consent should be sought for genetic testing even when used as a diagnostic means to determine the best drugs to prescribe, much as blood chemistry is used in diagnosis.

Quality of care concerns are related to the competence and knowledge of pharmacists and physicians regarding the value and challenges of pharmacogenetics. Pharmacists should assume an important responsibility for physician and patient education. Another quality of care concern has to do with the accuracy of genetic testing. The Food and Drug Administration has a responsibility for ensuring the quality of packaged test kits, and Clinical Laboratory Improvement Amendments (CLIA) regulations ensure the general quality of laboratories offering genetic tests that are not performed with kits. However, in the latter case, CLIA may not monitor specific tests. Further, CLIA has no role in monitoring tests that are used in research and not reported to patients or caregivers. This has the potential to compromise the quality of clinical trials.

The promise of pharmacogenetics is great. But that promise in some areas is of relative, not absolute, value. In other areas it is not certain and is fraught with ethical and policy challenges that we will be facing for many years as the science progresses.

CONCLUSION

Public policy initiatives do not necessarily represent what an individual would consider the best moral choice, even though enactment and implementation of policy by laws and regulations is intended to reflect the prevailing values of a society. Prevailing values often are not universally shared. Different people hold profoundly different ethical positions on matters of public importance. In such circumstances, there are certain to be political disagreements about some policies and consequent political struggles to establish or change policy.

We live in a diverse society in which individual autonomy and privacy are strongly held values. Conflicts become especially bitter when policies are made or proposed that coerce people to do things that are contrary to their values or prevent them from actions they believe to be moral or in their self-interest. We see this play out in the debates about abortion, stem cell research, and, in the case of pharmacists, conscientious objection.

This tension between ethics and the use of ethics in policy making is not going to go away. Policy debates inevitably involve clashes of values and morals. This is a characteristic of a free society. At best we can hope to keep the debates civil and respectful.

REFERENCES

1. Webster's new universal unabridged dictionary. 2nd ed. New York: Simon & Schuster, 1979.
2. Purtilo RB. Ethical dimensions in the health professions. 3rd ed. Philadelphia: WB Saunders, 1999:81-9.
3. Fieser J. Normative ethics. Internet Encyclopedia of Philosophy. (Accessed March 4, 2007, at www.iep.utm.edu/e/ethics.htm.)
4. Solomon WD. In: Post SG, ed. Encyclopedia of bioethics. 3rd ed. New York: Macmillan Reference USA, 2004:812-23.
5. Beauchamp TL, Childress JF. Principles of biomedical ethics. 5th ed. New York: Oxford University Press, 2001.
6. McCormick TR. Principles of bioethics. University of Washington School of Medicine. 1999. (Accessed March 4, 2007, at http://depts.washington.edu/bioethx/tools/princpl.html.)
7. Merriam-Webster's collegiate dictionary. 10th ed. Springfield, MA: Merriam-Webster, 1993.
8. Churchill LR. In: Post SG, ed. Encyclopedia of bioethics. 3rd ed. New York: Macmillan Reference USA, 2004:269-73.
9. Zalta EN, ed. Stanford encyclopedia of philosophy. The Metaphysical Research Lab, Stanford University. Available from: http://plato.stanford.edu/entries/contractarianism/. (Accessed March 5, 2007.)
10. Kelley M. In: Post SG, ed. Encyclopedia of bioethics. 3rd ed. New York: Macmillan Reference USA, 2004:523-7.
11. Sterba JP. In: Post SG, ed. Encyclopedia of bioethics. 3rd ed. New York: Macmillan Reference USA, 2004:1354-5.
12. Jonsen AR, Siegler M, Winslade WJ. Clinical ethics: a practical approach to ethical decisions in clinical medicine. 6th ed. New York: McGraw Hill, 2006.
13. Santa Clara University Markkula Center for Applied Ethics. A framework for thinking ethically. 1988. (Accessed March 5, 2007, at http://www.scu.edu/ethics/practicing/decision/framework.htm.)
14. Ethics Resource Center. The decision making process. (Accessed March 5, 2007, at http://www.ethics.org/resources/decision-making-process.asp.)
15. Bowling Green State University Computer Science Department. Procedural ethics chronological site index. (Accessed March 5, 2007, at http://www.cs.bgsu.edu/maner/heuristics/toc.htm.)
16. Smith S, Neaves W, Teitelbaum S. Adult stem cell treatments for diseases? Science 2006;313:439. (Supporting online material accessed February 27, 2007, at http://www.sciencemag.org/cgi/content/full/1129987/DC1.)
17. Prentice DA, Tarne G. Treating diseases with adult stem cells. Science 2007;315:328. (Supporting online material accessed February 27, 2007, at http://www.sciencemag.org/cgi/content/full/315/5810/328b/DC1.)
18. Glasier A. Emergency postcoital contraception. N Engl J Med 1997;337:1058-64.
19. Singer P. Practical ethics. 2nd ed. Cambridge: Cambridge University Press, 1993:175-217.
20. Zinaman MJ, Clegg ED, Brown CC, O'Connor J, Selevan SG. Estimates of human fertility and pregnancy loss. Fertil Steril 1996;65:503-9.
21. Kolstad HA, Bonde JP, Hjøllund NH, et al. Menstrual cycle patterns and fertility: a prospective follow-up study of pregnancy and early embryonal loss in 295 couples who were planning their first pregnancy. Fertil Steril 1999;71:490-6.

22. Wang X, Changzong C, Wang L, Chen D, Guang W, French J. Conception, early pregnancy loss, and time to clinical pregnancy: a population based prospective study. Fertil Steril 2003;79:577-84.

23. Dennis C, Check E. "Ethical" routes to stem cells highlight political divide. Nature 2005;437: 1076-7.

24. Vogel G. Embryo-free techniques gain momentum. Science 2005;309:240-1.

25. American Society of Health Systems Pharmacists. Pharmacist's right of conscience and patient's right of access to therapy. ASHP policy positions, statements, and guidelines—ethics. 2001. (Accessed February 28, 2007, at http://www.ashp.org/s_ashp/bin.asp?CID=6&DID=4011& DOC=FILE.PDF.)

26. Swartz MS. "Conscience clauses" or "unconscionable clauses": personal beliefs versus professional responsibilities. Yale J Health Pol Law Ethics 2006;6:269-350.

27. Wicclair MR. Pharmacies, pharmacists, and conscientious objection. Kennedy Inst Ethics J 2006;16:225-50.

28. Wall LL, Brown D. Refusals by pharmacists to dispense emergency contraception. Obstet Gynecol 2006;107:1148-51.

29. Savulescu J. Conscientious objection in medicine. BMJ 2006;332:294-7.

30. Davis JK. Conscientious refusal and doctor's right to quit. J Med Philos 2004;29:75-91.

31. Cantor J, Baum K. The limits of conscientious objection—may pharmacists refuse to fill prescriptions for emergency contraception? N Engl J Med 2004;351:2008-12.

32. Manasse HR. Conscientious objection and the pharmacist. Science 2005;308:1558-9.

33. Greenberger MD, Vogelstein R. Pharmacist refusals: a threat to women's health. Science 2005; 308:1557-8.

34. Dresser R. Professionals, conformity and conscience. Hasting Center Rep 2005;35:9-10.

35. Baergen R, Owens C. Revisiting pharmacists' refusals to dispense emergency contraception. Obstet Gynecol 2006;108:1277-82.

36. Pellegrino ED. The physician's conscience, conscience clauses, and religious belief: a Catholic perspective. Fordham Urban Law J 2002;30:221-44.

37. Fenton E, Lomasky L. Dispensing with liberty: conscientious refusal and the "morning-after pill." J Med Philos 2005;30:579-92.

38. Calis KA, Pucino F, Restrepo ML. Pharmacists and emergency contraception: letters to the editor. N Engl J Med 2005;352:942-3.

39. Giacalone RP, Cacciatore GG. HIPAA and its impact on pharmacy practice. Am J Health Syst Pharm 2003;60:433-45.

40. Bishop SK, Winckler SC. Implementing HIPAA privacy regulations in pharmacy practice. J Am Pharm Assoc 2002;42:836-44.

41. Annas GJ. HIPAA regulations: a new era of medical-record privacy? N Engl J Med 2003;348:1486-90.

42. Office of Citizen Services and Communication, U.S. General Services Administration. Latest information on Veterans Affairs data security. (Accessed March 5, 2007, at http://www.usa.gov/veteransinfo.)

43. Garis RI, Clark BE. Pilot study of an undocumented source of pharmacy benefit manager revenue. J Am Pharm Assoc 2004;44:15-21.

44. Garis RI, Clark BE, Siracuse MV, Makoid MC. Examining the value of pharmacy benefit management companies. Am J Health Syst Pharm 2004;61:81-5.
45. Wessel D, Wysocki B, Martinez B. As health middlemen thrive, employers try to tame them. Wall Street Journal, December 29, 2006, A1.
46. Claxon G, Gil I, Finder B, et al. Employer health benefits 2006 annual survey. Menlo Park, CA: Kaiser Family Foundation and Health Research and Educational Trust, 2006. (Accessed March 5, 2007, at http://www.kff.org/insurance/7527/upload/7527.pdf.)
47. Makoid MC, Garis RI. Inside the cost of prescription drugs. Creighton University Magazine 2001;16-23.
48. Freudenheim M. Drug middlemen are facing pressure over rising prices. New York Times, January 5, 2002. (Accessed March 5, 2007, at http://query.nytimes.com/gst/fullpage.html?res=9D01EEDD1F30F936A35752C0A9649C8B63&sec=health&spon=&pagewanted=all.)
49. Takeda Pharmaceuticals North America. The prescription drug benefit cost and plan design survey report. 2004 ed. Conducted for Takeda by the Pharmacy Benefit Management Institute. Albuquerque, NM: Wellman Publishing, 2004.
50. Buchanan A, Califano A, Kahn J, McPherson E, Robertson J, Brody B. Pharmacogenetics: ethical issues and policy options. Kennedy Inst Ethics J 2002;12:1-15.
51. Lipton P, Afshar H, Bobrow M, et al. Pharmacogenetics: ethical issues. London: Nuffield Council on Bioethics, 2003.
52. Haas DW. Human genetic variability and HIV treatment response. Curr HIV/AIDS Rep 2006;3:53-8.

Index

Italicized page locators indicate a figure; tables are noted with a *t*.